Study Guide for

Fundamentals of Nursing
The Art and Science of Person-Centered Care

Study Guide for

Fundamentals of Nursing
The Art and Science of Person-Centered Care

Tenth Edition

Andrea R. Mann, MSN, RN, CNE
Professor of Practice
Gwynedd Mercy University
Frances M. Maguire School of Nursing and Health Professions
Gwynedd Valley, Pennsylvania

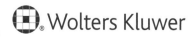 Wolters Kluwer

Philadelphia · Baltimore · New York · London
Buenos Aires · Hong Kong · Sydney · Tokyo

Vice President, Nursing Segment: Julie K. Stegman
Director, Nursing Education and Practice Content: Jamie Blum
Senior Acquisitions Editor: Jonathan Joyce
Senior Development Editor: Julie M. Vitale
Developmental Editor: Kelly Horvath
Editorial Coordinator: Erin Hernandez
Senior Content Editing Associate: Devika Kishore
Senior Production Project Manager: Frances M. Gunning
Marketing Manager: Greta Swanson
Manager, Graphic Arts & Design: Stephen Druding
Art Director, Illustration: Jennifer Clements
Manufacturing Coordinator: Margie Orzech-Zeranko
Prepress Vendor: Aptara, Inc.

10th Edition

10 9 8 7 6 5 4 3 2

Printed in Mexico

ISBN: 9781975168209

shop.lww.com

QUADM0324

Preface

Andrea Mann, in collaboration with the authors of the tenth edition of *Fundamentals of Nursing: The Art and Science of Person-Centered Care,* has thoughtfully developed this Study Guide. As nursing students, you must learn a great deal of complex foundational knowledge which will be used through your education and beyond. The goal of this study guide, in concert with the textbook, is to help nursing students reinforce content, synthesize information, and apply it to practice. To that end, the content in each chapter of the Study Guide is structured to guide you from simple to complex ideas to challenge you as you work toward integrating the art and science of nursing into your practice. A strong foundation will promote the clinical reasoning that leads to sound clinical judgment. To help you accomplish this goal, the following types of exercises are provided in each chapter of the Study Guide.

ASSESSING YOUR UNDERSTANDING

These exercises group similar types of questions together to help you learn the information in a variety of formats. The types of questions included follow the same format in each Study Guide chapter, but not every type of question is used in each chapter. The format includes:

- Identification Questions
- Fill in the Blanks
- Matching Exercises
- Correct the False Statements
- Short Answer

APPLYING YOUR KNOWLEDGE

These questions challenge you to reflect on the critical thinking and blended skills developed in the classroom and apply them to your own practice of the *art and science of person-centered nursing care.*

- Critical Thinking Questions: these questions offer an exciting and practical means to challenge the assumptions you bring to nursing and to "stretch" your application of new theoretical concepts.
- Reflective Practice: Cultivating QSEN Competencies: these exercises offer opportunities to use your critical thinking ability and knowledge of blended skills to respond to real-life scenarios, similar to those that may occur in your practice.
- Patient Care Studies: these studies in the clinical nursing care chapters provide a unique opportunity for you to "encounter" an actual patient, to use the nursing process to assess and diagnose the patient's nursing needs, and brainstorm ways to best meet these needs.

PRACTICING FOR NCLEX

Multiple-Choice Questions: Each chapter contains a section of multiple-choice questions presented in the NCLEX-RN exam format.
Alternate-Format Questions: The alternate-format-style questions for the NCLEX-RN exam include the types of questions described below. Several of these types are provided in each chapter to help you become familiar with this NCLEX format. They are:

- Multiple-Response Questions: questions with a detailed stem that require you to select more than one correct answer.
- Sequencing Questions: questions with a detailed stem that require you to place the options provided in the correct order.
- Prioritization Questions: questions that ask you to triage specific patient needs and attend to what is most urgent first.
- Hot Spot Questions: questions that require you to identify a specific area on an illustration or a graph.
- Chart/Exhibit Questions: multiple-choice questions with a detailed stem that require you to review information in a chart or an exhibit in order to select the correct answer.

ANSWER KEY

The answers to the Assessing Your Understanding, Reflective Practice, and Practicing for NCLEX questions are included in the Answer Key at the back of the book so that you can immediately assess your own learning as you complete each chapter.

The authors and Wolters Kluwer hope you find this Study Guide to be helpful and enjoyable, and we wish you every success as you begin the exciting journey toward becoming a nurse.

Contents

CHAPTER 1

Introduction to Nursing and Professional Formation

ASSESSING YOUR UNDERSTANDING

FILL IN THE BLANKS

1. Nursing is a _____ and an art; nurses skillfully apply the knowledge to help others achieve maximum health and quality of life.

2. The _____, founded in 1899, was the first international organization of professional women committed to maintaining high standards of nursing service and nursing education and ethics.

3. Founded in the late 1800s, the _____ is a professional organization for registered nurses in the United States whose mission is to advance the profession of nursing to improve health for all.

4. The ANA's *2021 Nursing:* _____ defines activities specific and unique to nursing and speaks to professional roles, protection for the nurse, the patient, and the health care institution.

5. _____ are laws established in each state in the United States to regulate the practice of nursing and protect the public.

6. A guideline for nursing practice, which informs critical thinking and clinical reasoning is known as the _____ integrates both the art and science of nursing.

7. The ANA defines _____ education as professional development experiences designed to enrich the nurse's contribution to health care.

8. _____ refers to the legal authority to practice nursing.

9. The four broad aims and competencies of nursing are to promote _____, prevent _____, restore _____, and facilitate _____.

10. The _____ of Nursing Practice is a terminal degree in nursing practice offering an alternative approach to research-focused terminal degrees such as the PhD.

11. Nurses provide care to people, families, groups, and _____.

12. The ability of people to obtain, process, and understand the basic information needed to make appropriate decisions about health is called _____.

13. _____ refers to a cumulative state of frustration with the work environment that develops over a long period of time.

1

CORRECT THE UNDERLINED WORDS

1. The Nurse Licensure Compact (NLC) provides licensure in the <u>resident</u> states. _____

2. <u>Clara Barton's</u> attention to maintaining accurate records is recognized as the beginning of nursing researcher. _____

3. The educational program that prepares nurses to deliver nursing care to patients at the bedside is referred to as a <u>nursing technician</u> program. _____

4. The government report *Healthy People 2030* establishes health promotion guidelines for <u>individual communities</u>. _____

5. <u>Restoration</u> refers to the aptitude for overcoming an adverse life circumstance with a hopeful attitude and utilizing healthy internal coping mechanisms among others. _____

SHORT ANSWER: THINKING LIKE A NURSE

Use your own words to explain the following aspects of nursing.

1. Thoughtful, person-centered care: _____

2. Name four roles in professional nursing that require a graduate degree: _____

3. In-service education versus the education received in a formal or collegiate nursing program: _____

4. Advantages of joining the National Student Nurses Association and/or a professional nursing organization: _____

5. Function of nurses in interprofessional teams and collaborative practice: _____

6. Two (of the four) broad elements in common with the nurse practice acts of each state: _____

7. Purpose of the nursing process: _____

8. Give an example in which a nurse may incorporate the following broad aims of nursing into a nursing care plan for a patient who is undergoing diagnostic tests for lung cancer and who smokes two packs of cigarettes a day.

   a. Promoting health: _____

   b. Preventing illness: _____

   c. Restoring health: _____

   d. Facilitating coping: _____

9. List the seven defining criteria for nursing as a profession. _____

10. Critical challenges to nursing practice in the 21st century are listed below. Briefly state how these trends may affect nursing practice and/or health care.

    a. Increasing cost of health care: _____

    b. Growing population of patients who are older and more acutely ill: _____

c. Changing demographics and increasing diversity: _____

_____

_____

d. Current nursing shortage: _____

_____

_____

e. Opportunities for lifelong learning and workforce development: _____

_____

_____

f. Growing need for interprofessional education for collaborative practice: _____

_____

_____

11. Critical challenges to nursing practice in the 21st century are listed below. Briefly state how these trends could affect nurses' practice and nursing education.
a. Need to remain current with technology:

_____

_____

b. Need to remain current with research:

_____

_____

c. Health policy and regulation: _____

_____

_____

d. Globalization of the world's economy and society: _____

_____

_____

e. Shift to population-based care and the increasing complexity of patient care:

_____

_____

f. Era of the educated consumer, alternative therapies and genomics, and palliative care: _____

_____

_____

12. Give an example of a nursing action that might be performed by a nurse relying on these four competencies:
a. Cognitive skills: _____

_____

_____

b. Technical skills: _____

_____

_____

c. Interpersonal skills: _____

_____

_____

d. Ethical/legal skills: _____

_____

_____

13. Nurses may not practice adequate self-care often due to competing priorities. State three early signs of fatigue and one action you can take to prevent this and combat burnout.

_____

_____

_____

_____

APPLYING YOUR KNOWLEDGE

CRITICAL THINKING QUESTIONS

1. Describe a situation in which you promoted these nursing aims.
a. Promoting health: _____

_____

_____

b. Preventing illness: _____

_____

_____

c. Restoring health: _____

_____

_____

d. Facilitating coping: _____

_____

_____

e. For one situation above, evaluate whether your nursing actions were successful and describe why or why not. _____

_____

_____

_____

2. The nurse manager of a medical-surgical unit notified all nurses whose licenses were going to expire the following month to submit their renewed licenses prior to expiration. One nurse did not produce proof of a current license and was sent home. Explain the purpose of the manager's action.

_____

_____

_____

REFLECTIVE PRACTICE: CULTIVATING QSEN COMPETENCIES

Use the following expanded scenario from Chapter 1 in your textbook to answer the questions below.

Scenario: Roberto is a 38-year-old man diagnosed with metastatic colon cancer. Having undergone radiation treatments and chemotherapy, he is extremely weak and malnourished. He is receiving intravenous fluids via a central venous catheter. He has two pressure injuries on his sacrum, each approximately 2 cm in diameter, requiring wound care. He also has a colostomy that he cannot care for independently.

1. Patient-centered care: What basic human needs should the nurse address to provide individualized, holistic care for Roberto?

_____

_____

_____

2. Patient-centered care: What would be a successful outcome for this patient?

_____

_____

_____

3. Patient-centered care: What technical, interpersonal, and ethical/legal competencies are most likely to bring about the desired outcome?

Intellectual: _____

_____

_____

Technical: _____

_____

_____

Interpersonal: _____

_____

_____

Ethical/legal: _____

_____

_____

4. Teamwork and collaboration: What resources might be helpful for Roberto?

_____

_____

5. Informatics/teamwork and collaboration: Which information will the nurse enter in the electronic health record as a means of communicating with the interprofessional team?

_____

_____

PRACTICING FOR NCLEX

MULTIPLE-CHOICE QUESTIONS

Circle the letter that corresponds to the best answer for each question.

1. A nurse is facilitating a patient's coping with disability. Which example best reflects this nursing aim?
   a. Assisting the patient in reviewing the positive experiences of their life
   b. Providing range-of-motion exercises to a client who has had a stroke
   c. Administering an influenza vaccination
   d. Teaching adolescents about water and diving safety

2. Florence Nightingale was a nursing pioneer who challenged prejudices against women and elevated the status of all nurses. Which is one of her most noted accomplishments?
   a. Establishing the fact that nursing is the same as medicine
   b. Promoting adding nursing education as part of a medical degree
   c. Establishing the tenets of the American Red Cross
   d. Maintaining statistics recognized as the beginning of nursing research

3. A nurse educator is discussing the role of nursing based on the American Nurses Association. Which statement best describes this role?
   a. Nursing is a profession dependent upon the medical community and works through a health care provider.
   b. It is the role of the health care provider, not the nurse, to assist patients in understanding their health problems.
   c. Nurses focus on the human experience and responses when caring for individuals, families, groups, and communities.
   d. The essential qualities of professional nursing care are resilience, strength, endurance, and compassion.

4. A community health nurse is planning health promotion activities for the year. Which document will best inform the nurse when formulating the plan and interventions?
   a. American Nurses Association's *Scope and Standards of Practice*
   b. *Healthy People 2030*
   c. World Health Organization's *State of the World's Nursing Report*
   d. State's Nurse Practice Act

5. A nurse is planning care for a group of patients in a long-term care facility. What is the nurse's focus of care?
   a. Nursing interventions provided
   b. Patients receiving the care
   c. Nurse as the caregiver
   d. Nursing as a profession

6. A nurse historian is researching influences on nursing practice in the mid-20th century. Which trend occurring during the 1950s will the research uncover?
   a. Large numbers of women began to work outside the home, asserting their independence.
   b. Nursing practice was broadened to include practice in a wide variety of health care settings.
   c. Male dominance in the health care profession slowed the progress of professionalism in the nursing practice.
   d. Hospital schools were established to provide more easily controlled and less expensive staff for the hospital.

7. A nurse on a medical-surgical unit is caring for a patient during a lengthy hospitalization related to the 2020 pandemic. Which of the four broad aims of nursing practice does this reflect?
   a. Promoting health
   b. Preventing illness
   c. Restoring health
   d. Facilitate coping

8. The nurse has gathered data on a client admitted for a surgical procedure. After collecting data from the client and electronic health record, the nurse will use which following step of the nursing process?
   a. Assessing
   b. Analyzing/diagnosing
   c. Implementing
   d. Developing outcomes

9. A client nearing the end of life tells a nurse they do not want to continue aggressive treatment despite their family's wishes. When the nurse supports the client during a family visit, the nurse is performing which nursing role?
   a. Counselor
   b. Communicator
   c. Collaborator
   d. Advocate

10. A nurse identifies a patient's health care needs and devises a care plan to meet them. Which framework is the nurse using?
   a. Nursing standards
   b. Nursing orders
   c. Nurse practice acts
   d. Nursing process

11. A community health nurse is developing strategies to increase patient health literacy. Which strategy will the nurse incorporate while planning care?
   a. Demonstrating the procedure, such as newborn care in a pregnancy class
   b. Ensuring that written educational materials reflect languages spoken in the community
   c. Making suggestions for handling increasing confusion with an elder family member
   d. Voting to support legislation that funds community-based clinics

ALTERNATE-FORMAT QUESTIONS

Multiple-Response Questions

Circle the letters that correspond to the best answers for each question.

1. Which nursing actions demonstrate the aim of professional nursing to promote health? Select all that apply.
   a. Providing education on sexually transmitted diseases at a college health center
   b. Performing blood pressure screenings at a community health fair
   c. Serving as a role model of health for patients by maintaining a healthy weight
   d. Helping a person with paraplegia learn how to use a wheelchair
   e. Discussing lifestyle decisions that would enhance the well-being of a teenager
   f. Administering an insulin injection to a patient with diabetes

2. Which nursing actions demonstrate the aim of nursing practice to facilitate coping? Select all that apply.
   a. Teaching a class on the nutritional needs of pregnant persons
   b. Performing a dressing change on a patient who has undergone surgery
   c. Teaching a patient and their family strategies for living with diabetes

   d. Assisting a patient and their family to prepare for death
   e. Initiating intravenous therapy for an older adult patient
   f. Providing counseling for the family of a teenager with an eating disorder

3. A group of nursing students are discussing how the Nurse Practice Act regulates practice. Which are examples of common elements of a Nurse Practice Act, regardless of state? Select all that apply.
   a. Defining the legal scope of nursing practice
   b. Enforcing federally regulated nursing legislation
   c. Excluding untrained and unlicensed people from practicing nursing
   d. Enforcing rules and regulations defined by the nurse practice act
   e. Establishing the criteria for the education and licensure of nurses
   f. Defining legal requirements and titles for RNs and LPNs

4. A graduate nurse applies for a professional nursing license in their state of residence. Which actions are examples of the jurisdiction of the state board of nursing? Select all that apply.
   a. Permitting graduates of approved schools of nursing to take the NCLEX
   b. Authorizing nurses to practice nursing in any state
   c. Granting licensure by endorsement to a registered nurse from another state
   d. Denying licensure based on previous criminal actions
   e. Protecting nurses from being suspended for professional misconduct
   f. Issuing specialty licenses to nurses practicing in long-term care facilities

Sequencing Question

Place the steps of the nursing process in the order they are conducted.
   a. Evaluating
   b. Diagnosing
   c. Assessing
   d. Outcome identification and planning
   e. Implementing

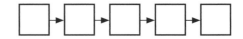

CHAPTER 2

Theory, Research, and Evidence-Based Practice

ASSESSING YOUR UNDERSTANDING

FILL IN THE BLANKS

1. _____ knowledge is that part of nursing practice passed down from generation to generation.

2. _____ in nursing is a problem-solving approach to making clinical decisions and to guide practice, using the best research outcomes.

3. _____ are abstract impressions organized into symbols of reality.

4. A _____ is composed of a group of concepts that describe a pattern of reality.

5. A group of concepts that follows an understandable pattern makes up a _____, or model.

6. The _____ theory describes the process by which living matter adjusts to other living things and to environmental conditions.

7. _____ outlines the process of growth and development of humans as orderly and predictable, beginning with conception and ending with death, and having unique stages.

8. _____ is the patient's right to agree knowledgeably, to participate in a study without coercion, or to refuse to participate without jeopardizing their care.

9. Erik Erikson based his theory of _____ on the process of socialization, emphasizing how people learn to interact with the world.

10. _____ developed a hierarchical theory of physical and psychosocial human needs considered essential to life.

11. _____ refers to nursing care that is supported by reliable research-based outcomes.

12. When using evidence-based practice the nurse integrates the evidence with clinical expertise and _____ and _____ preferences to make the best clinical decision.

MATCHING EXERCISES

Matching Exercise 1

Match the term in Part A with its definition in Part B.

PART A

a. Informed consent

b. Institutional review board

c. Quantitative research

d. Qualitative research

e. Research utilization

PART B

_____ **1.** Method of research conducted to gain insight by discovering meanings

_____ **2.** Involves the concepts of basic and applied research

_____ **3.** Patient's right to consent knowledgeably to participate in a study or treatment without coercion

_____ **4.** Reviews all studies conducted in an institution to determine their risk status and to ensure that ethical principles are followed

_____ **5.** Process of transforming research knowledge into practice, with knowledge referring to both conducting and analyzing research

Matching Exercise 2

Match the term in Part A with its definition in Part B.

PART A

a. General systems theory
b. Process
c. Nursing theory
d. Philosophy
e. Concept
f. Theory

PART B

_____ **1.** Set of interacting elements, all serving the common purpose of contributing to an overall goal

_____ **2.** Emphasizes relationships between the whole and the parts and describes how parts function and behave

_____ **3.** Study of wisdom, fundamental knowledge, and the processes used to develop and construct our perceptions of life

_____ **4.** Differentiates nursing from other disciplines and activities, serving the purposes of describing, explaining, predicting, and controlling desired outcomes of nursing care practices

_____ **5.** Statement that explains/characterizes an action, occurrence, or event that is based on observed facts but lacks absolute or direct proof

_____ **6.** Action phase of a conceptual framework; a series of actions, changes, or functions that bring about a desired goal

Matching Exercise 3

Match the term in Part A with its definition in Part B.

PART A

a. Systematic review
b. Meta-analysis

PART B

_____ **1.** Summarizes findings from multiple studies of a specific clinical practice question or topic, recommending practice change

_____ **2.** Uses statistical analysis of the effect of a specific intervention across multiple studies, providing stronger evidence than results from a single study

Matching Exercise 4

Match the term in Part A with its definition in Part B.

PART A

a. Study to examine the impact of healers on patients with cancer in a certain culture
b. Complications of births attended by midwives from the renaissance to the present
c. Study of beliefs regarding high blood pressure in the Hmong of Thailand
d. Experience of being dependent on kidney dialysis for survival

PART B

_____ **1.** Ethnography
_____ **2.** Phenomenology
_____ **3.** Grounded theory
_____ **4.** Historical

Matching Exercise 5

Match the term in Part A with its definition in Part B.

PART A

a. Abstract
b. Introduction
c. Method
d. Results
e. Discussion
f. References

PART B

_____ **1.** Discusses relevant studies that have been conducted in the same area of study

_____ **2.** Describes how the study was conducted, the type and number of subjects, the research design, what data were collected and how, and analysis done

_____ **3.** Presents this component using words, charts, tables, or graphs

_____ **4.** Reports what the meaning of the results related to the purpose of the study and the literature review

_____ **5.** List of articles and books used by the researcher

_____ **6.** Summarizes the entire article and usually provides the purpose of the study

SHORT ANSWER

1. State the four concepts that influence and determine nursing practice, placing a star beside the most important.

   a. _____

   b. _____

   c. _____

   d. _____

2. Briefly describe quality improvement.

   _____

   _____

   _____

3. Nursing theories are often based on, and influenced by, other broadly applicable processes and theories. Briefly describe the ideas and principles of the following theories that are basic to many nursing concepts.

   a. General systems theory: _____

   _____

   _____

   b. Adaptation theory: _____

   _____

   _____

   c. Developmental theory: _____

   _____

   _____

4. List four basic characteristics of nursing theories.

   a. _____

   b. _____

   c. _____

   d. _____

5. Explain how the following factors have influenced the nursing profession.

   a. Cultural influences on nursing: _____

   _____

   _____

   b. Educational influences on nursing: _____

   _____

   _____

   c. Research and publishing in nursing: _____

   _____

   _____

   d. Improved communication in nursing: ____

   _____

   _____

   e. Improved autonomy of nursing: _____

   _____

   _____

6. List four goals of nursing research according to the National Institute of Nursing Research (NINR).

   a. _____

   b. _____

   c. _____

   d. _____

7. Which nursing theorist(s) might best define your own personal beliefs about nursing practice and why?

   _____

   _____

   _____

8. State two perceived barriers to implementation of evidence-based practice (EBP).

   _____

   _____

   _____

9. During your clinical experience you observe an experienced nurse performing a procedure differently than you were taught. What might you say to understand the nurse's actions?

_____

_____

_____

APPLYING YOUR KNOWLEDGE

CRITICAL THINKING QUESTIONS

1. Select a nursing theory and describe how it would direct assessment and management of a patient's health/nursing needs.

2. Nurses in the intensive care unit studied a pressure relieving product on bedbound patients and found the product reduced sacral wounds by 20%. How will the nurses share their findings with other professionals?

REFLECTIVE PRACTICE: CULTIVATING QSEN COMPETENCIES

Use the following expanded scenario from Chapter 2 in your textbook to answer the questions below.

Scenario: Rachel, the daughter of a 57-year-old patient being discharged with an order for intermittent nasogastric tube feedings, is being taught how to perform the procedure. During one of the teaching sessions, Rachel asks, "How will I know that the tube is in the right place?"

1. Patient-centered care/evidence-based practice: How might the nurse respond to Rachel concerns regarding the care of her mother?

_____

_____

_____

2. Patient-centered care: What would be a successful outcome for this patient?

_____

_____

_____

3. Patient-centered care/safety: What intellectual, technical, interpersonal, and ethical/legal competencies are most likely to bring about the desired outcome?

Intellectual: _____

_____

_____

Technical: _____

_____

_____

Interpersonal: _____

_____

_____

Ethical/legal: _____

_____

_____

4. Teamwork and collaboration: What resources might be helpful for Rachel?

_____

_____

PRACTICING FOR NCLEX

MULTIPLE-CHOICE QUESTIONS

Circle the letter that corresponds to the best answer for each question.

1. A nurse researcher is studying the meaning of the lived experiences of breast cancer survivors. This nurse has used which method of qualitative research?
   a. Phenomenology
   b. Grounded theory
   c. Ethnography
   d. Historical

2. A nurse observes that several patients taking a new antibiotic have developed elevated kidney function tests. Based on this information, the nurse infers that the medication can cause kidney damage. Which type of reasoning is this?
   a. Inductive reasoning
   b. Nursing process
   c. Deductive reasoning
   d. General systems theory

3. A nursing theorist examines a hospital environment by studying the workings of each department individually then relates this information to the hospital as a whole. What type of theory is being used?
   a. Adaptation theory
   b. Developmental theory
   c. General systems theory
   d. Psychosocial theory

4. A nursing theorist studies health care systems in communities. Which statement accurately describes a characteristic of these systems?
   a. The system is an entity in itself and cannot communicate with or react to its environment.
   b. Boundaries separate health care systems both from each other and from the environment.
   c. The system is closed in that it does not allow energy, matter, or information to move between it and its boundaries.
   d. The system is independent of its subsystems in that a change in one element does not affect the whole.

5. A nurse working in a pediatric practice assesses the psychosocial development of children during wellness visits. Which theorist's work is the nurse using?
   a. Erikson
   b. Maslow
   c. Watson
   d. Rogers

6. Nurses plan care for their patients in a variety of settings. During all phases of the nursing process, what exemplifies the primary focus of nursing?
   a. Promoting health for a population of vulnerable elders
   b. Providing thoughtful, patient-centered care in all settings
   c. Performing medication reconciliation at each initial meeting
   d. Comforting a patient who received bad results from a test

7. A nurse frames their nursing care around the theory that nursing interventions should be instituted for patients demonstrating ineffective adaptive responses. This nurse has based their care on the work of which theorists?
   a. Imogene M. King
   b. Madeleine Leininger
   c. Sister Callista Roy
   d. Jean Watson

8. A nurse in a long-term care facility focuses care on helping patients adapt to their environment. This nurse is using the principles of which nursing theorist?
   a. Florence Nightingale
   b. Myra E. Levine
   c. Martha Rogers
   d. Dorothea Orem

9. Nurses on an oncology unit are conducting a study to determine which mouth rinse best improves oral comfort of patients receiving chemotherapy. The nurses identify the mouth rinses as which components of the study?
   a. Hypothesis
   b. Instrument
   c. Method
   d. Variable

ALTERNATE-FORMAT QUESTIONS

Multiple-Response Questions

Circle the letters that correspond to the best answers for each question.

1. A nurse is writing an article for a nursing journal describing a study of the emergency protocols in hospitals. Which statements accurately describe elements of this study? Select all that apply.
   a. The abstract summarizes the article and is found at the end of the article.
   b. The introduction reviews the literature and states the purpose of the article.
   c. The method section provides details of how the study was conducted.
   d. Results are often presented in words, charts, tables, or graphs.
   e. The discussion provides details about the subjects, design, and data collection.
   f. References are listed at the beginning and include articles and books cited.

2. A nurse is using the quantitative research process to study the cause of health care–associated infections and their prevention. Which actions are examples of the components of this process? Select all that apply.

   a. Collects data from subjects in the study

   b. Defines the purpose of the study after conclusions have been made

   c. Formulates a hypothesis and variables in the study

   d. Uses instruments to determine the variables in the study

   e. Uses grounded theory to discover the beliefs of the subjects

3. Nursing students enrolled in a research course have been asked to develop ideas for qualitative research. Which examples of qualitative research should be included in the discussion? Select all that apply.

   a. Nursing issues related to the Native American patient

   b. Historical nursing trends to understand the current profession

   c. Effect of nursing interventions on patient outcomes

   d. Cause-and-effect relationships between variables in a lab

   e. How people describe the effect of illness in their lives

4. Nurses in a large cardiology practice have suggested that an electronic record system will improve communication of the interprofessional team. When using the PICOT format to support their proposal, the nurses will choose which statements to illustrate the process? Select all that apply.

   a. P: The nurse manager purchases an electronic health record keeping system.

   b. P: The nurse chooses the population involved (cardiology patients).

   c. I: The nurse considers interventions to make the plan work.

   d. C: The nurse compares the written records to the computerized records.

   e. O: The nurse determines the occurrence of problems in the systems.

   f. T: The nurse finishes comparing the records and evaluates the outcome.

Sequencing Questions

1. A nurse researcher is using the steps of the quantitative research process to study the impact of managed care on the U.S. health care system. Place the following steps of this process in the order in which they will be performed.

   a. Defines the purpose of the study.

   b. Develops a plan to find answers to the questions of the study.

   c. Uses statistical procedures to analyze the data found.

   d. States the research problem.

   e. Reviews the literature already published on the topic.

   f. Formulates a hypothesis and defines the study variables.

   g. Selects the group to be studied and specific samples to use for data.

   h. Collects the data using interviews, questionnaires, and examinations.

   i. Publishes the study.

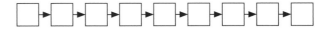

2. Place the steps of the evidence-based practice PICOT process in order.

   a. Usually judging one treatment or intervention against another or the usual standard of care

   b. May include exposure, treatment, patient perception, diagnostic test, or predicting factor

   c. Specifically identifying the outcome to enable a literature search for evidence that examined the same outcome, perhaps in different ways

   d. Need for explicit description; may include setting, limiting to subgroups (such as by age)

   e. When the comparison of interest is completed and the outcome can be evaluated

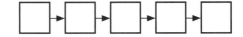

CHAPTER 3

Health, Wellness, and Health Disparities

ASSESSING YOUR UNDERSTANDING

FILL IN THE BLANKS

1. _____ is a medical term meaning that there is a pathologic change in the structure or function of the body or mind, whereas illness is the person's response to that disease.

2. Rheumatoid arthritis is an example of a(n) _____ illness.

3. A(n) _____ illness generally has a rapid onset of symptoms and lasts only a relatively short time.

4. The re-emergence of symptoms of a chronic disease in a patient who has been in remission is known as a(n) _____.

5. A landscaper's increased risk for developing skin cancer because of excessive exposure to the sun is considered a(n) _____ risk factor.

6. Health is a state of complete physical, mental, and social well-being, not merely the absence of _____ or _____.

7. That a newborn living in a zip code of an underserved, largely poor and minority population has a life expectancy 20 years shorter than a newborn in an affluent White area is an example of a(n) _____.

8. The health of the public is measured globally by _____; how frequently a disease occurs; and _____, the numbers of deaths resulting from a disease.

9. _____ is not about treating everyone the same, rather, it is about ensuring that everyone has access to the conditions they need to thrive.

10. _____ is welcoming individuals of different race, religion, nationality, culture, age, sexual orientation, and identity; _____ is giving everyone a sense of purpose and belonging, a feeling of being valued.

MATCHING EXERCISES

Match the risk factors listed below the table with their appropriate examples in the table. Identify the risk factor as modifiable or non-modifiable. Answers may be used more than once.

Matching Exercise 1

Example	Risk Factor	Modifiable or Non-modifiable
1. A mother and her school-aged child are concerned about increasing gang-related violence in their neighborhood		
2. An adolescent driver is admitted to the emergency room with multiple fractures after a car accident.		
3. A woman with multiple sex partners tests positive for HIV.		
4. A woman is worried about breast cancer because it "runs in the family."		
5. An overweight executive presents with high blood pressure.		
6. A man with alcoholism develops a liver abscess.		
7. A patient tells you his father died of colon cancer.		
8. A smoker develops a chronic cough.		
9. A toddler presents with a mild concussion following a fall.		
10. A pregnant person has toxemia in her fifth month.		
11. A 40-year-old man has a father and brother who died of heart attacks at an early age.		
12. An older adult fractured a hip and ankle bone when falling down a flight of stairs in his home.		

a. Age
b. Genetic composition
c. Physiologic factors
d. Health habits
e. Lifestyle
f. Environment

Matching Exercise 2

Match the model of health and illness listed in Part A with the correct definition in Part B.

PART A

a. Agent–host–environment model
b. Health belief model
c. Health–illness continuum
d. High-level wellness model
e. Health promotion model

PART B

_____ **1.** Views health as a constantly changing state, with high-level wellness and death being on opposite ends of a graduated scale.

_____ **2.** Dunn's model of health is based on a person functioning to maximum potential while maintaining balance and a purposeful direction in the environment.

_____ **3.** Leavell and Clark's model used in community health, examines the causes of disease by assessing and understanding risk factors.

_____ **4.** Rosenstock's model of health is based on three components of disease perception: (1) perceived susceptibility to a disease, (2) perceived seriousness of a disease, and (3) perceived benefits of action.

_____ **5.** Pender's model illustrates the multidimensional nature of people interacting with their environment as they pursue health.

Matching Exercise 3

Match the type of human dimension listed in Part A with the patient examples in Part B. Answers may be used more than once.

PART A

a. Emotional dimension
b. Sociocultural dimension
c. Spiritual dimension
d. Intellectual
e. Physical dimension

PART B

_____ **1.** An older adult must learn to manage his diabetes.

_____ **2.** Worried about losing his job, a middle-aged executive exacerbates his gastric ulcer.

_____ **3.** The mother of a toddler must learn how to childproof her house.

_____ **4.** An older adult obtains a raised toilet seat for the bathroom.

_____ **5.** A homeless man does not seek treatment for pneumonia.

_____ **6.** A patient refusing treatment for cancer arranges a pilgrimage to a holy site where miraculous cures have been recorded.

SHORT ANSWER

1. Give five examples of vulnerable populations.

   a. _____

   b. _____

   c. _____

   d. _____

   e. _____

2. Compare and contrast health equity and equality.

   _____

   _____

3. Describe how your own self-concept has been influenced by the following factors:

   a. Interpersonal interactions: _____

   _____

   _____

   b. Physical and cultural influences: _____

   _____

   _____

   c. Education: _____

   _____

   _____

   d. Illness: _____

   _____

   _____

4. Compare and contrast acute and chronic illness.

   _____

   _____

   _____

5. List two examples of nursing actions that would be performed at each of the following levels of health promotion and illness prevention.

   a. Primary: _____

   _____

   _____

   b. Secondary: _____

   _____

   _____

   c. Tertiary: _____

   _____

   _____

6. Describe the processes of Dunn's model of high-level wellness, a part of each person's perception of their wellness state, which helps them know who and what they are.

   a. Being: _____

   _____

   _____

   b. Belonging: _____

   _____

   _____

   c. Becoming: _____

   _____

   _____

   d. Befitting: _____

   _____

   _____

7. Describe where you personally fit on the health–illness continuum and why.

   _____

   _____

   _____

APPLYING YOUR KNOWLEDGE

CRITICAL THINKING QUESTIONS

1. Identify and compare the factors affecting the health and illness of the following patients:

   a. A 39-year-old pregnant person who has been in good health throughout her pregnancy is admitted to the obstetrics unit for vaginal bleeding in her 16th week of pregnancy. Her husband is at her bedside.

   b. A 20-year-old woman who is addicted to crack cocaine is brought to the emergency room by her boyfriend. She is in her 23rd week of pregnancy is having contractions.

   c. Determine the nurse's role in assisting these patients and their families.

2. Interview a person who has experienced an acute illness and one who is living with a chronic illness. Identify the health risk factors, basic human needs, and self-concepts of each person. Describe the different ways acute and chronic illnesses affect patients and their families.

REFLECTIVE PRACTICE: CULTIVATING QSEN COMPETENCIES

Use the following expanded scenario from Chapter 3 in your textbook to answer the questions below.

   Scenario: Ruth is a 62-year-old woman who was hospitalized after a "mini-stroke." She has now returned to her pre-event level of functioning and is being prepared for discharge. She states, "I know that I have an increased risk for a major stroke, so I want to do everything possible to stay as active and as healthy as I possibly can."

1. Patient-centered care/evidence-based practice: How might the nurse respond to Ruth's stated desire for a higher level of wellness?

   _____

   _____

   _____

2. Patient-centered care: What would be a successful outcome for this patient?

   _____

   _____

   _____

3. Patient-centered care: What intellectual, interpersonal, and ethical/legal competencies are most likely to bring about the desired outcome?

   Intellectual: _____

   _____

   _____

   Interpersonal: _____

   _____

   _____

   Ethical/legal: _____

   _____

   _____

4. Teamwork and collaboration: What resources might be helpful for this patient?

   _____

   _____

   _____

PRACTICING FOR NCLEX

MULTIPLE-CHOICE QUESTIONS

Circle the letter that corresponds to the best answer for each question.

1. A nurse is immunizing children against measles. At what level of preventive care is the nurse engaging?

   a. Primary

   b. Secondary

   c. Tertiary

   d. Quaternary

2. The nurse in the community is planning to include a program related to tertiary levels of health promotion. Which activities will the nurse include in this plan?

   a. Developing a support group for HIV-positive individuals

   b. Teaching breast self-examination at the women's center

   c. Providing a program to deter smoking for middle-school children

   d. Offering free tuberculin skin testing at the local community center

3. A nurse is caring for a patient with breast cancer. The patient tells the nurse: "I don't know why this happened to me, but I'm ready to move on and do whatever I need to do to get healthy again." This patient is in which stage of acute illness?
   a. Stage 1
   b. Stage 2
   c. Stage 3
   d. Stage 4

4. A nurse in a rheumatology clinic is assessing a patient with systemic lupus erythematosus, a chronic autoimmune disease affecting organs and joints. The patient asks what the health care provider meant by "being in remission." What will the nurse teach the patient is a remission of an illness?
   a. "Symptoms of the illness reappear abruptly"
   b. "The disease is no longer present."
   c. "New symptoms may occur at this time."
   d. "Symptoms are not currently experienced."

5. A nurse observes that a patient who has pneumonia is in the recovery and rehabilitation stage of the illness. What is the expected patient response in this stage of the illness?
   a. Gives up the dependent role
   b. Assumes a dependent role
   c. Seeks medical attention
   d. Recognizes symptoms of illness

6. Nurses provide holistic health care integrating patient needs with the human dimensions. Which needs are being met when a nurse recommends a community senior center for an older adult who is living alone?
   a. Spiritual needs
   b. Sociocultural needs
   c. Intellectual needs
   d. Emotional needs

ALTERNATE-FORMAT QUESTIONS
Multiple-Response Questions
Circle the letters that correspond to the best answers for each question.

1. A nurse is using Leavell and Clark's Agent–Host–Environment Health Model to help plan nursing interventions for patients in a hospital setting. Which nursing actions to prevent health care–associated infections (HAIs) in these patients best illustrate the principles of this model? Select all that apply.
   a. The nurse should assess the patients for risk factors for infection when planning nursing care.
   b. The nurse should assess patients' ability to fight off infection by using a graduated scale with high-level wellness on one end and death on the other.
   c. The nurse should consider the patients' family history and age when assessing risk factors for infection.
   d. The nurse should consider patients' past behavior when determining goals for recovery.
   e. The nurse should assess what the patients believe to be true about themselves and their illnesses when developing a nursing plan to prevent HAIs.
   f. The nurse should examine environmental stressors in patients' lives to see how they might affect their recovery and ability to ward off infection.

2. A nurse is performing health promotion activities for patients at a local health care clinic. Which nursing actions exemplify the focus of secondary preventive care? Select all that apply.
   a. Scheduling immunizations for a child
   b. Teaching parents about child safety in the home
   c. Performing range-of-motion exercises on a patient
   d. Screening patients for hypertension
   e. Scheduling a mammogram for a patient
   f. Referring a patient to family counseling

3. A nurse provides interventions for patients in a long-term care facility to help them meet their intellectual needs. Which nursing actions promote these needs? Select all that apply.

a. Providing patient teaching about foot care to a patient with diabetes

b. Shutting down a cafeteria to investigate cases of food poisoning

c. Referring a patient experiencing dysfunctional grief to a grief counselor

d. Explaining the benefits of following a healthy diet to a patient with obesity

e. Showing residents a video discussing modified activities for older adults

f. Setting up a pet therapy program for residents

Sequencing Question

Place the stages of Suchman's stages of illness in the order they occur.

a. Achieving recovery and rehabilitation; may transition from hospital to home

b. Assuming the dependent role, accepting the diagnosis, and following the prescribed treatment plan.

c. Recognizing one or more symptoms that are incompatible with their personal definition of health.

d. Defining themselves as sick, validating this experience from others, and giving up normal activities

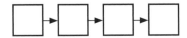

CHAPTER 4

Health of the Individual, Family, Community, and Environment

ASSESSING YOUR UNDERSTANDING

FILL IN THE BLANKS

1. According to Maslow, the most essential of all basic human needs is _____.

2. Using Maslow's hierarchy of needs hygiene and aseptic techniques to prevent infection are categorized as _____ and _____ needs.

3. Family is composed of interdependent members, related or _____ who affect one another.

4. A community is a specific population or group of people living in the same geographic area under similar regulations and having common _____, _____, and needs.

5. _____ health refers to the aspect of human health determined by physical, chemical, biologic, and psychosocial factors in the environment (WHO).

6. Nurses must be aware of the change in climate as it is anticipated that as temperatures increase there will be an increase in _____ and food _____.

7. When the human need for love and belonging is not met, people may report feeling _____ or _____.

8. Based on Maslow's hierarchy of needs, a woman recovering from a mastectomy may experience a change in _____.

9. _____ nursing care considers all human dimensions affecting how the patient's basic needs are met.

10. A person's social _____ are made up of all the people who help meet financial, personal, physical, and emotional needs.

MATCHING EXERCISES

Matching Exercise 1

Match the term in Part A with the definition in Part B.

PART A

a. Physiologic needs

b. Safety and security needs

c. Love and belonging

d. Self-esteem needs

e. Self-actualization

PART B

____ **1.** Need for people to reach their full potential through development of their unique capabilities

____ **2.** Need for a person to feel good about themselves, feel pride and a sense of accomplishment, and be respected and appreciated for those accomplishments

____ **3.** Need for oxygen, water, food, elimination, temperature, sexuality, physical activity, and rest-the minimum to maintain life

____ **4.** Protection from potential or actual harm physically and emotionally

____ **5.** Giving and receiving love, and the feeling of belonging to groups such as families, peers, friends, a neighborhood, and a community

Matching Exercise 2

Match the term in Part A with the description in Part B.

PART A

a. Lifestyle

b. Psychosocial

c. Developmental

d. Environmental

e. Biologic

PART B

____ **1.** A family has a child with severe birth defects.

____ **2.** The parents of an adolescent are notified that drugs have been found in the child's school locker.

____ **3.** A single parent of a preschool child must return to work but cannot afford adequate childcare.

____ **4.** A family whose water has been deemed unsafe due to contaminants.

____ **5.** An older adult living with family cannot tolerate what they feels is inadequate discipline of her grandchildren.

SHORT ANSWER

1. Compare and contrast community health nursing to community-based nursing.

_____

_____

2. List at least three typical questions that should be part of a family assessment.

_____

_____

3. Briefly describe the provisions of the Patient Protection and Affordable Care Act (PPACA) and two instances in which its repeal (without equivalent coverage) could be detrimental.

_____

_____

4. Describe how nurses can be/become environmentally aware.

_____

_____

5. Give an example of the following optimal family functions and explain how each meets the needs of individual family members and society as a whole.

a. Physical: _____

_____

_____

b. Economic: _____

_____

_____

c. Reproductive: _____

_____

_____

d. Affective and coping: _____

_____

e. Socialization: _____

_____

_____

6. A first-time mother-to-be is rushed to the operating room for an emergency cesarean birth. Her partner is nearby with a look of confusion and apprehension on their face. Give an example of how each of the following basic needs can be met by the nurse caring for this family.

a. Physiologic needs: _____

_____

_____

b. Safety and security needs: _____

_____

_____

c. Love and belonging needs: _____

_____

_____

d. Self-esteem needs: _____

_____

_____

e. Self-actualization needs: _____

_____

_____

APPLYING YOUR KNOWLEDGE

CRITICAL THINKING QUESTIONS

1. You are the nurse at a corrections facility for adjudicated adolescents. What can be done to promote health in these adolescents? Explain how you could attempt to provide the following basic needs.

a. Physiologic needs: _____

_____

_____

b. Safety and security needs: _____

_____

_____

c. Love and belonging needs: _____

_____

_____

d. Self-esteem needs: _____

_____

_____

e. Self-actualization needs: _____

_____

_____

2. A 25-year-old student in the local health clinic states he doesn't know if he'll be able to return if the PPACA is repealed. Knowing this student has asthma what patient-centered, political, and community actions might you take?

REFLECTIVE PRACTICE: CULTIVATING QSEN COMPETENCIES

Use the following expanded scenario from Chapter 4 in your textbook to answer the questions below.

Scenario: Samuel is the 80-year-old husband of a 76-year-old woman who was diagnosed with Alzheimer disease 1 year ago. Visibly tearful, he states, "I don't think that I can continue to care for my wife at home anymore. But how can I even consider putting her in a nursing home?"

1. Patient-centered care/safety: What basic human needs should be addressed by the nurse to provide individualized, holistic care for Samuel and his wife?

_____

_____

_____

2. Patient-centered care/safety: What would a successful outcome be for this patient?

_____

_____

3. Patient-centered care/evidence-based practice: What intellectual, interpersonal, and ethical/legal competencies are most likely to bring about the desired outcome?

Intellectual: _____

_____

Interpersonal: _____

_____

Ethical/legal: _____

_____

_____

4. Teamwork and collaboration: What resources might be helpful for Samuel?

_____

_____

_____

PRACTICING FOR NCLEX

MULTIPLE-CHOICE QUESTIONS

Circle the letter that corresponds to the best answer for each question.

1. A nurse is caring for a patient who has been admitted to the hospital for a stroke. The nurse uses the hierarchy of human basic needs to prioritize which intervention?
   a. Ensuring that the patient has family and friends visit him
   b. Helping the patient to fill out an advanced directives form
   c. Finding a safe environment for the patient upon discharge
   d. Teaching the patient to call for help before ambulating

2. A nurse is working at a community clinic that serves mostly families with young children. What would be a priority intervention for patients in this developmental stage?
   a. Setting up parenting classes
   b. Providing alcohol and drug information
   c. Screening for congenital defects
   d. Providing sex education

3. A nurse is caring for an adolescent with a traumatic lower extremity amputation secondary to a motor vehicle accident. Which human needs will the nurse set as a priority for this adolescent?
   a. Love and belonging needs
   b. Safety and security needs
   c. Self-actualization needs
   d. Self-esteem needs

4. A home health care nurse working in a low-income community assesses the risk factors and barriers to health. What is an example of a community risk factor?
   a. A community member finds out they are genetically predisposed to develop arthritis.
   b. An older adult is at risk for falls in the home due to clutter in hallways and on stairs.
   c. Children are kept inside on a sunny days because of lack of recreational opportunities.
   d. A child is born with severe intellectual disability.

5. The nurse in the medical clinic is caring for an older adult who has a long-term life partner. What will the nurse screen for?
   a. Environmental risk factors
   b. Sexual abuse
   c. Family conflict
   d. Chronic illnesses

ALTERNATE-FORMAT QUESTIONS

Multiple-Response Questions

Circle the letters that correspond to the best answers for each question.

1. A nurse prioritizes meeting the physiologic needs of patients. Which are examples of physiologic needs according to Maslow's hierarchy of needs? Select all that apply.
   a. Washing hands and donning sterile gloves before inserting a catheter
   b. Inviting a patient's estranged son to visit him
   c. Applying oxygen to a patient with chest pain
   d. Assisting a student with food insecurity in obtaining meals
   e. Restricting visitors for 2 hours so her patient can rest

2. A community health nurse is assessing factors in the community that affect health. Which situations will the nurse identify for follow-up? Select all that apply.

   a. Local school has a playground

   b. Few grocery stores or stores with fresh produce

   c. Area water contains lead

   d. There is a nearby factory that employs many local residents

   e. One health clinic serves the entire county

   f. Area is known for its high rate of gun violence

3. A nurse is providing family-centered care to patients in a community health care clinic. Which statements about the family unit are accurate? Select all that apply.

   a. Residents of a group home would not be considered a family.

   b. The family is a buffer between the needs of individual members and society.

   c. The family should not be concerned with meeting the needs of society.

   d. Duvall (1985) identified critical family developmental tasks and stages in the family life cycle.

   e. The nuclear family is composed of two parents and their children.

   f. A blended family exists when parents adopt a child from another culture.

4. A nurse is caring for a family consisting of three middle-aged adults. Which examples describe developmental tasks of this type of family structure? Select all that apply.

   a. Adjust to the cost of family life

   b. Maintain ties with younger and older generations

   c. Prepare for retirement

   d. Adjust to loss of spouse

   e. Support moral and ethical family values

   f. Cope with loss of energy and privacy

5. A nurse is planning an educational offering focusing on lifestyle risk factors. What will the nurse include in the discussion? Select all that apply.

   a. Teen pregnancy

   b. Sexually transmitted disease

   c. Substance abuse

   d. Older adults living on a fixed income

   e. Environmental pollution

Prioritization Questions

1. A nurse in a hospital setting is prioritizing care for patients based on Maslow's hierarchy. Place the following examples of interventions to meet human needs in order from highest-level needs to lower-level needs:

   a. Including family members in the care of a patient.

   b. Placing a No Smoking sign on the door of a patient who is receiving oxygen.

   c. Providing nutrition for a patient through a feeding tube.

   d. Preparing a room for the patient to meet with their religious leader.

   e. Helping a patient focus on her strengths following a diagnosis of breast cancer.

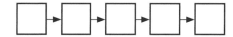

2. A community health nurse has an assignment to visit three patients. Place the nurse's visits in the appropriate order:

   a. Elderly patient who experienced a fall and whose back and flank are painful

   b. Patient whose daughter took the day off to receive education on their illness

   c. Patient with emphysema who reports more shortness of breath than usual

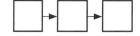

CHAPTER 5

Culturally Respectful Care

ASSESSING YOUR UNDERSTANDING

FILL IN THE BLANKS

1. Culture is a shared system of _____, values, and _____ that provides structure of daily living.

2. A group of nurses work in a freestanding surgical center on the grounds of a larger health care system. The clinic is considered a(n) _____ of the larger cultural group.

3. An example of _____ refers to a group of people with a common heritage, living in a neighborhood where they maintain their own language, food preferences, and cultural practices.

4. _____ refers to behavior of a minority group or person living within a dominant group, who has taken on the characteristics of the dominant culture and may lose the cultural features and practices that made them unique.

5. _____ occurs when people become aware of cultural differences, feel threatened, and respond by denigrating the beliefs and traditions of others to make themselves feel more secure about their own values.

6. _____ occurs when a nurse ignores differences in the cultures of patients and proceeds as though they do not exist.

7. A nurse who practiced in another country immigrates to the United States. The psychological feelings this nurse might experience when practicing in the new culture is termed culture _____.

8. A nurse assumes that all Native American patients use a shaman for healing practices. This is an example of _____.

9. To provide culturally respectful care and obtain information about the patient's beliefs related to health care the nurse should use _____ questions.

10. Accommodating patient's cultural dietary practices into the plan of care, where possible, may improve _____ to the prescribed therapy.

MATCHING EXERCISE

Match the term in Part A with the cultural group in Part B.

PART A

a. Sickle cell anemia

b. Cancer of the liver

c. Breast cancer

d. Lactose intolerance

e. Fetal alcohol syndrome

f. Tay–Sachs disease

PART B

____ 1. Native Americans and Alaska Natives

____ 2. African Americans

____ 3. Asians

____ 4. Hispanics

____ 5. Whites

____ 6. Eastern European Jews

SHORT ANSWER

1. State three changes occurring in the U.S. population over the last several decades that may affect nursing care.

   a. _____

   b. _____

   c. _____

2. Briefly discuss nursing concerns for people living in poverty.

   _____

   _____

3. Describe how you would advise impoverished patients who are not meeting their health care needs due to the following conditions:

   a. Lack of transportation to clinic, hospital, or health care provider's office: _____

   _____

   _____

   b. Living in overcrowded conditions; absence of running water and adequate sanitation:

   _____

   _____

   _____

   c. Lack of health insurance: _____

   _____

   _____

4. Explain why the following groups of people are at high risk for living in poverty.

   a. Families headed by single women: _____

   _____

   _____

   b. Older adults: _____

   _____

   _____

   c. Future generations of those now in poverty:

   _____

   _____

   _____

5. List five characteristics the nurse should be aware of when planning care, often found in people living within the culture of poverty.

   a. _____

   b. _____

   c. _____

   d. _____

   e. _____

APPLYING YOUR KNOWLEDGE

CRITICAL THINKING QUESTIONS

1. How would you respond to the individual nursing needs of the following patients?

   a. An Orthodox Jewish man refuses to let a female nurse perform a nursing assessment and asks for a male doctor to examine him instead.

   _____

   _____

   _____

   b. A girl, age 13, delivers her first baby. She tells you she had an abortion earlier but is ready for this new baby.

   _____

   _____

   _____

   c. A man who speaks limited English brings his non–English speaking grandfather to the emergency room, with signs of a myocardial infarction.

   _____

   _____

   _____

2. Interview a classmate about their cultural background. Ask them what cultural practices are important at home and how culture might influence their beliefs about health care.

REFLECTIVE PRACTICE: CULTIVATING QSEN COMPETENCIES

Use the following expanded scenario from Chapter 5 in your textbook to answer the questions below.

Scenario: Danielle is an immigrant from Haiti who has been in the United States for approximately 8 months. She recently had surgical repair of a fractured femur and is now confined to a hospital bed in skeletal traction. She asks that a Haitian folk healer from her neighborhood be allowed to come to the hospital to help heal her broken leg.

1. Patient-centered care/safety: How might the nurse respond to Danielle's request for a Haitian folk healer?

   _____

   _____

   _____

2. Patient-centered care: What would be a successful outcome for this patient?

   _____

   _____

   _____

3. Patient-centered care/evidence-based practice: What intellectual, interpersonal, and ethical/legal competencies are most likely to bring about the desired outcome?

   Intellectual: _____

   _____

   Interpersonal: _____

   _____

   Ethical/legal: _____

   _____

4. Teamwork and collaboration: What resources might be helpful for the nurse to better plan care for Danielle?

   _____

   _____

   _____

PRACTICING FOR NCLEX

MULTIPLE-CHOICE QUESTIONS

Circle the letter that corresponds to the best answer for each question.

1. A patient's daughter tells the nurse that her mother received pork their meal tray, but their culture prohibits consuming pork. Which of the following responses represents the most culturally respectful response by the nurse?
   a. "I'll take the tray away right away and order a new one."
   b. "Are there other dietary restrictions we should be aware of?"
   c. "I'll have the dietician come to speak to you about her diet."
   d. "I will enter this preference in the electronic health record?"

2. A nurse is planning an ice cream social for multicultural residents of a long-term care facility. For which of the following groups will the nurse offer an alternate treat due to increased incidence of lactose intolerance?
   a. African Americans
   b. White females
   c. Native Americans
   d. Hispanics

3. The nurse is performing a pain assessment on a patient from another culture. Which statement reflects the most accurate documentation of pain?
   a. Absence of grimacing or guarding
   b. Pain rating of 8 on a scale of 1–10
   c. Spouse stating the patient is having moderate pain
   d. Getting out of bed to eat their meal

4. A nurse is caring for a non–English speaking patient who is scheduled for an MRI. Which action will the nurse take when communicating about the test?
   a. Speaking louder so the patient can hear you
   b. Asking the patient's daughter to translate
   c. Using a professional translator
   d. Providing written instructions

5. A prison nurse is caring for a new prisoner brought to the infirmary. The prisoner appears disoriented and complains about the noise, bright lights, and lack of privacy. The nurse documents which of the following problems in the electronic health record?
   a. Culture assimilation
   b. Culture disorientation
   c. Culture blindness
   d. Culture shock

6. A patient who emigrated from Southeast Asia tells the nurse she would like her family to bring in an herbal tea to help with postoperative constipation. Which response by the nurse is most appropriate?
   a. "We do not permit any food or beverages prepared outside the facility."
   b. "Tell me about the use of this herb in your culture."
   c. "I'll check with the health care provider for medication interactions
   d. "You'll be going home in 3 days; could you take it then?"

7. A nurse is caring for a patient with a leaking aneurysm and low blood pressure, for whom several units of packed red blood cells are prescribed. The patient states their culture prohibits receiving any blood products, even though they know they will die, or they are barred from "paradise" after death. How should the nurse prioritize care?
   a. Administer the prescribed blood transfusions as a life saving measure.
   b. Tell the patient they will discuss IV fluids and comfort care with the medical team.
   c. Suggest the patient speak with her religious leader prior to making this decision.
   d. Tell the patient that their family needs them and to reconsider this action.

ALTERNATE-FORMAT QUESTIONS
Multiple-Response Questions
Circle the letters that correspond to the best answers for each question.

1. A nurse is providing care for patients of multiple cultures in a community clinic. Which characteristics of culture should the nurse consider when planning culturally competent care? Select all that apply.
   a. Culture guides behavior into acceptable ways for people in a specific group.
   b. Culture is not affected by a group's social and physical environment.
   c. Cultural practices and beliefs are constantly evolving and changing over time to satisfy a group's needs.
   d. Culture influences the way people of a group view themselves.
   e. There are differences both within cultures and among cultures.
   f. Subcultures exist within most cultures.

2. A nurse in a long-term care facility performs which actions when practicing culturally respectful care? Select all that apply.
   a. Asking open-ended questions when performing cultural assessments on patients
   b. Using past experiences of members of a culture exclusively to solve cultural issues that may arise
   c. Ignoring personal beliefs, values, practices, and family experiences that may cause biases that affect the nursing care of culturally diverse patients
   d. Using observation and listening to acquire knowledge of the beliefs and values of patients
   e. Discouraging families from bringing food from home for the patient to help the patient adapt to the food provided by the facility
   f. Incorporating the suggestions of a patient's folk medicine practitioner into the care plan

3. A nurse working in a free community clinic serving low-income patients recognizes a culture of poverty may exist. Which factors support a culture of poverty? Select all that apply.

   a. Not bothering to look for work anymore

   b. Abusive home environment

   c. Working 30 hours weekly at a local store

   d. Supportive community in their place of worship

   e. Widowed parent living with their parents

4. During post-conference, nursing students enrolled in a community health course are discussing ways for health care organizations to become and remain culturally competent. Which recommendations will the students include in the discussion? Select all that apply.

   a. Delivering care compatible with cultural beliefs and preferences

   b. Hiring a majority of staff who speak the languages of the community

   c. Recruiting a culturally diverse staff reflective of the service area

   d. Providing the staff with education on using linguistic services

   e. Documenting ethnicity and spoken language in the electronic health record

CHAPTER 6

Values, Ethics, and Advocacy

ASSESSING YOUR UNDERSTANDING

FILL IN THE BLANKS

1. When a young boy is left to explore values on his own with no guidance from his parents, the parents are using a(n) _____ approach to value transmission.

2. A(n) _____ of _____ is a set of principles that reflect the primary goals, values, and obligations of the profession.

3. A nurse supports a patient making a treatment decision to analyze personal preferences, goals, and the anticipated outcome of each choice. This nurse is helping the patient by engaging them in _____.

4. A nurse who is proud and happy about a decision to obtain further education is involved in the _____ step of the process of valuing.

5. A nurse reflects on their personal values, ranking them along a continuum of importance leading to a personal code of conduct. This is the nurse's _____.

6. A nurse who is committed to protecting the right of an adolescent minor to refuse medical treatment is practicing patient _____.

7. _____ occurs when there has been a betrayal of what is right by someone who holds legitimate authority, or by oneself.

8. Nurses have a duty to report unsafe care, which may be referred to as _____.

9. Students who succumb to the high pressure to succeed by resorting to plagiarism or academic dishonesty may be _____ likely to continue this behavior when working as a nurse.

10. The nurse who upholds moral, legal, and humanistic principles to ensure equal treatment under the law and equal access to quality health care is engaged in a quest for _____.

MATCHING EXERCISES

Match the term in Part A with the definition in Part B.

Matching Exercise 1

PART A

a. Value

b. Advocacy

c. Values clarification

d. Ethical dilemma

e. Ethics

f. Ethical distress

PART B

_____ **1.** Occurring when two or more clear moral principles apply, but they support mutually inconsistent courses of action

_____ **2.** Process of discovery allowing a person to choose between alternatives and to identify whether the choices are the result of previous conditioning

_____ **3.** Ethical problem in which the person knows the right thing to do, but institutional constraints make it nearly impossible to pursue the right actions

_____ **4.** Systematic inquiry into the principles of right and wrong conduct, of virtue and vice, and of good and evil, as they relate to conduct

_____ **5.** Protection and support of another's rights

_____ **6.** Personal belief about worth that acts as a standard to guide behavior

Matching Exercise 2

Match the term in Part A with the mode of value transmission Part B.

PART A

a. Modeling

b. Moralizing

c. Laissez-faire

d. Rewarding and punishing

e. Responsible choice

PART B

_____ **1.** Child is taught by teachers and parents that premarital sex is sinful

_____ **2.** Child is sent to his room following an altercation with his sibling

_____ **3.** Child is allowed to determine his own bedtime

_____ **4.** Child observes his parents interact with people of various cultures

_____ **5.** Child is encouraged by their parents to explore all aspects of their personal code of ethics

SHORT ANSWER

1. The mother of a school-aged child with cystic fibrosis works during the day as a cashier and is enrolled in an evening nursing. Her husband's employment requires constant overnight travel. The child needs more attention than the mother has time to supply, and the mother feels guilty that her child needs more attention than she can provide and feels guilty for taking time to better herself. She cannot afford to hire a full-time caretaker for her child. Describe how the nurse could help the patient's mother define their values and choose a plan of action.

   a. Values clarification: _____

   _____

   _____

   b. Choosing: _____

   _____

   _____

   c. Prizing: _____

   _____

   _____

   d. Acting: _____

   _____

   _____

2. Identify four ethical issues confronted by nurses in their daily nursing practice. How would you deal with these issues in your own practice?

   a. _____

   _____

   b. _____

   _____

   c. _____

   _____

   d. _____

   _____

3. Briefly describe the five principles of bioethics and give an example of each.

   a. Autonomy: _____

   b. Nonmaleficence: _____

   c. Beneficence: _____

   d. Justice: _____

   e. Fidelity: _____

4. Describe how you, as a nurse, would act as an advocate for the following patients:

   a. Infant born addicted to crack cocaine whose mother wants to take him home: _____

   b. 12-year-old girl who seeks a pregnancy test at a Planned Parenthood clinic without her parents' knowledge: _____

   c. 15-year-old girl who has anorexia nervosa and refuses to eat anything during her hospital stay: _____

   d. 28-year-old man who contracted AIDS from an infected male partner, and who tells you that the other nurses have been avoiding him: _____

   e. 48-year-old mother with emphysema who refuses to quit smoking: _____

   f. 78-year-old woman in a long-term care facility who is dying of cancer and asks you to help her "end the pain" through assisted suicide: _____

5. List the qualities you possess that you feel are most important in developing your own personal code of ethics. _____

6. Use the five-step model of ethical decision making to resolve the following moral distress. You recommend a psychiatric evaluation for a homeless patient, diagnosed with high blood pressure. The patient appears confused, withdrawn or alternately combative, and unable to engage in self-care or manage their discharge medications. Suspecting early Alzheimer disease, advocate for the consultation, but the health care provider insists the patient be discharged without additional interventions.

   a. Assess the situation: _____

   b. Diagnose/identify the ethical problem: ____

   c. Plan: _____

   d. Implement your decision: _____

   e. Evaluate your decision: _____

7. Give an example of an ethical problem that may occur among the following health care personnel, patients, and institutions.

   a. Nurse/patient: _____

   _____

   _____

   b. Nurse/nurse: _____

   _____

   _____

   c. Nurse/health care provider: _____

   _____

   _____

   d. Nurse/institution: _____

   _____

   _____

APPLYING YOUR KNOWLEDGE

CRITICAL THINKING QUESTIONS

1. Describe how you would respond in an ethical manner to the following patient requests:

   a. The anxious father of a 17-year-old gay patient asks you to perform an HIV test on his son without his son's knowledge.

   _____

   _____

   _____

   _____

   b. A woman who presents with contusions and marks consistent with domestic abuse tells you that her husband pushed her down the steps. She asks you not to tell anyone. When her husband arrives, he hovers over her in an obsessive and overly protective manner.

   _____

   _____

   _____

   _____

2. Describe what you would do in the following situations:

   a. A doctor asks you to falsify a report that he prescribed medicine contraindicated for a patient's condition.

   _____

   _____

   _____

   b. A nurse coworker refuses to bathe an HIV-positive patient.

   _____

   _____

   _____

   c. Due to administrative cutbacks, not enough nurses are scheduled to cover the critical care unit in which you work.

   _____

   _____

   _____

Share your responses with a classmate and explore the difference in your responses. What competencies and character traits promote ethical behavior?

REFLECTIVE PRACTICE: CULTIVATING QSEN COMPETENCIES

Use the following expanded scenario from Chapter 6 in your textbook to answer the questions below.

Scenario: Mr. Raines, a homeless, 68-year-old indigent man diagnosed with schizophrenia, developmental delays, and uncontrolled hypertension, was admitted for control of moderately severe elevated blood pressure. A review of his medical record reveals that Mr. Raines was getting samples of medications for blood pressure treatment from the pharmaceutical representatives at the clinic, but recent policy changes stopped this practice approximately 4 weeks ago. Mr. Raines is about to be discharged with several prescriptions for medications but no way to fill them.

1. Patient-centered care: How might the nurse react to Mr. Raines response to filling his prescriptions?

   _____

   _____

   _____

2. Patient-centered care: What would be a successful outcome for this patient?

_____

_____

_____

3. Safety: What intellectual, technical, interpersonal, and ethical/legal competencies are most likely to bring about the desired outcome?

Intellectual: _____

_____

Technical: _____

_____

_____

Interpersonal: _____

_____

_____

Ethical/legal: _____

_____

_____

4. Teamwork and collaboration: What resources might be helpful for Mr. Raines?

_____

_____

_____

PRACTICING FOR NCLEX

MULTIPLE-CHOICE QUESTIONS

Circle the letter that corresponds to the best answer for each question.

1. Hospital policy dictates that mother and baby be discharged 24 hours after delivery. The nurse caring for the mother identifies that the woman is not prepared to go home and recognizes this represents what problem?
   a. Ethical uncertainty
   b. Ethical distress
   c. Ethical dilemma
   d. Ethical dissatisfaction

2. An adolescent with anorexia nervosa has stopped eating and is slowly starving to death. The parents insist the nurse obtain a prescription to place a feeding tube for nourishment. Which example demonstrates the nurse's use of the utilitarian theory of ethics?
   a. The nurse obtains a prescription to provide tube feedings for the adolescent as the end result is good and will save the patient's life.
   b. The nurse refuses to force feed the patient because the nurse believes ignoring the patient's wishes is wrong.
   c. The nurse believes that force feeding a patient could be right or wrong depending on the process used to accomplish the action.
   d. The nurse believes that forcing nourishment on a patient violates the principles of autonomy and nonmaleficence.

3. A nurse demonstrates the professional value known as altruism when caring for patients in a long-term care facility. Which nursing action is based on this value?
   a. Consulting a patient when planning nursing care to determine priorities
   b. Advocating for the right of an adult patient with intellectual disability to refuse surgery
   c. Helping an older adult patient fill out an informed consent form
   d. Promoting universal access to health care for underserved populations

4. A nurse cultivates dispositions that enable practicing nursing in a way they believe. This nurse is displaying what essential element of moral facility?
   a. Moral sensibility
   b. Moral responsiveness
   c. Moral capacity
   d. Moral valuing

5. A nurse who provides information and support for patients and their families to make health care decisions is practicing which principle of bioethics?

   a. Autonomy
   b. Nonmaleficence
   c. Justice
   d. Fidelity

6. Nurses who value patient advocacy follow what guideline?

   a. Valuing loyalty to an employing institution or to a colleague over their commitment to their patient
   b. Prioritizing the good of the individual patient rather than to the good of society in general
   c. Choosing the claims of the patient's well-being over the claims of the patient's autonomy
   d. Making decisions for patients who are uninformed concerning their rights and opportunities

7. A nursing instructor is teaching students about the use of moral agency in nursing practice. Which action most accurately represents this principle?

   a. Teaching a patient and family members the purpose of an advanced directive and do not resuscitate order
   b. Advocating for organ donation, verified by the patient's driver's license, after documented brain death
   c. Teaching a client about surgical options for gastric bypass and their recovery times
   d. Promoting dignity and respect of all patients by using proper draping for the patient's privacy

8. A nurse is preparing to transfer a patient to the operating room when the patient states, "I no longer want to have this surgery." After ensuring that the patient understands the consequence of canceling the surgery and notifying the surgeon, which ethical principle takes priority?

   a. Social justice
   b. Human dignity
   c. Integrity
   d. Advocacy

ALTERNATE-FORMAT QUESTIONS

Multiple-Response Questions

Circle the letters that correspond to the best answers for each question.

1. A school nurse interviewing parents of a child who is doing poorly in school determines that the parents practice a laissez-faire method of discipline. What does the nurse identity as examples of this form of value transmission? Select all that apply.

   a. A child says a prayer before meals that he learned from his parents.
   b. A child is taken for ice cream to celebrate his good report card.
   c. An adolescent explores religions of friends in hopes of developing his own faith.
   d. An adolescent is punished for staying out too late with her friends.
   e. An adolescent tries alcohol at a party with her friends.

2. Nurses practice the professional value of autonomy when providing nursing care for patients. Which nursing actions best describe the use of this value? Select all that apply.

   a. Staying later than their shift to continue caring for a patient in critical condition
   b. Researching a new procedure that would benefit their patient
   c. Keeping a promise to call a patient's doctor regarding pain relief
   d. Reading the Patient Bill of Rights to a visually impaired patient
   e. Communicating patient hesitancy about canceling an impending surgery

3. Which nursing actions best demonstrate the use of the professional value of altruism? Select all that apply.

   a. Demonstrating an understanding of the culture of their patient
   b. Becoming a mentor to a nursing student working on their unit
   c. Being accountable for the care provided to a mentally challenged patient
   d. Lobbying for universal access to health care
   e. Respecting the right of a Native American to call in a shaman for a consultation
   f. Protecting the privacy of a patient with AIDS

4. Which nursing actions best demonstrate the use of the professional value of human dignity? Select all that apply.
   a. Completing the nursing care plan in anticipation of the patient's transfer from the ED
   b. Providing honest information to a patient about their illness
   c. Providing privacy for an older adult patient
   d. Reporting an error made by an incompetent coworker
   e. Developing individualized nursing care plans for their patients
   f. Refusing to discuss a patient with a curious friend

5. Nursing students enrolled in a leadership class are discussing the principle of nonmaleficence with their professor. Which examples will be included in their discussion? Select all that apply.
   a. Performing regular patient assessments for pressure injuries
   b. Following "medication rights" when administering medicine to patients
   c. Providing information to patients to help them make decisions about treatment options
   d. Arranging for hospice for a patient who is terminally ill
   e. Removing an IV due to redness and warmth at the site
   f. Acting fairly when allocating time and resources to patients

CHAPTER 7

Legal Dimensions of Nursing Practice

ASSESSING YOUR UNDERSTANDING

FILL IN THE BLANKS

1. Standards or rules of conduct established and enforced by the government that is intended to protect the rights of the public refers to _____ laws.

2. A state's _____ protects the public by broadly defining the legal scope of nursing practice.

3. _____ is a specialized form of credentialing based on laws passed by a state legislature.

4. A nurse who reviews the heath record and explains to the judge and jury whether nursing care met acceptable standards is called a(n) _____.

5. When nurses participate in a group that is establishing, maintaining, and improving conditions of employment and the health care environment they are participating in the practice of _____.

6. When a nurse documents the fall of an older adult patient for purposes of risk management, the nurse is filing a(n) _____ report.

7. The Joint Commission defines an unexpected occurrence involving death, serious or psychological injury, or the risk thereof as a(n) _____ event.

8. A(n) _____ also called a variance or occurrence report, is used by health care facilities to document anything out of the ordinary that results in, or has the potential to result in, harm to a patient, employee, or visitor.

9. _____ is a method of ensuring professional competencies.

10. It is important to note that licensure is not a right after completing a nursing education program; rather, it is a _____.

MATCHING EXERCISES

Matching Exercise 1

Match the tort listed in Part A with the definition in Part B.

PART A

a. Assault

b. Battery

c. False imprisonment

d. Fraud

e. Negligence

f. Libel

PART B

____ 1. A nurse strikes a patient who complains that she is not being cared for properly.

____ 2. A nurse shares a rumor with their colleagues that a patient is a compulsive gambler.

___ **3.** A nurse threatens to slap an older adult patient who refuses to clean up after themselves.

___ **4.** A nurse forgets to replace an IV bag that is empty.

___ **5.** A nurse seeking a position in long-term care claims to be certified in gerontologic nursing, which is untrue.

___ **6.** A nurse uses restraints on a patient unnecessarily.

Matching Exercise 2

Match the term listed in Part A with the definition in Part B.

PART A

a. Litigation
b. Defendant
c. Felony
d. Tort
e. Contract
f. Precedent

PART B

___ **1.** Exchange of promises between two parties

___ **2.** Process of a lawsuit

___ **3.** Party being accused in a lawsuit

___ **4.** First case that sets down the rule by decision

___ **5.** Crime punishable by imprisonment in a state or federal penitentiary for more than 1 year

___ **6.** Wrong committed by a person against another person or their property that generally results in a civil trial

Matching Exercise 3

Match the type of law listed in Part A with its definition/example listed in Part B.

PART A

a. Administrative law
b. Common law
c. Public law
d. Civil law
e. Criminal law
f. Statutory law

PART B

___ **1.** Nurse practice acts

___ **2.** Rules and regulations of boards of nursing

___ **3.** Malpractice law

___ **4.** Laws regulating relationships among people

___ **5.** Laws involving murder, manslaughter, criminal negligence, theft, and illegal possession of drugs

___ **6.** Laws regulating relationships between people and the government

Matching Exercise 4

Match the legal term listed in Part A with its definition in Part B.

PART A

a. False imprisonment
b. Fraud
c. Libel
d. Malpractice
e. Negligence

PART B

___ **1.** Willful and purposeful misrepresentation that could or has caused loss or harm to a person or property

___ **2.** Failure to meet the standard of care

___ **3.** Negligence by professional personnel

___ **4.** Unjustified retention or prevention of the movement of another person without proper consent

___ **5.** Written defamation of character

SHORT ANSWER

1. Give an example of how nurses can avoid the following common allegations of malpractice.

a. Failure to ensure patient safety: _____

_____

b. Improper treatment or performance of treatment: _____

_____

c. Failure to monitor, report, and rescue: _____

_____

_____

d. Medication errors and reactions: _____

_____

_____

e. Failure to follow facility procedure: _____

_____

_____

f. Adverse incidents: _____

_____

_____

2. Define voluntary standards of nursing practice and legal standards and give an example of each.

   a. Voluntary standards: _____

_____

_____

   b. Legal standards: _____

_____

_____

3. List three cases in which informed consent is needed from a patient:

   a. _____

   b. _____

   c. _____

4. Give three examples of invasion of privacy in a nurse–patient relationship:

   a. _____

   b. _____

   c. _____

5. List three strengths a nurse must possess to testify competently as an expert witness:

   a. _____

   b. _____

   c. _____

6. Describe under what conditions a nurse would accept a telephone order from a health care provider:

_____

_____

_____

7. List two cases in which it would be appropriate to question a health care provider's order.

   a. _____

   b. _____

8. When bathing a patient who has had a hip replacement, the nurse does not replace the side rails, and the patient falls out of bed. The patient is shaken up and sore from the fall, but there appears to be no further damage to their hip.

   a. What is the nurse's liability in this situation?

_____

_____

   b. What information should be included in the incident report?

_____

_____

   c. Do you feel the patient has a case for negligence? Explain why or why not, using the four elements of liability that must be present to prove that negligence has occurred (duty, breach of duty, causation, damages).

_____

_____

9. What is the purpose of the nurse carrying liability insurance?

_____

_____

APPLYING YOUR KNOWLEDGE

CRITICAL THINKING QUESTIONS

1. Think about how you would respond in the following situation and discuss your responsibilities with your classmates. Are there ever differences between the legally prudent and morally right response?

   a. Another student tells you they inadvertently gave medications to the wrong patient. The student says they are terrified of the nursing instructor and has decided not to inform anyone.

   b. An older adult resident in a long-term care facility tells you the evening nurses sometimes push and hit the residents, but begs you not to tell anyone.

   c. You observe a surgeon contaminate a sterile field; when you inform him, he tells you not to be so squeamish.

2. Meet the risk manager of the institution where you attend clinical or research their role. Discuss how the nurse and risk manager work together.

REFLECTIVE PRACTICE: CULTIVATING QSEN COMPETENCIES

Use the following expanded scenario from Chapter 7 in your textbook to answer the questions below.

Scenario: Meredith is the mother of a terminally ill child with a brain tumor who is admitted to a residential hospice for better pain and symptom management. One morning she tells the nurse, "I'm very unhappy with the care my son is receiving. I'm going to talk with my attorney as soon as possible to press charges against the hospice."

1. Teamwork and collaboration: How might the nurses involved in this scenario respond to Meredith's disclosure that she will be pressing charges against the hospital?

   _____

   _____

   _____

2. Safety/teamwork and collaboration: What intellectual, technical, interpersonal, and ethical/legal competencies are most likely to be used in this situation?

   Intellectual: _____

   _____

   _____

   Technical: _____

   _____

   _____

   Interpersonal: _____

   _____

   _____

   Ethical/legal: _____

   _____

   _____

3. Safety/teamwork and collaboration: What resources might be helpful for the nurses in this case?

   _____

   _____

   _____

PRACTICING FOR NCLEX

MULTIPLE-CHOICE QUESTIONS

Circle the letter that corresponds to the best answer for each question.

1. The nurse attends a seminar on Health Insurance Portability and Accountability Act (HIPAA) learns that patients' rights to which of the following is covered under that law?
   a. Copying their health records
   b. Documenting errors of care in their medical record
   c. Seeking damages for unsatisfactory care
   d. Rating the quality of care received

2. A nurse's colleague appears sedated and has an odor of alcohol on their breath during handoff report. What is the nurse's best course of action?
   a. Warning the nurse that you will report her if it happens again
   b. Reporting the nurse to the state's board of nursing
   c. Sharing your suspicions with the nurse manager
   d. Beginning to keep a log of suspicious behaviors

3. Nurses practicing in a critical care unit must acquire additional, specialized skills, and knowledge to provide care to the critically ill patient. These nurses can validate this specialty competence through what process?
   a. Certification
   b. Accreditation
   c. Licensure
   d. Litigation

4. The nurse is assisting the health care provider with obtaining informed consent from a non–English speaking patient. Which of the following actions is essential?
   a. Asking the family member that is present to step outside
   b. Ensuring the client signs the form prior to the procedure
   c. Witnessing the patient's consent form by affixing your signature
   d. Validating that the patient can describe the procedure they have agreed to

5. In some cases, the act of providing nursing care in unexpected situations is covered by the Good Samaritan laws. Which nursing actions would most likely be covered by these laws?

   a. Providing emergency care where consent is given

   b. Performing negligent acts in an emergency situation

   c. Giving medical advice to a neighbor regarding a rash

   d. Providing emergency care to someone choking in a restaurant

6. A nursing student is assisting a patient to ambulate following hip replacement surgery when the patient falls, reinjuring the hip. Who is potentially responsible for the injury to this patient?

   a. Nursing student

   b. Nurse instructor

   c. Hospital

   d. All of the above

7. A nurse who comments to her coworkers at lunch that her patient with a sexually transmitted disease has been sexually active in the community may be guilty of what tort?

   a. Slander

   b. Libel

   c. Fraud

   d. Assault

8. A nurse is named as a defendant in a malpractice lawsuit. Which action would be recommended for this nurse?

   a. Discussing the case with the plaintiff to ensure understanding of each other's positions

   b. If a mistake was made on a chart, changing it to read appropriately

   c. Being prepared to tell your side to the press, if necessary

   d. Not volunteering any information on the witness stand

9. A nurse is preparing to administer an intravenous antibiotic to a postoperative patient. When performing the final check of the medication the nurse recognizes it is a similar sounding medication, but not the correct one. After administering the correct medication, which of the following actions will the nurse take?

   a. Calling the pharmacy to report that the wrong medication was delivered

   b. Explaining to the patient that a potential error occurred

   c. Completing an event report describing the near miss

   d. Informing the pharmacy manager of the error

ALTERNATE-FORMAT QUESTIONS

Multiple-Response Questions

Circle the letters that correspond to the best answers for each question.

1. A nurse is writing an email to a U.S. Congressman to support the promotion of health care issues. Which guidelines will the nurse use to ensure a properly written email? Select all that apply.

   a. Stating the purpose of the email briefly and clearly in the first paragraph

   b. Naming the city and state where they live and vote

   c. Avoiding using specific examples from the workplace to support the position

   d. Asking the legislator to vote for/support what is being asked

   e. Keeping the email to two pages and include a cover page with contact information

   f. Addressing the email to as many legislators as possible

2. As part of interprofessional education, a group of leadership students and law students participate in a mock malpractice trial. The participants must correctly apply which statements related to this process? Select all that apply.

   a. "The defendant is the person who is initiating the lawsuit."

   b. "The process of bringing and trying this lawsuit is called litigation."

   c. "The defendant is presumed guilty until proven innocent."

   d. "The opinions of appellate judges are published and become common law."

   e. "Malpractice is the term generally used to describe negligence by professional personnel."

3. Nursing students have been taught that nurses practice within the legal and mandatory standards of the nursing profession. To which mandatory standards must they adhere upon graduation? Select all that apply.
   a. State nurse practice acts
   b. Organization's procedure manual
   c. American Nurses Association Standards of Practice
   d. Certification
   e. Licensure

4. Nurses follow nursing practice rules when working within the profession. What are examples of state-mandated rules? Select all that apply.
   a. Nurse practice acts
   b. Medicare provisions reimbursement of nursing services
   c. Nursing educational requirements
   d. Delegation trees
   e. Disciplinary authority of board of nursing
   f. Medication administration

5. Nurses may commit both intentional and unintentional torts when practicing within the profession. Which are examples of intentional torts? Select all that apply.
   a. Forgetting to put the side rails up on a crib and the toddler falls out
   b. Not reporting a change in patient's condition in a timely manner
   c. Threatening to hit an older adult patient who has dementia and is wailing
   d. Seeking employment in a hospital after falsifying credentials on a resume
   e. Placing a patient who is a fall risk in restraints without the proper order

6. Legal counsel for a nurse being sued for malpractice explains that what must be established to prove that malpractice or negligence occurred? Select all that apply.
   a. Duty
   b. Intent to harm
   c. Breach of duty
   d. Causation
   e. Damages
   f. Fraud

7. Nurses use legal safeguards to protect themselves from exposure to legal risks and protect the patient from harm. What are examples of these safeguards? Select all that apply.
   a. Obtaining consent from a patient prior to performing a procedure
   b. Health care providers bearing responsibility for administration of an incorrect prescription
   c. Educating the patient about the Patient Bill of Rights
   d. Carrying out health care provider prescriptions without questioning them
   e. Documenting all patient care in a timely manner

Sequencing Question

1. Place the following steps involved in malpractice litigation in the order in which they would normally occur:
   a. A decision or verdict is reached.
   b. The basis for the claim is appropriate and timely; all elements of liability are present.
   c. The trial takes place.
   d. Pretrial discovery activities and review of medical records and deposition of plaintiff, defendants, and witnesses are performed.
   e. All parties named as defendants, as well as insurance companies and attorneys, work toward a fair settlement.
   f. If the verdict is not accepted by both sides, it may be appealed to an appellate court.
   g. The case is presented to a malpractice arbitration panel. The panel's decision is either accepted or rejected, in which case a complaint is filed in trial court.
   h. The defendants contest allegations.

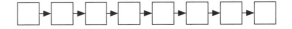

Communication

ASSESSING YOUR UNDERSTANDING

FILL IN THE BLANKS

1. A nurse initiates the communication process by addressing a patient need. This patient need becomes a(n) _____ for conversation.

2. The channel of communication is the medium the sender has selected to send the message. These channels include _____, _____, and _____.

3. When using nonverbal communication, the nurse recognizes that the _____ is the most expressive part of the body.

4. Effective communication supports collaborative relationships and continuous improvement in patient _____ and quality of care.

5. A patient who verbally explains their understanding of discharge instructions is providing _____ to the caregiver.

6. A patient who expresses anger at a diagnosis by slamming a food tray on the table is using _____ communication.

7. When a nurse helps a patient achieve goals that allow their human needs to be satisfied, the nurse and patient are involved in a(n) _____ relationship.

8. When a nurse and patient meet, introduce themselves, and clarify their roles, they are in the _____ phase of the helping relationship.

9. A nurse is using a(n) _____ comment/question when she says to her patient, "I understand a high-fiber diet was recommended. Are you able to get enough fiber with the foods you've been eating?"

10. Anger and aggressive behavior between nurses, or nurse-to-nurse hostility, has been labeled _____.

11. Referring to a patient by room number on a social media post may result in a sanction by the _____ of Nursing.

MATCHING EXERCISES

Matching Exercise 1

Match the type of communication in Part A with the definition in Part B.

PART A

a. Intrapersonal communication

b. Interpersonal communication

c. Small-group communication

d. Organizational communication

PART B

_____ 1. Occurs within a person

_____ 2. Occurs between two or more people with a goal to exchange messages

_____ 3. Occurs when nurses interact with two or more people

_____ 4. Occurs among groups within the workplace to achieve established goals

Matching Exercise 2

Match the term in Part A with the definition in Part B.

PART A

a. Message
b. Receiver
c. Channel
d. Noise
e. Source
f. Feedback

PART B

___ 1. Actual product of the encoder

___ 2. Translates and makes a decision about the product

___ 3. Verbal and nonverbal evidence that the patient received and understood the product

___ 4. Medium selected to convey the product

___ 5. Factors that distort the quality of the product

___ 6. Prepares and sends the product

Matching Exercise 3

Match the term in Part A with the definition in Part B.

PART A

a. Orientation phase
b. Working phase
c. Termination phase

PART B

___ 1. Patient demonstrates ability to maneuver on crutches

___ 2. Patient acknowledges the goals they have accomplished in physical therapy

___ 3. Patient learns the name of the physical therapist and addresses them by name

Matching Exercise 4

Match the type of interviewing technique in Part A with the statement that reflects it in Part B.

PART A

a. Validating question/comment
b. Clarifying question/comment
c. Reflective question/comment
d. Sequencing question/comment
e. Directing question/comment

PART B

___ 1. "You say you've always been healthy and active. Is this the first time you've been hospitalized?"

___ 2. "You expressed concern about your children at home…"

___ 3. "You've been on your present medication for 3 years. Have you experience any side effects?"

___ 4. "Your chest pain began after exercising on a bicycle?"

___ 5. "You've been upset about taking medication…have you continued?"

SHORT ANSWER

1. Rewrite the following statements to reflect therapeutic nursing communication.

    a. You didn't eat any candy today, did you?

    _____

    _____

    b. Are you having pain?

    _____

    _____

    c. Please don't cry.

    _____

    _____

    d. What are you so annoyed about?

    _____

    _____

    e. "Don't worry, I'm sure the surgery will go without a hitch."

    _____

    _____

2. Give an example of the following nonverbal forms of communication a patient might display and explain how they can provide clues to the patient's health status.

    a. Touch: _____

    _____

    _____

    b. Eye contact: _____

    _____

    _____

c. Facial expressions: _____

_____

_____

d. Posture: _____

_____

_____

e. Gait: _____

_____

_____

f. Gestures: _____

_____

_____

g. General physical appearance: _____

_____

_____

h. Mode of dress and grooming: _____

_____

_____

i. Sounds: _____

_____

_____

j. Silence: _____

_____

_____

3. Briefly describe how you would alter your explanation of a surgical procedure to account for the developmental considerations of the following patients:

a. School-aged child: _____

_____

_____

b. Adolescent: _____

_____

_____

c. Older adult with a hearing impairment:

_____

_____

_____

4. A nurse is meeting a patient for the first time. What clues to a person's identity can sometimes be determined by knowing that person's occupation?

_____

_____

5. Briefly explain the role communication plays in the following steps of the nursing process.

a. Assessing: _____

_____

_____

b. Diagnosing: _____

_____

_____

c. Planning: _____

_____

_____

d. Implementing: _____

_____

_____

e. Evaluating: _____

_____

_____

f. Documenting: _____

_____

_____

6. Explain why the following variables must be considered when establishing rapport between the nurse and patient.

a. Providing privacy: _____

_____

_____

b. Maintaining confidentiality: _____

_____

_____

c. Developing therapeutic communication skills: _____

_____

_____

d. Using silence as a tool: _____

_____

_____

7. Underline the nonverbal communication by the nurse and patient in the following scenario:

A patient is recovering the day after a mastectomy. She is married with two school-aged children. When the nurse enters the patient's room, she finds the patient with tears in her eyes and a worried expression on her face. When asked how she is feeling, the patient replies "fine," although her face is rigid, and her mouth is drawn in a firm line. She is moving her foot back and forth under the covers. On further investigation, the nurse finds that the patient is worried about her children and her ability to be a healthy, functioning wife and mother again. After prompting, the patient says, "I don't know if my husband will still love me like this." She sighs and falls silent, reflecting upon her recovery. The nurse repositions the patient and puts her hand over the patient's hand. She establishes eye contact and suggests that things have a way of working out over time.

8. An older adult with early signs of Alzheimer disease, requiring supervision begins to attend a daycare center while their daughter is working. The nurse enters into a helping relationship with the patient, cognizant she will be leaving the organization at the end of the month. Write two patient goals the nurse could establish to help the patient with dementia navigate this change in personnel.

a. Orientation phase: _____

_____

_____

b. Working phase: _____

_____

_____

c. Termination phase: _____

_____

_____

9. Give an example statement or behavior for the following interpersonal skills necessary used to promote a healthy nurse–patient relationship.

a. Warmth and friendliness: _____

_____

_____

b. Openness and respect: _____

_____

_____

c. Empathy: _____

_____

_____

d. Competence: _____

_____

_____

e. Consideration of patient variables: _____

_____

_____

10. List five common blocks/obstacles to communication and describe nursing's role in overcoming these obstacles.

a. _____

_____

_____

b. _____

_____

_____

c. _____

_____

_____

d. _____

_____

_____

e. _____

_____

_____

11. Discuss how bullying may impact nursing care in health care facilities and the optimal organizational response to these disruptive behaviors.

    a. Bullying: _____

    _____

    _____

    b. Organizational response: _____

    _____

    _____

APPLYING YOUR KNOWLEDGE

CRITICAL THINKING QUESTIONS

1. Write a general script for communicating with a middle-aged adult with a history of strokes with some expressive aphasia was brought to the emergency department with left-sided paralysis. Begin with, "Hello, my name is..." to the end of the conversation.

    _____

    _____

    _____

2. How competent and comfortable are you in each situation? What skills do you need to develop?

    _____

    _____

    _____

3. Reflect on the importance of nonverbal communication.

    _____

    _____

    _____

4. Get feedback from someone you trust on the following attributes that stimulate a healthy nurse–patient relationship: warmth and friendliness, openness, empathy, competence, and consideration of patient variables. Compare this to your perceptions and further develop areas where growth is needed.

REFLECTIVE PRACTICE: CULTIVATING QSEN COMPETENCIES

Use the following expanded scenario from Chapter 8 in your textbook to answer the questions below.

Scenario: Irwina, a 75-year-old woman, has been transferred to a long-term care facility from the hospital after being diagnosed and treated for pneumonia. Her health record reveals that she is hard of hearing, "pleasantly confused" at times, and speaks "broken English." An initial nursing assessment is needed.

1. Patient-centered care: What communication skills might the nurse use to complete an assessment of Irwina?

    _____

    _____

    _____

2. Patient-centered care/safety. What would be a successful outcome for this patient?

    _____

    _____

    _____

3. Patient-centered care/safety. What intellectual, interpersonal, and ethical/legal competencies are most likely to bring about the desired outcome?

    Intellectual: _____

    _____

    Interpersonal: _____

    _____

    Ethical/legal: _____

    _____

4. Teamwork and collaboration: What resources might be helpful?

    _____

    _____

    _____

PRACTICING FOR NCLEX

MULTIPLE-CHOICE QUESTIONS

Circle the letter that corresponds to the best answer for each question.

1. A client's family member becomes loud and verbally abusive to the nurse. Which response by the nurse is most therapeutic?
   a. "I am going to notify the security department about your abusive behavior."
   b. "If you can't calm down, I won't be able to speak with you."
   c. "Please leave the nursing unit and return when you are not yelling."
   d. "You seem concerned about your loved one; can I help you understand something?"

2. Nurses may use social media to share ideas, develop professional connections, and investigate evidence-based practices. Which example reflects the most appropriate use of social media by a nurse?
   a. Describing a coworker on Twitter by giving their title rather than their name
   b. Posting pictures of a patient who lost 100 lb and later deleting the photo
   c. Describing a patient on Facebook by giving their diagnosis rather than their name
   d. Basing their posts on Facebook on their employer's policies

3. A home care nurse and patient discuss the frequency and duration of visits. In which phases of the helping relationship is this type of agreement established?
   a. Orientation phase
   b. Acceptance phase
   c. Working phase
   d. Termination phase

4. A nurse says to a nursing assistant, "It looks like you forgot to wash your hands between patients. Let's discuss a reminder you could use to help you remember." This communication is an example of which type of speech?
   a. Aggressive
   b. Assertive
   c. Nonassertive
   d. Therapeutic

5. A nurse is attempting to communicate with a patient who has limited ability to speak and understand English. Which nursing action will best facilitate the communication process?
   a. Speaking slowly and distinctly in a moderate volume
   b. Repeating the message multiple times until understood
   c. Using medical terms and abbreviations
   d. Avoiding using a dictionary to help maintain focus on the patient

6. A nurse is caring for a patient with advanced dementia who is nonverbal. Which type of communication will the nurse rely on when conducting a pain assessment?
   a. Picture communication chart
   b. Patient's body language
   c. Therapeutic communication
   d. Sympathetic communication

7. In a helping relationship, the nurse will typically perform which action?
   a. Encouraging the patient to independently explore goals that allow their human needs to be satisfied
   b. Setting up a reciprocal relationship in which patient and nurse are both helper and person being helped
   c. Establishing a dynamic relationship in which active communication is reciprocal
   d. Establishing goals for the patient that are not set in a specific timeframe

8. A nurse plans to deliver care to newborns by stimulating the sense most highly developed at birth. Which action will the nurse use?
   a. Speaking to the infant in a loud voice to get attention
   b. Playing "peek-a-boo" with the infant
   c. Wearing colorful clothing to stimulate the infant
   d. Gently stroking the baby's cheek to facilitate feeding

9. A nursing student tells the professor their primary nurse keeps saying, "you should have read the chart; I don't have time to give you report." What is the student experiencing?

   a. Rite of passage
   b. Incivility
   c. Scapegoating
   d. Violent behavior

10. A patient who underwent a hysterectomy 4 days ago says to the nurse, "I wonder if I'll still feel like a woman." Which response by the nurse will encourage the patient to more fully express her concerns?

    a. "When did you begin to wonder about this?"
    b. "Do you want more children?"
    c. "Feel like a woman…"
    d. Remain silent

11. Nursing students learn about incivility, which is considered rude, intimidating verbal or nonverbal behavior. Which response observed by the students can be considered uncivil?

    a. "These students don't know anything," said with an eye roll to a colleague.
    b. "Your orientation is 12 weeks; what do you think you need to focus on?"
    c. "That health care provider was very demeaning; would you like to talk about it?"
    d. "I know you are upset," said a nurse to a patient. "I'd like to help."

ALTERNATE-FORMAT QUESTIONS

Multiple-Response Questions

Circle the letters that correspond to the best answers for each question.

1. A nursing instructor suggests that students engaging in which behaviors should reflect on their communication skills? Select all that apply.

   a. Speaking to the patient from the doorway
   b. Avoiding periods of silence during conversations
   c. Listening to the themes in the patient's comments
   d. Standing close to the patient and maintaining eye contact
   e. Thinking for a moment before responding to the patient
   f. Nodding affirmatively while the patient is speaking

2. A nurse is communicating the care plan to a patient who is cognitively impaired. Which nursing actions will facilitate this process? Select all that apply.

   a. Maintaining eye contact with the patient
   b. Giving the patient time to respond
   c. Communicating in a quiet environment with few distractions
   d. Keeping communication simple and concrete
   e. Giving an in-depth explanation of the plan of care
   f. Taking a break if there is no response

3. A nurse is administering medications to a client who is unconscious after a head injury. Which communication strategies will the nurse use? Select all that apply.

   a. Speak to the patient in a louder-than-normal voice.
   b. Taking care with what is said, since hearing is the last sense lost
   c. Assuming the patient can hear and discussing their care with their family
   d. Playing preferred music to help stimulate the patient
   e. Avoiding the use of touch to communicate with the patient
   f. Speaking to the patient before touching them

4. Nurses on a burn unit meet as a group to discuss revisions to the dressing change policies. Which statements accurately describe the functions of group dynamics? Select all that apply.

   a. The group leader solely uses their talents and interpersonal strengths to assist the group to accomplish goals.
   b. Effective groups possess members who elicit mutually respectful relationships.
   c. The group's ability to function at a high level depends only on the group leader's sensitivity to the needs of the group and its individual members.
   d. When a group member dominates or thwarts the group process, the leader or other group members must confront them to promote the needed collegial relationship.
   e. Power is used to "fix" immediate problems without considering the needs of the powerless.
   f. In an effective group, members support, praise, and critique one another.

5. A nurse is caring for a patient who had a laryngectomy for cancer and can no longer speak. Which communication techniques will the nurse plan to use while delivering care? Select all that apply.

   a. Asking yes–no questions

   b. Providing a pad of paper or magic slate

   c. Notifying the operator and those who answer the call bell that the patient cannot speak

   d. Providing a 1:1 patient sitter

   e. Ensuring the family remains with the patient during the hospitalization

   f. Making sure the call bell is within reach at all times

6. Which nursing actions will improve communication with patients and promote an effective helping relationship? Select all that apply.

   a. Controlling their tone of voice to convey exactly what is meant

   b. Keeping the patient focused on the topic at hand without diverging to another topic

   c. Communicating as simply as possible, gearing conversation to the patient's level

   d. Using words that might have different interpretations, such as feeling "blue"

   e. Avoiding admitting to a lack of knowledge, which could undermine the patient's confidence in the helping relationship

   f. Finding opportunities to communicate information to patients during routine care

7. Which nursing actions help improve listening skills when engaging in therapeutic communication with patients? Select all that apply.

   a. Sitting with their arms and legs crossed in a relaxed position

   b. Maintaining eye contact with the patient in a face-to-face pose

   c. Using facial expressions and gestures indicate they are paying attention

   d. Allowing a lull in the conversation while considering a response to the patient

   e. Pretending to listen, while performing a procedure, rather than interrupt the patient

8. A nurse is providing care to a patient who is legally blind. When communicating with the patient, which techniques will be most effective? Select all that apply.

   a. Speaking louder than usual

   b. Touching the patient to indicate your presence

   c. Placing the call bell in the patient's hand and explain its use

   d. Cleaning the patient's eyeglasses as part of their care

   e. Stating your name clearly

Sequencing Questions

1. A nurse is using the SBAR technique for hand-off communication when transferring a patient from the operating room to the medical surgical unit. Place the following components of the SBAR communication (Situation, Background, Assessment, and Recommendations) in the proper order.

   a. This 20-year-old patient presented to the ER with right lower quadrant pain, fever, and an elevated WBC count.

   b. The patient is postlaparoscopic appendectomy.

   c. The patient is sleepy, but responsive. There are five small dressings on the abdomen that are clean and dry.

   d. The patient may need pain medication in 30 minutes.

   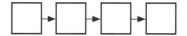

2. The nurse is using SBAR communication when notifying the health care provider about a patient fall. Place the following components of the SBAR communication in the proper order.

   a. The patient was admitted for change in mental status and shortness of breath.

   b. The patient was found sitting on the floor and states she doesn't know what happened.

   c. We can apply a bed alarm to alert us if she gets up and get a patient sitter to watch her.

   d. The vital signs are T 98.8°F, pulse 88, respirations 20, and blood pressure 118/70.

   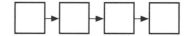

3. Place the phases of therapeutic relationship between patient and nurse in order.

   a. Working phase

   b. Termination phase

   c. Orientation phase

   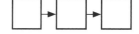

CHAPTER 9

Teaching and Counseling

ASSESSING YOUR UNDERSTANDING

FILL IN THE BLANKS

1. The aim of patient education for a nurse who counsels a teenager wanting to lose weight to eat a healthy diet and exercise is an example of _____ health.

2. When a nurse and a patient form a relationship in which mutual respect and trust are established, they have developed a(n) _____ relationship.

3. The _____ domain of learning is the process by which a person acquires or increases knowledge in a measurable way as a result of teaching.

4. A positive outcome in the _____ domain of learning occurs when a patient expresses a desire to control binge eating and to value eating a healthy diet.

5. The best source of assessment information is generally elicited from the _____.

6. _____ is an internal impulse (such as emotion or physical pain) that encourages the patient to take action or change behavior.

7. Content for the teaching plan that is supported by nursing research and that reflects the most accurate and clinically supported information is called _____.

8. When a nurse assists a patient to decide to quit smoking, the nurse is fulfilling the role of _____.

9. A nurse _____ establishes a partnership with a patient and uses discovery to identify the patient's personal goals and agenda in a way that will result in change rather than using teaching and education strategies directed by the nurse as the expert.

10. The Speak Up initiative, sponsored by The Joint Commission, aims to _____ and educate patients by making them a partner in their care.

MATCHING EXERCISES

Matching Exercise 1

Match the type of teaching strategy in Part A with the definition in Part B. Answers may be used more than once

PART A

a. Written material

b. Lecture

c. Demonstration

d. Discovery

e. Role modeling

PART B

____ 1. A nurse speaks to a group of patients about the dangers of smoking.

____ 2. A nurse performs a newborn bath for a group of new mothers to observe.

____ 3. A nurse provides a pamphlet to an adolescent that describes how STIs are transmitted

___ **4.** A nursing student acts as a patient, while the nursing instructor conducts a nursing interview.

___ **5.** A nurse talks with a patient about their feelings of powerlessness following a transient ischemic attack.

Matching Exercise 2

Match the nursing aim in Part A with the teaching strategy in Part B. Answers may be used more than once.

PART A

a. Promoting health

b. Preventing illness

c. Restoring health

d. Facilitating coping

PART B

___ **1.** A nurse demonstrates surgical dressing change to a postoperative patient.

___ **2.** A nurse teaches a new mother the importance of keeping up to date with childhood immunizations.

___ **3.** A nurse teaches a young athlete stretching exercises to be used before running track.

___ **4.** A hospice nurse refers the daughter of a terminally ill patient to a support group.

___ **5.** A nurse presents a lecture on baby-proofing the home to a group of parents.

___ **6.** A nurse refers a recovering alcoholic to a local recovery group.

Matching Exercise 3

Match the learning domain listed in Part A to the example in Part B. Answers may be used more than once.

PART A

a. Affective learning

b. Cognitive learning

c. Psychomotor learning

PART B

___ **1.** A patient redemonstrates self-administration of insulin.

___ **2.** A patient explains how eating a heart prudent diet will lower cholesterol level.

___ **3.** A patient learns how to perform range-of-motion exercises after surgery.

___ **4.** A patient expresses self-confidence after she completes a class to stop smoking.

___ **5.** A patient decides to get dressed in the morning following treatment for depression.

___ **6.** A new mother demonstrates circumcision care on her baby prior to discharge.

Matching Exercise 4

Match the type of learner listed in Part A to the age-appropriate teaching strategy in Part B.

PART A

a. Preschool-aged child

b. School-aged child

c. Adolescent learner

d. Adult learner

PART B

___ **1.** Learning is useful immediately, allows self-concept of independence

___ **2.** Logical reasoning, reasons for procedures; parents reinforce teaching

___ **3.** Manipulate equipment, short attention span, use simple words; focus on parents

___ **4.** Piaget's state of formal operations, supports need for independence

SHORT ANSWER

1. Give a brief example of actions or interventions the nurse may use to facilitate the following goals.

a. Promoting health: _____

_____

b. Preventing illness: _____

_____

c. Restoring health: _____

_____

d. Facilitating coping: _____

_____

2. How would you modify your teaching plan to motivate the following patients to learn a new skill?

   a. Adult who has a fear of failure: _____

   _____

   _____

   b. Adult who resists learning because of preconceived ideas about the process and your expectations of them: _____

   _____

   _____

   c. Older adult who is afraid to learn something new: _____

   _____

   _____

3. The home care nurse is visiting an older adult recovering from a stroke that resulted in left hemiparesis. List three teaching strategies you can use to teach exercises for rehabilitation, giving an example of each.

   a. _____

   _____

   _____

   b. _____

   _____

   _____

   c. _____

   _____

   _____

4. List two solutions to the problem that time constraints place on the nurse when planning patient learning.

   a. _____

   _____

   _____

   b. _____

   _____

   _____

5. Briefly describe the following types of teaching and give an example of each.

   a. Formal: _____

   _____

   _____

b. Informal: _____

_____

_____

6. Give an example of a strategy that could be used to evaluate the following types of learning.

   a. Cognitive domain: _____

   _____

   _____

   b. Affective domain: _____

   _____

   _____

   c. Psychomotor domain: _____

   _____

   _____

7. Define the following types of counseling and give an example of a case in which each type would be used by the nurse.

   a. Short-term counseling: _____

   _____

   _____

   b. Long-term counseling: _____

   _____

   _____

   c. Motivational counseling: _____

   _____

   _____

8. List four elements that should be considered in each assessment of patient learning needs.

   a. _____

   _____

   _____

   b. _____

   _____

   _____

   c. _____

   _____

   _____

   d. _____

   _____

   _____

9. Give an example of the following teaching strategies that you have experienced in your personal life. Which strategies do you feel were most effective for you and why?

a. Role modeling: _____

_____

_____

b. Lecture/discussion: _____

_____

_____

c. Demonstration: _____

_____

_____

d. Discovery: _____

_____

_____

e. Role-playing: _____

_____

_____

f. Audiovisual materials: _____

_____

_____

10. List four measures that promote patient and family adherence to the treatment plan.

a. _____

_____

_____

b. _____

_____

_____

c. _____

_____

_____

d. _____

_____

_____

11. List three of the five common mistakes that hinder patient teaching.

a. _____

_____

_____

b. _____

_____

_____

_____

c. _____

_____

_____

APPLYING YOUR KNOWLEDGE

CRITICAL THINKING QUESTIONS

1. Devise a teaching plan for a patient with painful arthritis on weight reduction and exercise.

a. What is the first step the nurse will take?

_____

_____

_____

b. Give an example of how the nurse could use these teaching strategies:

Lecture/discussion: _____

_____

_____

Demonstration/role-playing: _____

_____

_____

c. What method do you believe will be most advantageous and why?

_____

_____

_____

2. As a child, you learned many things from your parents or guardians. Consider the teaching strategies they used and how you could use both formal and informal teaching to help children accomplish the following goals.

a. Avoiding drugs and alcohol: _____

_____

_____

b. Learning how to cook a healthy meal: _____

_____

_____

c. Dealing with peer pressure: _____

_____

_____

3. Observe nurses teaching and counseling patients and family members to promote health, prevent illness, restore health, or facilitate coping. How did the nurse identify each patient's learning needs? Was the nurse successful in teaching this patient? How would you have handled the teaching process differently? Assess each patient's knowledge, attitudes, and skills needed to independently manage their own health care.

_____

_____

_____

REFLECTIVE PRACTICE: CULTIVATING QSEN COMPETENCIES

Use the following expanded scenario from Chapter 9 in your textbook to answer the questions below.

Scenario: Marco accompanies his wife, Claudia, to the antepartal clinic for a routine visit. They are expecting their first child in 5 months. He reports that they are happy and excited but also scared and very nervous. They are planning for a home birth, asking lots of questions about childbirth and their new responsibilities as parents, and are both wondering if they will be good parents.

1. Patient-centered care/safety: What should be the focus of patient teaching for this couple?

_____

_____

_____

2. Patient-centered care/safety: What would be a successful outcome for Marco and Claudia?

_____

_____

_____

3. Patient-centered care: What intellectual, interpersonal, and ethical/legal competencies are most likely to bring about the desired outcome?

Intellectual: _____

_____

_____

Interpersonal: _____

_____

_____

Ethical/legal: _____

_____

_____

4. Teamwork and collaboration/informatics: What resources might be helpful for this couple?

_____

_____

_____

PRACTICING FOR NCLEX

MULTIPLE-CHOICE QUESTIONS

Circle the letter that corresponds to the best answer for each question.

1. The nurse determines a school-aged child who is having an ECG would most likely benefit from which of these explanations?
   a. "This test will determine if your heart is beating in a normal rhythm."
   b. We are taking a picture of your heart; here is a picture of what the machine will show us.
   c. "This test won't hurt at all. I will explain it to your parents."
   d. "I will attach these leads to your legs and chest to check out your heart."

2. A nurse recognizes a patient with a new diagnosis of COPD requires teaching to learn how to use the prescribed inhalers. What will the nurse do first?
   a. Write up the teaching plan
   b. Determine the patient's learning needs
   c. Ensure the patient will adhere to the medication regimen
   d. Develop learning outcomes

3. A nurse is writing learning outcomes for a patient who was recently diagnosed with type 2 diabetes. Which methods will the nurse use?

   a. Writing one or two broad objectives rather than several specific outcomes

   b. Writing general statements that could be accomplished in any amount of time

   c. Planning learner objectives with another nurse before obtaining input from the patient and family

   d. Collaborating with the patient to determining the overall need, followed by specific outcomes

4. A nurse is developing a teaching plan for a school-aged child who will have surgery tomorrow. Which instructional materials will be best for the nurse to use?

   a. Discussion

   b. Games with a doll

   c. Video of the procedure

   d. Self-learning module

5. A nurse is planning a bereavement program for parents who have lost a child to suicide. Which type of counseling session would the nurse plan to use in for this group?

   a. Long-term counseling

   b. Motivational counseling

   c. Short-term counseling

   d. Professional counseling

6. When a patient says, "I don't care if I get better; I have nothing to live for, anyway," which type of counseling will the nurse initiate?

   a. Long-term counseling

   b. Motivational counseling

   c. Short-term counseling

   d. Professional counseling

7. When teaching an adult patient how to control stress through relaxation techniques, the nurse should consider which qualities of the adult learner?

   a. As adults mature, their self-concept becomes more dependent; therefore, this patient must be made aware of the importance of reducing stress.

   b. The adult learner is less concerned with how immediately useful the material is as they are with the quality of the material.

   c. As patients, adults are the least likely to resist learning because of preconceived ideas about the teaching–learning process.

   d. The nurse can help the patient draw from their previous experiences as a resource to reduce stress.

8. When documenting a teaching session on diabetes management, the nurse wrote, "the patient has been unable to learn the material and needs more education." Which statements should the nurse include to further clarify progress toward the learning outcome?

   a. The patent and spouse asked many questions during the teaching session.

   b. The patient refused to make eye contact during the teaching session.

   c. The patient asked that their spouse be included in the session due to their poor memory.

   d. The patient stated that diabetes causes elevated blood glucose but is unable to state normal values.

9. After giving the patient and spouse written materials on a low-sodium diet for heart failure, they are unable to state specific foods to avoid. Which modification to the plan may be most helpful to meet the goal for dietary management?

   a. Reading the material to the patient and spouse

   b. Obtaining a prescription for a consult with a dietician

   c. Requesting that they read the material before you return

   d. Assisting them to select appropriate food from the menu

10. A nurse in a diabetes clinic is developing teaching materials for patient education. Which of reflects the most current evidence-based practice for using printed material?

   a. Developing materials at the 4th- to 6th-grade level

   b. Limiting the number of graphics and pictures

   c. Providing learning materials in English

   d. Avoiding interactive materials

ALTERNATE-FORMAT QUESTIONS

Multiple-Response Questions

Circle the letters that correspond to the best answers for each question.

1. A nurse in a short-term rehabilitation facility is providing teaching to patients. Which actions will the nurse use to promote teaching effectiveness? Select all that apply.

   a. Accepting that patients have the right to change their minds
   b. Planning goals with the patient
   c. Using medical terminology frequently while teaching
   d. Avoiding modifying restrictions of the patient's environment
   e. Evaluating what the patient has learned
   f. Reviewing educational media when planning learner objectives

2. A nurse in a trauma center focuses on restoring health. Which topics would the nurse likely explore? Select all that apply.

   a. Immunizations
   b. Patient and nurse's expectations of one another
   c. Community resources
   d. Hygiene
   e. How the patient will participate in care

3. A nurse uses the acronym TEACH when planning care for hospitalized patients. Which intervention accurately represents an aspect of this acronym? Select all that apply.

   a. T—The nurse turns to the health care provider for support.
   b. E—The nurse educates the patient before treatment.
   c. A—The nurse acts on every teaching moment.
   d. C—The nurse clarifies often.
   e. H—The nurse helps the patient cope when education fails.
   f. H—The nurse honors the patient as a partner in the education process.

4. A nurse is using the teaching–learning process to teach new parents how to care for their infants. Which nursing actions by the nurse reflect recommended steps of this process? Select all that apply.

   a. Assessing the learning needs and learning readiness of the parents
   b. Identifies general, attainable, measurable, and long-term goals for patient learning
   c. Includes group teaching and formal teaching in every teaching plan
   d. Not allow time constraints, schedules, and the physical environment to influence the choice of teaching strategies.
   e. Formulates a verbal or written contract with the patient.
   f. Relates new learning material to the parent's life experiences to promote assimilation of new information.

5. A nurse working in a family medical practice plans teaching based on the patient's developmental stage. Which actions best reflect this consideration? Select all that apply.

   a. Directing the health teaching for a 3-year-old to the parents
   b. Providing lengthy explanations of a procedure to a preschool-aged child
   c. Including a school-aged child in the teaching–learning process
   d. Using the same learning strategies for an adolescent as for an adult
   e. Providing material that is useful immediately to adult patients

6. A nurse in the community assesses a community member's motivation to prevent COVID-19 infections. Based on the health belief model, which individuals would be most motivated to learn this information? Select all that apply.

   a. Someone who does not view themselves as susceptible to the disease
   b. Someone who views a disease as a serious threat
   c. Someone who states that certain actions will reduce the probability of contracting the disease

d. Someone who believes that the threat of taking actions against a disease is not as great as the disease itself

e. Someone who believes that noncompliance is not an option

f. Someone who believes that doing nothing is preferable to painful treatments

7. During patient education, what should the Ask Me 3 questions the nurse answers during a teaching session address?

   a. "How will my insurance cover this treatment?"

   b. "What is my main problem?"

   c. "What do I need to do?"

   d. "Why is it important for me to do this?"

   e. "Is English your primary language?"

8. A nurse is planning a teaching session at the local community center and acknowledges the group's social determinants of health to maximize learning. Which social determinants of health will the nurse consider? Select all that apply.

   a. Cultural influences and language deficits

   b. Family support networks

   c. Financial resources

   d. Health literacy level

   e. Patient's age and developmental level

Prioritization Questions

1. When does the nurse begin planning and implementing patient education?

   _____

   _____

   _____

2. When planning patient education, which patient information will the nurse prioritize?

   a. Concurrent illnesses

   b. Age of the learner

   c. Readiness to learn

   d. Preferred learning style

Leading, Managing, and Delegating

ASSESSING YOUR UNDERSTANDING

FILL IN THE BLANKS

1. _____ is described as the ability to direct or motivate a person or group to achieve set goals.

2. A nurse manager possesses _____ power attained by virtue of their position, while an experienced nurse on the unit influences team members with their _____ power.

3. The qualities of self-management, self-awareness, social awareness, and relationship management belong to successful leaders who demonstrate _____ intelligence.

4. A charge nurse who makes decisions for the nursing team without considering their feelings or ideas is using the _____ style of leadership.

5. In hospitals, the autocratic style of leadership has been gradually replaced by the _____ style of leadership.

6. Leadership as a philosophy and set of practices that enrich the lives of individuals, focus on relationships, build better organizations, and create a more just and caring world, is referred to as _____.

7. _____ leadership theory views an organization and its members as interconnected and collaborative, helpful in this age

in which change is conceived as dynamic, ever present, and continually unfolding.

8. A manager using the style of leadership based rewarding good behavior or punishing detrimental behavior is termed _____ leadership.

9. _____ leaders are often charismatic risk takers, create intellectually stimulating practice environments, focus others on a common vision, and demonstrate honest communication and vulnerability.

10. A _____ hospital employs transformational leaders, promotes structural empowerment, exemplary professional practice, new knowledge, innovation, and improvements, leading to quality results.

11. When nurses are encouraged to disclose clinical (or potential) errors turning them into opportunities for improvement without the fear of punitive actions, the organization has created a _____.

12. The role of _____ is involved with planning, organizing, directing, and controlling available human, material, and financial resources to deliver quality care to patients and families.

13. A practice empowering nurses to have as much influence over their work environment as possible is referred to as _____,

14. A nurse _____ is selected (and generally paid) to introduce a new employee to

responsibilities through teaching, support, and guidance, ensuring the nurse gains the appropriate knowledge and skills for safe and efficient patient care.

MATCHING EXERCISE

Match the type of leadership in Part A with the definition in Part B. Some answers may not be used.

PART A

a. Autocratic leadership

b. Democratic leadership

c. Laissez-faire leadership

d. Transformational leadership

e. Transactional leadership

f. Servant leadership

PART B

_____ 1. A nurse manager uses a reward and punishment system to ensure employees to meet work goals and deadlines.

_____ 2. A nurse manager desires to serve the population, enrich people's lives, build better organizations, and ultimately create a more just and caring world.

_____ 3. A nurse takes control during a "code blue" and directs all personnel during resuscitation efforts.

_____ 4. A nurse in charge of scheduling suggests that the nurses meet and work out the schedule on their own.

_____ 5. A director of nursing develops a budget to support additional education for nurses.

_____ 6. A nurse leads other nurses in developing a schedule to cook meals for the homeless.

SHORT ANSWER

1. After several years of practice you transfer to the transplant unit where you meet a nurse who is dynamic, person-centered and admired for their collaboration with the interprofessional team. You invite her to coffee and ask her to be your mentor. What are the expectations you should have of a mentor?

2. List the steps you would employ to change visiting hours from a few hours daily to open visitation, 24 hours a day. How would you handle people who resist the change?

3. Briefly describe the following reasons why people resist change and state how you would confront the problem in your own practice.

   a. Threat to self: _____

   b. Lack of understanding: _____

   c. Limited tolerance to change: _____

   d. Disagreements about the benefits of change: _____

   e. Fear of increased responsibility: _____

4. Briefly explain the following conflict resolution strategies and the consequences of using each.

   a. Avoiding: _____

   b. Collaborating: _____

   c. Competing: _____

   d. Compromising: _____

e. Cooperating/accommodating: _____

_____

_____

f. Smoothing: _____

_____

_____

5. Leaders have five major sources of power in their arsenals. Define the type of power listed below and state the typical reason they fail or succeed.

a. Coercive power: _____

_____

_____

b. Legitimate power: _____

_____

_____

c. Reward power: _____

_____

_____

d. Expert power: _____

_____

_____

e. Referent or relationship power: _____

_____

_____

APPLYING YOUR KNOWLEDGE

CRITICAL THINKING QUESTIONS

1. Imagine you are the charge nurse on a surgical unit where a nurse calls out sick with no replacement available. After handing out patient assignments for the shift, several nurses are grumbling about that their assignments are too heavy. You overhear one nurse say they would rather quit than start taking on additional duties.

a. As a leader, how would you handle this situation?

b. What type of leadership style would you feel most comfortable using?

c. What do you anticipate the outcome will be or should be?

2. Consider the leadership styles of a primary nurse or nurse you have worked with in the past. What makes them effective or ineffective leaders? Which of their styles or behaviors do you plan to incorporate into your practice?

3. Describe how you can use the following leadership qualities in your current practice.

a. Dynamism: _____

_____

_____

b. Enthusiasm: _____

_____

_____

c. Ability to be self-directed: _____

_____

_____

d. Displaying a positive self-image: _____

_____

_____

e. Being a role model: _____

_____

_____

f. Having a vision: _____

_____

_____

4. When assigned to a patient with end-stage lung cancer who is receiving hospice care, discuss how you would use the following leaderships skills to provide holistic, thoughtful, person-centered care.

a. Communication: _____

_____

_____

b. Problem-solving: _____

_____

_____

c. Management: _____

_____

_____

d. Self-evaluation: _____

_____

_____

REFLECTIVE PRACTICE: CULTIVATING QSEN COMPETENCIES

Use the following scenario from Chapter 10 in your textbook to answer the questions below.

Scenario: Rehema is a college sophomore who comes to the health care center requesting information about sexually transmitted infections (STIs). During the visit, she says, "So many of my friends are concerned about STIs. They all say we should start a group on campus to discuss this problem, and they want me to set it up and be the leader. But I wouldn't know where to start or what to do!"

1. Patient-centered care/safety: How might the nurse empower Rehema with the knowledge and ability to be a leader of her peers?

   _____

   _____

   _____

2. Patient-centered care/teamwork and collaboration: What would be a successful outcome for Rehema?

   _____

   _____

   _____

3. Patient-centered care/teamwork and collaboration: What intellectual, interpersonal, and/or ethical/legal competencies are most likely to bring about the desired outcome?

   _____

   _____

   _____

4. Teamwork and collaboration: What resources might be helpful for Rehema?

   _____

   _____

   _____

PRACTICING FOR NCLEX

MULTIPLE-CHOICE QUESTIONS

Circle the letter that corresponds to the best answer for each question.

1. A nurse manager who values employee satisfaction uses a variety of activities to motivate the staff to be the best nurses possible. In which style of leadership are group satisfaction and motivation primary benefits?

   a. Democratic

   b. Autocratic

   c. Laissez-faire

   d. Transformational

2. A new nurse manager is considering which leadership style they should adopt. The manger avoids which style, recognizing resentment, high staff turnover, and burnout can result?

   a. Democratic

   b. Autocratic

   c. Laissez-faire

   d. Transformational

3. A nurse on an oncology unit believes administering and monitoring chemotherapy while carrying a full patient assignment creates a potentially unsafe situation. The nurse manager disagrees, stating that assignments are consistent with other local oncology units. What reflects the nurse's best use of the chain of command?

   a. Notifying the state board of nursing

   b. Speaking to the attending oncology provider

   c. Making an appointment to speak to the director of nursing

   d. Asking to meet with the president of the hospital

4. A nurse manager of a hospital unit is working within a decentralized management structure. Which description best exemplifies this type of system?

   a. Senior managers make all the decisions.

   b. Nurses are not intimately involved in decisions involving patient care.

   c. Decisions are made by those who are most knowledgeable about the issue.

   d. Nurse managers are not accountable for patient, staffing, supplies, or budgets.

5. A nurse manager is using Lewin's change theory when revising the staff's scheduling procedure on a critical care unit. The manager is in the process of changing the schedules and announcing the changes. Which action reflects the current stage of change?

   a. Moving

   b. Freezing

   c. Unfreezing

   d. Transforming

6. The most experienced, collaborative nurse on the unit begins displaying low energy and emotional exhaustion and feels she no longer provides effective care. The nurse's colleagues are concerned that she is displaying which response?

   a. Laissez-faire attitude

   b. Resilience

   c. Poor attitude

   d. Clinician burnout

ALTERNATE-FORMAT QUESTIONS

Multiple-Response Questions

Circle the letters that correspond to the best answers for each question.

1. A nursing student enrolled in a leadership course is observing staff members on a pediatric unit to determine who has explicit or implied power. Which are examples of those with implied power? Select all that apply.

   a. Nurse preceptor

   b. Nurse manager

   c. Popular nurse

   d. Charge nurse

   e. Nurse who knows everyone

   f. Nurse with 20 years' experience

2. A graduate nurse applies for a job working in a hospital that has achieved Magnet status. Which conditions would this nurse expect? Select all that apply.

   a. Focus on positive patient care outcomes

   b. Centralized decision making

   c. Autonomous, accountable, professional nursing practice

   d. Higher staff turnover

   e. Staff burnout and exodus from the bedside

   f. Supportive nurse managers

3. A nurse manager of a health care provider's office uses the laissez-faire style of leadership with the staff. Which descriptions exemplify this management style? Select all that apply.

   a. The nurse manager is the authority on all issues.

   b. The nurse manager allows the staff to choose their own schedules.

   c. The nurse manager allows dominant staff members to direct the group activities.

   d. The manager and staff work independently, making task accomplishment difficult.

   e. The manager views staff as equal partners in the practice.

   f. The nurse manager inspires and motivates staff to provide excellent patient care.

4. A registered nurse is delegating activities to assistive personnel (APs) on a hospital unit. Which activities could this nurse safely delegate? Select all that apply.

   a. Changing a stage 3 pressure wound dressing

   b. Bathing a comatose patient

   c. Teaching a patient with a colostomy care

   d. Taking vital signs every four hours

   e. Administering oral acetaminophen

   f. Transporting a transfer patient to another unit

5. Registered nurses follow the American Nurses Association (ANA) regulations prior to delegating tasks to APs. Which principles regarding the regulation, education, and use of the AP are recommended by the ANA? Select all that apply.

   a. It is the health care institution that determines the scope of nursing practice.

   b. An LPN supervises any assistant involved in providing direct patient care.

   c. The purpose of assistive personnel to work in a supportive role to the registered nurse.

   d. APs carry out tasks allowing the RN to concentrate on more complex patient care.

   e. The role of the LPN is to assign nursing duties to the AP.

   f. The registered nurse is responsible and accountable for nursing practice.

Sequencing Question

1. Place the steps of Lewin's change theory in the order the steps occur.

   a. Moving

   b. Refreezing

   c. Unfreezing

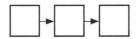

CHAPTER 11

Health Care Delivery System

ASSESSING YOUR UNDERSTANDING

FILL IN THE BLANKS

1. While some patients enter a hospital and stay overnight, much diagnostic testing, some surgeries, treatments, and therapies, often occur on a/an _____ basis.

2. _____ centers are often located in convenient areas and may offer "walk-in" services and accessibility outside of traditional office hours.

3. _____ care is a type of care provided for caregivers of homebound ill, disabled, or older adults.

4. _____ is a program of palliative and supportive care services providing physical, psychological, social, and spiritual care for dying people and their families and loved ones.

5. Alcoholics Anonymous is an example of an organization/service where attendance is _____.

6. A respiratory _____ is a member of the interprofessional team educated to improve pulmonary function and oxygenation.

7. Twenty percent of Americans lack access to _____ health care due to a lack of providers.

8. Although nursing is currently one of the fastest growing occupations in the country, demand is rapidly outpacing _____.

9. The American Nurses Association plans to reject legislation that would increase the number of _____ individuals.

10. The 1999 IOM report (IOM now known as the National Academies of Sciences, Engineering, and Medicine), *To Err is Human,* focused on the number of deaths in U.S. hospitals as a result of preventable medical _____.

11. _____ organizations operate in complex, high-hazard domains for extended periods without serious accidents or catastrophic failures.

12. _____ health care is designed to provide care for common health problems/minor illnesses; performing minor surgical procedures; and providing obstetric care, well-child care, counseling, and referrals.

13. Health care _____ (patients or clients) are increasingly knowledgeable about health, prefer to control and make decisions about their own health, and seek to be active participants in their health care.

MATCHING EXERCISES

Matching Exercise 1

Match the type of health care setting in Part A with its definition in Part B.

PART A

a. Respite care
b. Hospice services
c. Mental health/behavioral centers
d. Daycare centers
e. Industry
f. Ambulatory care centers

PART B

____ 1. Nurses in this setting are often the major source of health assessment, health education, and emergency care for the nation's children

____ 2. Care for infants and children whose parents work, older adults who cannot be home alone, and patients with special needs who do not need to be in a health care institution

____ 3. Care provided to homebound ill, disabled, or older adult patients to provide the primary caregiver with time away from the responsibilities of day-to-day care

____ 4. Palliative and supportive inpatient or home care services for terminally ill people and their families, committed to maintaining quality of life and dignity in the dying process

____ 5. Occupational health nurses in these settings focus on preventing work-related illnesses and injuries by conducting health assessments, teaching health promotion, and caring for minor injuries and illnesses

____ 6. Crisis-centered, long-term counseling, or outpatient care through individual and group counseling, medications, and assistance with independent living.

Matching Exercise 2

Match the title of the member of the interprofessional health care team in Part A with their role described in Part B.

PART A

a. Physical therapist
b. Occupational therapist
c. Assistive personnel (AP)
d. Social worker
e. Chaplain/spiritual care provider
f. Speech therapist

PART B

____ 1. Diagnose and treat swallowing problems in patients who have had, for example, a head injury or a stroke

____ 2. Providers identify and respond to the spiritual needs of patients, families, and other members of the interdisciplinary team

____ 3. Help nurses provide direct care to patients

____ 4. Counsels patients and family members and assist with health care finances and in obtaining community resources and equipment

____ 5. Evaluate the patient's functional level and teaching activities to promote self-care in activities of daily living. Assess the home for safety and provide adaptive equipment as necessary

____ 6. Restore function or prevent further disability in a patient after an injury or illness

SHORT ANSWER

1. List four factors that have influenced the need for increased home health care.

    a. _____
    b. _____
    c. _____
    d. _____

2. Describe the role of the nurse in the following health care centers:

    a. Primary care offices: _____

    b. Ambulatory care centers and clinics: _____

    c. Mental health centers: _____

    d. Rehabilitation centers: _____

    e. Long-term care centers: _____

3. List six services that can be performed during outpatient care.

a. _____

b. _____

c. _____

d. _____

e. _____

f. _____

4. Explain the term *DRG* and its implication for hospitals.

_____

_____

_____

_____

5. Define the term *fragmentation of care* and its effect on the health care system.

_____

_____

_____

_____

APPLYING YOUR KNOWLEDGE

CRITICAL THINKING QUESTIONS

1. Think about a group of people in your community that is underserved and lacks access to nursing resources. How might the nurse address the needs of this group?

2. Visit a health care clinic in your community. Find out what types of services are performed and the backgrounds of the patients seeking these services. Research how the clinic is funded and how the staff is reimbursed for its services. Would you feel comfortable being cared for in this clinic? Explain why or why not.

3. Look at the promotional materials for a local health care plan and interview people on the plan. Which features of the plan are most important for the insured? What does the plan lack? Is the insured party free to choose their own doctors or treatment plans?

4. Compare and contrast the roles and responsibilities of a physical therapist (PT) versus an occupational therapist (OT), a physician versus a physician assistant (PA), and a social worker versus a chaplain. Consider where

they overlap to provide continuity of care for the patient. How will this information help you as a nurse to coordinate the efforts of the interdisciplinary team?

5. Is health care a right, privilege, or an obligation of a moral society?

REFLECTIVE PRACTICE: CULTIVATING QSEN COMPETENCIES

Use the following expanded scenario from Chapter 11 in your textbook to answer the questions below.

Scenario: Margaret, a 63-year-old woman, is caring at home for her 67-year-old husband who has been diagnosed with amyotrophic lateral sclerosis (ALS, or Lou Gehrig disease). She states, "All of the help from the home care facility has been a blessing. But I need more help and some equipment now that our insurance won't cover. Plus, now the doctor says that his condition has really worsened, and he probably has 6 months or less to live."

1. Patient-centered care/safety: What nursing interventions might the nurse employ to assist Margaret with her caregiver duties?

_____

_____

_____

2. Patient-centered care/safety: What would be a successful outcome for this patient and his wife?

_____

_____

3. Patient-centered care: What intellectual, technical, interpersonal, and/or ethical/legal competencies are most likely to bring about the desired outcome?

_____

_____

_____

4. Patient-centered care/teamwork and collaboration: What resources might be helpful for Margaret?

_____

_____

_____

PRACTICING FOR NCLEX

MULTIPLE-CHOICE QUESTIONS

Circle the letter that corresponds to the best answer for each question.

1. Nursing students in a leadership course are learning about health delivery systems. Which factor reflects a source of conflict in health care today?

   a. Insufficient specialty medical providers

   b. Limited access to health care for high-wage earners

   c. Improving health with simultaneous cost reduction

   d. Availability of Medicare for those older than age 65 years

2. A nurse is caring for a patient who has a PPO health care plan. What is the greatest advantage of this type of plan?

   a. Ease of referrals

   b. Cost-effectiveness

   c. Care coordination

   d. Improved health outcomes

3. A group of nursing students are discussing tertiary health care in postconference. Which members of the health care team do the students identify as tertiary care providers?

   a. Radiology technician working in mammography suite

   b. Health care provider that sutured a wound in urgent care

   c. Staff nurse practicing in the intensive care unit

   d. Nurse practitioner in a specialized oncology hospital

4. A nurse in the emergency department is discharging a patient who was in a motor vehicle accident. The patient is a single parent with a child with developmental delays, who is living in a new community. Which services would be an appropriate referral for this patient?

   a. Respite care

   b. Hospice care

   c. Medical home

   d. Parish nursing

5. A nurse manager in a mental health facility with a crisis intervention center is interviewing nurses for employment. Which skills does the manager prioritize in a new nurse?

   a. Technical skills

   b. Decision-making ability

   c. Communication and counseling skills

   d. Relating to coworkers on a professional level

6. A nurse discusses palliative care with a patient who has been hospitalized multiple times following a diagnosis of advanced cancer. What is the focus of this type of care?

   a. Provision of a dignified death experience

   b. Physical rehabilitation

   c. Relief from physical, mental, and spiritual distress

   d. Occupational therapy

7. Nurses in various health care settings provide services to prevent the fragmentation of health care occurring in today's society. Which nursing role is most important in preventing this effect?

   a. Care provision

   b. Counselor

   c. Teacher

   d. Care coordinator

8. Which patient would a nurse suggest should enroll in Medicare services?

   a. Patient with cancer

   b. Infant needing immunizations in a low-income family

   c. Patient with a disability

   d. Older adult patient with diabetes

9. A patient who had an internal fixation of a fractured hip tells the nursing student that they will not be able to pay for their new medication after discharge. To which of the interprofessional members of the health care team does the student refer the patient?

   a. Health care provider

   b. Social worker

   c. Pharmacist

   d. Physical therapist

10. Nurses on a surgical unit make every effort to ambulate surgical patients, ensure they participate in PT, and are discharged in a timely manner. In addition to using best practices, why does the organization put forth this effort?

    a. Patients who stay longer than treatment for the diagnosis will absorb the additional cost.
    b. Medicare does not reimburse a hospital for the increased cost of falls or delayed discharge.
    c. Evidence shows these activities lead to greater patient satisfaction and higher HCAHPS scores.
    d. Patients will be discharged based on whether they are able to demonstrate self-care.

11. As a care coordinator for patients in an oncology practice, with what will the nurse likely assist patients?

    a. Psychological support for situational depression
    b. Setting up infusions for chemotherapy
    c. Basic care, hygiene, and ADLs
    d. Providing prescriptions for antiemetic medications

ALTERNATE-FORMAT QUESTIONS

Multiple-Response Questions

Circle the letters that correspond to the best answers for each question.

1. Nurses provide care for patients throughout the health care system. Which methods are used to ensure continuity and cost-effective care during this process? Select all that apply.

    a. Managed care
    b. Case management
    c. Rural health centers
    d. Parish nursing
    e. Primary health care
    f. Primary care centers

2. As a student, you are assigned to shadow a nurse provider in a primary care clinic. Which typical roles of a nurse will you expect to observe? Select all that apply.

    a. Managing members of the health care team
    b. Performing in-service education
    c. Making health assessments
    d. Performing technical procedures
    e. Researching nursing issues
    f. Providing health education

3. Home health care is one of the most rapidly growing areas of the health care system. What are the chief functions of the home health care nurse? Select all that apply.

    a. Developing a nursing care plan
    b. Providing for a dignified death at home
    c. Providing patient teaching and counseling
    d. Providing continuity of care
    e. Administering medications
    f. Collecting payment for nursing care

4. A new graduate nurse is excited to be accepted for a position at a magnet hospital. This nurse expects what from this organization? Select all that apply.

    a. High-quality patient care, nursing excellence
    b. Creativity among the staff
    c. Application of best evidence to practice
    d. Nursing innovations
    e. Charting with the PICOT format
    f. Innovations in practice

5. In an issues and trends course, nursing students learn that increasing advanced practice nursing roles will best assist with which health care issues?

    a. Primary health care for older adults
    b. Access to health care in rural areas
    c. Ability to receive eye and dental exams
    d. Improved preventative care for children
    e. Access to respite care

6. The nurse and AP on a neurosurgical unit are caring for a group of patients. Which activities will the nurse prioritize for the AP to complete? Select all that apply.

    a. Administering an oral medication
    b. Repositioning a bedbound patient
    c. Inserting an indwelling urinary catheter
    d. Completing a sterile dressing change
    e. Documenting output from an indwelling catheter
    f. Feeding a patient who has had a stroke

Interprofessional Collaborative Practice and Care Coordination Across Settings

ASSESSING YOUR UNDERSTANDING

FILL IN THE BLANKS

1. A nurse is providing health care for people in a small neighborhood clinic. This type of care is termed _____ nursing.

2. A community is typically defined by a geographic area but can also be based on shared interests or characteristics such as _____, _____, _____, or _____.

3. _____ 2030 defines objectives for the nation, selected to drive action toward improving health and well-being.

4. Short interprofessional safety _____ held at the beginning of each shift focus on input about safety and quality concerns or information.

5. A patient who refuses treatment and leaves a hospital must sign a form releasing the health care provider and institution from legal responsibility for their health status. This patient is said to be leaving the hospital _____.

6. Discharge planning begins on _____ or the first patient encounter.

7. The home care nurse engages in a _____ phase and an entry phase when planning visits.

8. _____ care facilities are those in which the patient receives health care services but does not remain overnight.

9. _____ of _____ is the process by which health care providers give appropriate, uninterrupted care and facilitate the patient's smooth transition between different settings and levels of care.

10. When advocating for a patient, the nurse may use the mnemonic CUS to emphasize the need for attention to the matter. Using this model, the nurse states, "I am _____, I am _____, and I believe _____ is at risk."

11. The nurse _____ is a care coordinator who guides the patient through all phases of treatment, identifies and removes barriers, interacts with the interprofessional team, and acts as the central point of contact for the patient.

12. The patient's _____ is an essential to safety during a patient's stay. It is one of two identifiers, required by the Joint Commission national safety standards, used to accurately identify the patient prior to a procedure.

CORRECT THE FALSE STATEMENTS

Mark the statement "T" if true or "F" if false. If false, replace the underlined word or words to make the statement true.

____ **1.** The <u>health care provider</u> is the person who most often is responsible for helping the patient make a smooth transition from one type of care setting to another.

_____

____ **2.** Hospital admissions and lengths of hospital stay are <u>increasing</u>. _____

____ **3.** Discharge planning <u>is indicated</u> when a patient is to be placed in a long-term care facility or other continuing care setting.

_____

____ **4.** When <u>goals</u> are established with the patient, compliance with the treatment regimen is more likely. _____

____ **5.** When transferring a patient to a long-term facility for care, the <u>original</u> chart is sent with the patient. _____

____ **6.** Your patient says, "I'm going home today!" You verify this by checking the <u>nursing care plan</u>. _____

SHORT ANSWER

1. Describe interventions to reduce anxiety for a patient who expresses the following concerns:

a. "Who will take care of my children when I'm in here?"

_____

_____

b. "Will the procedure be painful?"

_____

_____

c. "Will I be able to afford this?"

_____

_____

2. Briefly describe the purpose, process, and timing of medication reconciliation.

_____

_____

3. Describe how the following activities help provide continuity of care for patients:

a. Discharge planning: _____

_____

_____

b. Interprofessional collaboration: _____

_____

_____

c. Involving patient and family in planning:

_____

_____

4. State factors the nurse should consider during discharge planning.

_____

_____

_____

_____

_____

5. Describe the appropriate nursing actions that would be performed during the following patient transfers:

a. Transfer within the hospital setting: _____

_____

_____

b. Transfer to a long-term facility: _____

_____

_____

c. Discharge from a health care setting: _____

_____

_____

6. What is the proper procedure for discharging a patient against medical advice (AMA)?

_____

_____

_____

7. Describe how you would prepare a hospital room for admission of a patient arriving by stretcher and is receiving oxygen.

_____

_____

_____

8. Give an example of the following skills needed to practice community-based nursing:

   a. Knowledgeable and skilled: _____

   _____

   _____

   b. Independent in making decisions: _____

   _____

   _____

   c. Accountable: _____

   _____

   _____

9. Briefly differentiate how SBAR communications differ from ISBARQ.

   _____

   _____

   _____

   _____

   _____

APPLYING YOUR KNOWLEDGE

CRITICAL THINKING QUESTIONS

1. Hospital services are increasingly performed on an outpatient basis, and nurses must bridge the gap from institution to home. How would you use this knowledge to plan discharge a patient who will leave the hospital after a same-day hip replacement?

2. Imagine that your older adult parent or grandparent is being discharged from the hospital post stroke with partial paralysis, and they are no longer capable of living alone. Community living options include a life-care community, a live-in companion, living with you and or your family, or living in a long-term care facility. What information and support would you need to make this decision? How might this knowledge influence your nursing practice?

REFLECTIVE PRACTICE: CULTIVATING QSEN COMPETENCIES

Use the following expanded scenario from Chapter 12 in your textbook to answer the questions below.

   Scenario: Jeff is a 9-year-old boy with a genetic disease that includes severe intellectual disability. He is transferred from the state home for children to the hospital for respiratory complications.

1. Patient-centered care/safety: How might the admitting nurse respond to the patient's admission and condition?

   _____

   _____

   _____

2. Patient-centered care/safety: What would be a successful outcome for this patient?

   _____

   _____

   _____

3. Patient-centered care: What intellectual, interpersonal, and/or ethical/legal competencies are most likely to bring about the desired outcome?

   _____

   _____

   _____

4. Teamwork and collaboration/informatics: What resources might be helpful for the nurse working with this patient?

   _____

   _____

   _____

PRACTICING FOR NCLEX

MULTIPLE-CHOICE QUESTIONS

Circle the letter that corresponds to the best answer for each question.

1. A nurse is caring for a patient who presented with acute respiratory distress from pneumonia but refuses to stay for treatment. What best reflects the nurse's responsibility?

a. Telling the patient they cannot leave until the health care provider explains the potential results of their actions

b. Requesting a psychiatric consultation to determine if the patient is mentally competent

c. Notifying the health care provider and asking the patient to sign an AMA discharge form

d. Calling the patient's family to ask them to discourage the patient from leaving

2. A nurse is preparing to discharge a patient from an acute care facility to their home. Which action must be performed by the nurse upon discharge of this patient?

a. Performing medication reconciliation

b. Writing a discharge order for the patient

c. Obtaining orders for future home visits that may be necessary

d. Sending the patient's records to the health care provider

3. A nurse is transferring a patient from a hospital setting to an extended care facility. Which action is most important to ensure continuity of care for this patient?

a. Notifying all departments of the room change

b. Carefully moving all the patient's personal items

c. Asking family members to take home the patient's money and valuables

d. Providing accurate and complete handoff communication to the new facility

4. A patient who is being discharged with a wound infection requiring long-term antibiotics needs skilled home care nursing. For which care will the nurse and care manager plan?

a. Ventilator management

b. Chemotherapy

c. Intravenous therapy

d. Oxygen therapy

5. A nurse is preparing a patient for discharge from the hospital to home health care. Which action will the nurse perform during this process?

a. Determining who should be able to visit the home

b. Obtaining supplies for the patient's use at home

c. Scheduling a follow-up visit with the health care provider

d. Providing a handoff report to the home care nurse

6. A nurse manager is interviewing candidates for a position as a care coordinator for a large hospital system, offering multiple levels of service. Which skill must the nurse possess to ensure continuity of care?

a. Ability to provide technical nursing assistance to meet the needs of patients and their families

b. Ability to establish trusting professional relationships with patients, family/caregivers, and health care professionals in all practice settings

c. Ability to provide clear, concise communication of patient priorities and the plan of care as a patient moves between different settings

d. Commitment to securing the best care settings and coordination of resources to support the level of care needed

ALTERNATE-FORMAT QUESTIONS

Multiple-Response Questions

Circle the letters that correspond to the best answers for each question.

1. A nurse is using the ISBARQ framework for handoff communication. Which examples accurately represent this process? Select all that apply.

a. The people involved in the process identify themselves, their roles, and their jobs.

b. The nurse introduces the patient to the health care professionals who will be involved in the new facility.

c. The nurse reports the patient's vital signs, mental and code status, medications, and lab results.

d. The nurse makes arrangements for future home health care visits for the patient who is being discharged from the hospital.

e. The nurse explains the patient's chief complaint, diagnosis, treatment plan, and patient preferences.

f. The nurse reports the current provider's assessment of the patient and need for further services.

2. A nurse is preparing a room for patient admission. Which actions follow recommended guidelines for this process? Select all that apply.

   a. Keeping the door open and positioning the bed in the highest position

   b. Folding back the top bed linens

   c. Assembling the necessary equipment and supplies, including a hospital gown and admission pack

   d. Waiting to supply pajamas or a hospital gown until the patient states whether they will wear their own

   e. Asking the health care provider to set up oxygen, suction, or special equipment

   f. Adjusting the physical environment of the room, including lighting and temperature

3. A nurse is admitting a patient to a hospital. Which actions will the nurse initially perform? Select all that apply.

   a. Making sure the patient's name and address and the name of their closest relative are printed on an identification wristband

   b. Informing the patient that they must sign consent to treatment forms and allow the hospital to contact insurance companies as needed

   c. Obtaining patient information, which is entered in the admission section of the patient's permanent electronic record

   d. Asking the patient about prepared advance directives or giving the appropriate form to the patient if none has been made

   e. Giving the patient a form explaining the Patient Care Partnership

4. During nursing orientation to a hospital, a nurse learns about the nursing policy when transferring patients. Which actions will the nurse expect to perform during this process? Select all that apply.

   a. Informing the patient's family of the change and asking them to remove the patient's personal belongings

   b. Asking the family of a patient moved to a critical care unit to take home the patient's personal belongings

   c. Formally discharging a patient who is being transferred from the hospital to the intensive care unit.

   d. Sending the original chart to the new facility when a patient is being transferred to a long-term care facility

   e. Carefully packing the belongings of a patient being discharged and sending them to the new facility

   f. Preparing a detailed assessment and care plan to send to the long-term facility to which a patient is transferred

5. A nurse is discharging a patient from the hospital. Which actions should occur when a patient is discharged from a health care setting? Select all that apply.

   a. The nurse performs discharge planning, beginning on admission to the facility.

   b. A hospital administrator coordinates and performs an approved handoff for the new facility.

   c. The nurse ensures that the family members are taught the knowledge and skills needed to care for the patient.

   d. The health care provider ensures that referrals are made to such facilities as home health care or social services.

   e. The nurse who conducts the initial nursing assessment will determine the special needs of the patient being discharged.

   f. Preferably, the nurse who conducts the initial nursing assessment will determine the special needs of the patient being discharged.

Sequencing Question

1. A nurse is using the ISBARQ technique for handoff communication when transferring a patient. Place the following information in the proper order for documentation.

   a. Mr. Anderson has a history of COPD and smoking for 50 years.

   b. Mr. Anderson is currently wheezing, and his last pulse oximetry reading was 91%; currently, he is receiving albuterol nebulizers every 4 hours as needed.

   c. Mr. Anderson is being transferred from the telemetry unit. He was admitted with shortness of breath and hypoxemia.

   d. Mr. Anderson may need a nebulizer treatment when he arrives; it is due in half an hour.

   e. Do you have any questions?

   f. My name is Susan Smith, calling a report on Mr. Anderson.

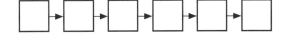

Blended Competencies, Clinical Reasoning, and Processes of Person-Centered Care

ASSESSING YOUR UNDERSTANDING

FILL IN THE BLANKS

1. A nurse committed to providing _____ care promotes humanity, dignity, and well-being of the patient, using a holistic and individualized approach.

2. When a nurse assists a patient to achieve desired goals such as promoting wellness, preventing disease and illness, restoring health, or facilitating coping with altered functioning, the nurse is using the _____ step of the nursing process.

3. The overall goal of the _____ project is to meet the challenge of preparing future nurses who will have the knowledge, skills, and attitudes (KSAs) necessary to continuously improve the quality and safety of health care systems.

4. A nurse who is considerate and compassionate and who keeps the person at the center of all deliberations in order to promote the humanity, dignity, and well-being of the person being cared for is engaging in _____ practice.

5. In Gibbs' Model of Reflection, making value judgments about what was good or bad about an experience occurs in the _____ step.

6. Nurses engaged in critical thinking must determine if the _____ they have is accurate, complete, factual, timely, and relevant.

7. When describing the nursing process using the ADPIE acronym, the nurse engages in assessing, _____, planning, implementing, and evaluating.

8. Clinical _____ refers to the outcome of critical thinking, clinical reasoning, and decision making after analyzing a situation.

9. Tanner's Clinical Judgment Model used to ground nurses practice includes the following steps: _____, _____, _____, _____.

10. A concept _____ is a strategy that promotes critical thinking, self-directed learning, and relationship analysis.

11. _____ practice is a purposeful activity that leads to action, improvement of practice, and better patient outcomes.

MATCHING EXERCISES

Matching Exercise 1

Match the name of the step of the nursing process in Part A with the appropriate example of the steps of the nursing process in Part B. Answers will be used more than once.

PART A

a. Assessing
b. Diagnosing
c. Planning
d. Implementing
e. Evaluating

PART B

_____ 1. A nurse performs an initial patient interview.

_____ 2. A home care nurse helps the physical therapist exercise the patient's limbs.

_____ 3. A nurse and interprofessional health care team determine how effective the treatment has been.

_____ 4. A nurse analyzes data to determine what health problems might exist.

_____ 5. A nurse sets a goal with an overweight adolescent to lose 1 lb a week.

_____ 6. A nurse consults with a patient's support people and other health care professionals to learn more about the patient's problem.

_____ 7. A nurse decides whether to continue, modify, or terminate the health care plan.

_____ 8. A nurse identifies the strengths that a patient with cancer possesses.

_____ 9. A home care nurse determines the nursing care needed by an older adult who had a stroke and lives with her daughter.

_____10. A nurse weighs a patient to determine whether their diet has been effective.

_____11. A nurse documents respiratory care performed on a patient.

_____12. A nurse reviews a patient's history in the electronic health records.

Matching Exercise 2

Match the type of skill in Part A with the appropriate example of the skill in Part B.

PART A

a. Cognitive
b. Technical
c. Interpersonal
d. Ethical/legal

PART B.

_____ 1. A nurse uses critical thinking skills to plan care for a patient.

_____ 2. A nurse correctly administers IV saline to a patient who is dehydrated.

_____ 3. A nurse witnesses a patient's signature on an informed consent form.

_____ 4. A nurse explains the need for auscultating the lungs to a patient with pneumonia.

_____ 5. A nurse comforts and supports parents whose baby was born with Down syndrome.

_____ 6. A nurse inserts an indwelling catheter using aseptic technique.

SHORT ANSWER

1. In order to engage in purposeful critical thinking to make sound nursing judgments, state three resources you could use to avoid "sloppy decisions."

   a. _____
   b. _____
   c. _____

2. List three patient and three nursing benefits of using the nursing process correctly.

   Patient:
   a. _____
   b. _____
   c. _____

   Nursing:
   a. _____
   b. _____
   c. _____

3. Describe how the nurse and patient work together to accomplish the following tasks of the nursing process:

a. Determining the need for nursing care:

_____

_____

b. Planning and implementing the care:

_____

_____

c. Evaluating the results of the nursing care:

_____

_____

4. Define the nursing process.

a. What are the primary goals of the nursing process?

_____

_____

b. What skills are necessary to use the nursing process successfully?

_____

_____

c. Which of these skills do you personally possess, and which do you need to develop in your practice?

_____

_____

5. Describe what the following words mean to you and how they apply to your use of the nursing process:

a. Systematic: _____

_____

b. Dynamic: _____

_____

c. Interpersonal: _____

_____

d. Outcome oriented: _____

_____

e. Universally applicable in nursing situations:

_____

_____

6. Briefly explain how the following considerations are relevant to the successful use of critical thinking competencies:

a. Purpose of thinking: _____

_____

b. Adequacy of knowledge: _____

_____

c. Potential problems: _____

_____

d. Helpful resources: _____

_____

e. Critique of judgment/decision: _____

_____

7. List four good habits nurses should develop to help them master the psychomotor skills essential to quality nursing process.

a. _____

b. _____

c. _____

d. _____

8. Think of three people you know personally, of different ages, professions, or cultures. What is it about each of these people that causes you to respect their human dignity? Are some people more deserving of respect than others? How do you show respect for them in your daily contact with them?

_____

_____

9. Follow several nurses on their daily rounds, noticing how they relate to their patients. Does their attitude indicate caring or "I don't have time for you"? Note what each nurse said or did to display this attitude.

a. Nurse 1: _____

_____

b. Nurse 2: _____

_____

c. Nurse 3: _____

_____

10. Nurses skilled in developing caring relationships often need to direct conversations with their patients. Develop four opening statements/questions designed to elicit information from a patient that you could use in your own practice.

   a. _____

   b. _____

   c. _____

   d. _____

11. List four areas a nurse should consider when seeking to develop a sense of legal and ethical accountability to a patient.

   a. _____

   b. _____

   c. _____

   d. _____

12. Give an example of how the following personal attributes of the professional nurse assist the nurse in planning and delivering person-centered care. Consider how each personal attribute affects each step of the nursing process.

   a. Open-mindedness: _____

   _____

   b. Profound sense of the value of the person:

   _____

   _____

   c. Self-awareness and knowledge of own beliefs and values: _____

   _____

   d. Sense of personal responsibility for actions:

   _____

   _____

   e. Caring about well-being of patients and acting accordingly: _____

   _____

   f. Leadership skills: _____

   _____

   g. Bravery to question the "system": _____

   _____

APPLYING YOUR KNOWLEDGE

CRITICAL THINKING QUESTIONS

1. Assess your personal blend of the skills nurses need: cognitive, technical, interpersonal, and ethical/legal. Would you want you to be your nurse? What skills do you need to develop to meet the needs of those entrusted to your care?

2. Think about major health problems on campus. How might a school of nursing use the nursing process to address one or more of these problems? Do you as a nursing student have an obligation to address the health problems you encounter?

3. Considering qualities you admire and respect in your friends/family and some qualities you do not. How can you use this knowledge to understand patients with different personality traits? Are some patients more worthy of your respect than others? Can your attitude toward a patient affect the outcome of treatment?

REFLECTIVE PRACTICE: CULTIVATING QSEN COMPETENCIES

Use the following expanded scenario from Chapter 13 in your textbook to answer the questions below.

   Scenario: Charlotte is a single mother whose 5-year-old daughter will be discharged soon. Charlotte is to learn how to perform wound care for her daughter at home. However, she has missed every planned teaching session thus far.

1. Patient-centered care/safety: How might the nurse use blended nursing skills to respond to this patient situation?

   _____

   _____

2. Patient-centered care/safety: What would be a successful outcome for this patient and her family?

   _____

   _____

   _____

3. Patient-centered care: What intellectual, technical, interpersonal, and/or ethical/legal competencies are most likely to bring about the desired outcome?

_____

_____

_____

4. Teamwork and collaboration/informatics: What resources might be helpful for Charlotte?

_____

_____

_____

PRACTICING FOR NCLEX

MULTIPLE-CHOICE QUESTIONS

Circle the letter that corresponds to the best answer for each question.

1. A nurse is using the QSEN competency of evidence-based practice when caring for patients. What is an example of this competency?
   a. Working with an interprofessional team to provide care for a patient with Alzheimer's disease
   b. Holding an in-service for staff to teach them the safe operation of a new piece of equipment
   c. Researching best practices to prevent the spread of infection in health care provider offices
   d. Using computer-generated care plans for patient care

2. A nurse is engaged in the assessment phase of the nursing process. What action will the nurse include in this phase?
   a. Determining if pain relief measures were successful
   b. Formulating a nursing diagnosis of grief for the patient who has cancer
   c. Using meticulous aseptic technique to insert a catheter
   d. Taking vital signs for the patient who returned from the operating room

3. Nursing students state that the steps of the nursing process seem to overlap, with each step flowing into the next. What descriptor does the nursing professor use to explain this characteristic of the nursing process?
   a. Interpersonal
   b. Dynamic
   c. Systematic
   d. Universally applicable

4. After administering pain medications to a patient, which action will the nurse perform next?
   a. Assess the patient's ability to move about and eat their meal
   b. Create the nursing diagnosis of pain
   c. After 30 minutes, ask the patient if their pain is relieved
   d. Tell the patient next dose of pain medication is due in 2 hours

5. The nurse on an oncology unit is attentive and responsive to the health care needs of individual patients and ensures the continuity of care when leaving the patient. Which interpersonal skill is the nurse displaying?
   a. Establishing caring relationships
   b. Enjoying mutual interchange
   c. Developing accountability
   d. Developing ethical/legal skills

6. A nurse uses the QSEN competency of Informatics when planning care for patients. What is an example of the use of this skill?
   a. Working collaboratively with a dietician to devise a patient meal plan
   b. Orienting a visually impaired patient to the hospital room
   c. Checking with the patient for priorities when planning patient care
   d. Researching new technologic advances in the treatment of cancer

7. A nurse is weighing the pros and cons of various interventions to relieve a patient's complex cancer pain, including medications and counseling. Which phrase best characterizes this process?
   a. Critical thinking
   b. Clinical reasoning
   c. Nursing judgment
   d. Pain management

8. A nursing student who prides herself on excellent communication skills received feedback from the clinical faculty citing her need to improve communication. Which statement is consistent with the comment?

   a. Assisted patient to select meals based on their cultural dietary observances

   b. Delivered nursing care based on patient's needs and preferences

   c. Documentation in the electronic health record included partial lists of interventions

   d. Reported a low fingerstick blood glucose to the primary nurse

9. A nursing student is caring for a patient who states that they have been living on the street for a year, since losing their job. Which response by the student best reflects a person-centered response?

   a. "I'm sorry to hear you've had this experience."

   b. "Tell me about your experience this past year."

   c. "Let's get you bathed; it must be dirty where you've been."

   d. "How do you pay for your food?"

10. While packing an infected abdominal wound, the patient shouts at the nurse and screams that the nurse is incompetent. Which person-centered practice could the nurse use to revise their approach to the patient?

    a. Requesting another nurse perform the dressing change next time

    b. Researching decision making

    c. Engaging in reflective practice

    d. Applying cognitive skills related to the surgical procedure

11. A nursing student enters the patient's room to find the patient on the floor in a puddle of urine. Which statement best reflects the student's use of clinical reasoning?

    a. "Mr. Jones, are you hurt?"

    b. "I reminded you not to get out of bed!"

    c. "Did you need to get to the bathroom quickly?"

    d. "Shall I call your family?"

12. A nursing student admires a nurse on the clinical unit whose critical thinking indicators (CTIs) the student would like to develop. Which behavior of the nurse best demonstrates using CTIs?

    a. Adhering to the medication administration record when telling the patient it is not yet time for pain medication

    b. Determining a patient with diabetes is not adhering to the treatment plan when hyperglycemia is present

    c. Demanding the lab returns to draw a patient's blood

    d. Identifying patients receiving anticoagulants who are at risk for bleeding

ALTERNATE-FORMAT QUESTIONS

Multiple-Response Questions

Circle the letters that correspond to the best answers for each question.

1. Nurses are expected to have the KSAs necessary to continually improve the quality and safety of the health care system where they work. Which KSAs are examples of nursing actions based on the QSEN competency of quality improvement? Select all that apply.

   a. A nurse manager schedules a staff meeting to review patient outcomes on the hospital unit.

   b. A nurse schedules a meeting with the nurse manager to review and update the policies for patient admissions.

   c. A nurse administrator sets up a committee to review the procedure manual and recommend any needed changes.

   d. A nurse coordinator calls a meeting of all the health care professionals involved in the care of a patient.

   e. A nurse uses the Internet to find new evidence-based recommendations for care of patients with cystic fibrosis.

   f. A nurse listens to a patient who is having trouble adjusting to a long-term care facility and treats the patient with compassion and respect.

2. Nurses use the nursing process as a problem-solving framework for their practices. Which statements describe characteristics of this process? Select all that apply.

   a. The trial-and-error problem-solving method is used extensively in the nursing process.

   b. The trial-and-error problem-solving method is recommended as a guide for nursing practice.

   c. The scientific problem-solving method is closely related to the nursing process.

   d. Nurse theorists and educators advocate basing clinical judgments on data alone in an attempt to establish nursing as a respected science.

   e. Today, nurses acknowledge the positive role of intuitive thinking in clinical decision making.

   f. Critical thinking in nursing can be intuitive or logical or a combination of both.

3. The ability to communicate clearly through documentation is a critical nursing skill. Which statements accurately describe the role of documentation in the nursing process? Select all that apply.

   a. The patient health record is the chief means of communication among members of the interdisciplinary team.

   b. If a nurse is accused of negligence, the nurse's word that they used the nursing process and carried out an effective plan of care is their best defense.

   c. Legally speaking, a nursing action not documented is a nursing action not performed.

   d. It is helpful to practice documentation while learning any given nursing activity.

   e. The content of the patient report and nursing documentation reflects nursing priorities in a practice setting.

   f. Data collection which is ongoing and responsive to changes in the patient's condition should be documented in the final step of the nursing process.

4. Nurses are sensitive to the ethical and legal implications of nursing practice. Which are examples of these ethical/legal skills? Select all that apply.

   a. Working collaboratively with the health care team as a respected and credible colleague to reach valued goals

   b. Being trusted to act in ways that advance the interests of patients

   c. Using technical equipment with competence and ease to achieve goals with minimal distress to patients

   d. Selecting nursing interventions that are most likely to yield the desired outcomes

   e. Being accountable for practice to oneself, the patient, the caregiving team, and society

   f. Acting as an effective patient advocate

5. Cognitively skilled nurses are critical thinkers. What are the characteristics of a critical thinker? Select all that apply.

   a. Thinking based on the opinions of others

   b. Being open to all points of view

   c. Acting like a "know-it-all"

   d. Resisting "easy answers" to patient problems

   e. Thinking "outside the box"

   f. Accepting the status quo

6. Nurses use the nursing process as a framework to plan care for patients. In which cases is the nursing process applicable? Select all that apply.

   a. When nurses work with patients who are able to participate in their care

   b. When families are clearly supportive and wish to participate in care

   c. When patients are totally dependent on the nurse for care

   d. When there are children as part of the family

   e. When there is a mental health issue

   f. When care is provided in an industrial setting

Sequencing Questions

1. Place the nursing activities in the order that they would occur when using the nursing process.

   a. Modifying the plan of care (if indicated)

   b. Carrying out the plan of care

   c. Establishing the database

   d. Interpreting and analyzing patient data

   e. Establishing priorities

   f. Measuring how well the patient has achieved desired outcomes

   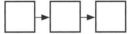

2. Place the following actions in order:

   a. Clinical judgment

   b. Clinical reasoning

   c. Critical thinking

   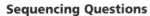

3. Place the steps of Tanner's Clinical Judgment Model in order:

   a. Noticing

   b. Reflecting

   c. Responding

   d. Interpreting

   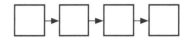

Clinical Judgment

ASSESSING YOUR UNDERSTANDING

FILL IN THE BLANKS

1. _____ thinking is the intellectually disciplined process of actively and skillfully conceptualizing, applying, analyzing, synthesizing, and/or evaluating information gathered from, or generated by, observation, experience, reflection, reasoning, or communication, as a guide to belief and action (Scriven and Paul, 1987).

2. Backward or _____ reasoning applies widely accepted knowledge and principles to a model to solve problems.

3. The type of reasoning which uses observation followed by drawing conclusions is referred to as forward reasoning or _____ reasoning.

4. Clinical _____ is defined as "thought processes that allow healthcare providers to arrive at a conclusion" (AACN, 2021, p. 62). Alfaro-LeFevre (2020) defines it as "the process you use to think about patient problems in the clinical setting," (p. 8) which results in a clinical judgment.

5. Clinical _____ is the result or observed outcome of critical thinking and decision making (NCSBN, 2019a) or "the skill of recognizing cues regarding a clinical situation, generating and weighing hypotheses, taking action, and evaluating outcomes for the purpose of arriving at a satisfactory clinical outcome" (AACN, 2021).

6. _____ awareness is "the perception of the elements in the environment in a volume of time and space, the comprehension of their meaning and the projection of their status in the near future."

7. Tanner's Clinical Judgment Model (2006) includes the nursing behaviors of _____, interpreting, responding, and reflecting.

8. Nursing education programs prepare students for licensure as a professional registered nurse by making them eligible to sit for the _____-RN.

9. The nursing _____ outlines the way nurses think and organize their thoughts.

10. Learning is _____, built upon lessons from prerequisite courses.

11. _____ is "an expected level of performance that integrates knowledge, skills, abilities, and judgment."

12. The Quality and Safety Education for Nurses (QSEN) outlines the _____, skills, and attitudes (KSAs) essential for prelicensure (and graduate) nurses, including teamwork and collaboration.

13. Benner's novice to expert model of development suggests that new nurses function at the novice level, then progress to the advanced _____ phase.

14. Nursing students are quick to learn that _____ are in charge of their learning.

15. When practicing NCLEX style questions, the nurse can use the _____ framework, meaning airway, breathing, and circulation to prioritize life-threatening things first.

MATCHING EXERCISES

Match the term in Part A with its definition in Part B.

PART A

a. Nursing process

b. Nursing judgment

c. Framework

d. Expert (Benner)

e. ANA Code

f. Reflection

PART B

_____ **1.** Intuitive responses that seamlessly sort data and consider a holistic approach

_____ **2.** Provides ethical guidance as a framework for professional nursing

_____ **3.** All NCLEX questions require this ability

_____ **4.** Occurs both in-action (in the moment) and on-action (after the situation)

_____ **5.** Framework outlining the way nurses think

_____ **6.** Conceptional structure (as of ideas) that template for thinking

SHORT ANSWER

1. Briefly describe critical thinking.

_____

_____

2. Briefly describe clinical reasoning.

_____

_____

3. Briefly describe clinical judgment.

_____

_____

4. Explain how Tanner's Clinical Judgment Model correlates to the nursing process.

_____

_____

5. Give an example of several ways a nursing student can prepare for nursing examinations and NCLEX-RN testing that requires clinical judgment.

_____

_____

APPLYING YOUR KNOWLEDGE

CRITICAL THINKING QUESTIONS

1. Underline cues you notice in the following scenario.

You receive a report on a patient admitted with a change in mental status and syncope. The patient has a history of diabetes, and their blood glucose was low upon arrival.

2. Give examples of questions and approaches you would further use when interviewing and planning care for this patient.

_____

_____

_____

REFLECTIVE PRACTICE: CULTIVATING QSEN COMPETENCIES

Use the following expanded scenario from Chapter 14 in your textbook to answer the questions below.

Scenario: Ashley came to nursing school after completing high school. She has no clinical experience of no legacy of nursing in her family or circle of friends. She wants to be a nurse and is interested in pediatrics but is open to exploring different possibilities in nursing. Ashley is focused on developing her critical thinking skills before she begins her first clinical rotation.

1. Discuss how Ashley might focus on knowledge, attitudes, and skill to be a nurse?

_____

_____

_____

2. Patient-centered care: How can this student provide patient-centered care?

_____

_____

_____

3. Teamwork and collaboration: What roles and communication could the student plan to observe and utilize?

_____

_____

_____

4. How can the student keep their focus on safety/evidence-based practice?

_____

_____

_____

5. How can Ashley begin to use informatics to make sound clinical judgments?

_____

_____

_____

PRACTICING FOR NCLEX

MULTIPLE-CHOICE QUESTIONS

Circle the letter that corresponds to the best answer for each question.

1. The nurse is using clinical reasoning to make the best nursing judgment. Which action best reflects a nursing judgment?
    a. Assessing that a patient receiving chemotherapy reports nausea
    b. Instructing a patient with a BP of 88/50 who reports dizziness to call before ambulating
    c. Documenting the patient's vital signs in the electronic health record
    d. Recording the patient has vesicular breath sounds in the electronic health record

2. After performing an initial assessment on a patient who complains of abdominal distress, the nurse determines the patient has been having diarrhea. When formulating the health problem of altered bowel elimination, the nurse is using which skill?
    a. Assessment skills
    b. Clinical reasoning
    c. Clinical judgment
    d. Informatics

3. A nurse is preparing to administer an intravenous medication that must be reconstituted. Which QSEN competency is the nurse using when consulting with the pharmacist about the appropriate diluent?
    a. Quality
    b. Teamwork and collaboration
    c. Informatics
    d. Evidence-based practice

4. A nursing student would like to improve their critical thinking skills. Which statement is most true regarding critical thinking?
    a. Critical thinking cannot be learned.
    b. Critical thinking is reserved for use with acutely ill patients.
    c. Critical thinking involves applying, analyzing, synthesizing, and evaluating information.
    d. Critical thinking can be used in place of the nursing process.

5. A nursing student makes a conscious effort to improve their clinical reasoning. Which of these actions demonstrates clinical reasoning?
    a. Recording vital signs and assessments in the electronic health record
    b. Determining which assessments should be performed immediately postoperatively
    c. Reading an evidence-based protocol in the facility's procedure manual
    d. Documenting medication administration in the electronic health record

6. Nursing students are learning about clinical judgment. Which action best reflects clinical judgment?
    a. Recognizing cues, weighing hypotheses, acting, and reaching a satisfactory clinical outcome
    b. Writing a paper on evidence-based practice for perioperative patients
    c. Obtaining a detailed head-to-toe assessment of the assigned
    d. Stating scientific rationales for nursing actions and medications

7. Nursing students learn the importance of situation awareness. What action best reflects this type of awareness?
    a. Performing the eight rights when administering medications.
    b. Including a patient's partner when providing education.
    c. Noting scatter rugs, dim lighting, and multiple cats as a fall risk during a home visit.
    d. Providing thoughtful, patient-centered care for each patient.

8. Nursing students working with Tanner's Clinical Judgment Model will expect the final step of this process to consist of what action?
   a. Assessing
   b. Interpreting
   c. Intervening
   d. Reflecting

9. In order to practice as a registered nurse, what must each nurse do to prove their ability to practice safely and make sound clinical judgments?
   a. Successfully complete the NCLEX-RN examination
   b. Show proof of graduation to their state board of nursing
   c. Pass a practical clinical examination at their place of employment
   d. Register for multistate licensure

10. In Tanner's Clinical Judgment Model, the reflecting step focuses on what?
   a. Whether the patient recovered
   b. Analyzing the in-action and on-action
   c. How test taking abilities can be improved
   d. Patient satisfaction scores

ALTERNATE-FORMAT QUESTIONS
Multiple-Response Questions
Circle the letters that correspond to the best answers for each question.

1. When studying for the NCLEX-RN, the graduate prepares for questions based on the Clinical Judgment Action Model (CJAM). Which cognitive operations are included in this model? Select all that apply.
   a. Interpreting statistical data
   b. Recognizing cues
   c. Restating facts from nursing textbooks
   d. Taking appropriate nursing actions
   e. Reflecting on actions
   f. Analyzing data

2. Nurses use the nursing process to develop, deliver, and evaluate care. What additional uses does this process have? Select all that apply.
   a. Representing a mental model, an organized way of thinking
   b. Formulating the framework for a predictable approach to reviewing best practices
   c. Identifying etiologies for diagnosing actual and potential health problems
   d. Culminating in a concept map integrating pathophysiology and laboratory values
   e. Expanding on the ANA's Scope and Standards of Practice

3. What do the Eight Core Competency Outcomes and Performance Assessment Model (COPA) include? Select all that apply.
   a. Pharmacology knowledge
   b. Communication skills
   c. Critical thinking
   d. Teaching skills
   e. Leadership skills
   f. Ability to pass the licensure exam

Prioritization Question

1. Nursing students are introduced to use of the QSEN competency of evidence-based practice when caring for patients. What competency takes priority when entering the patient room? Circle the letter that corresponds to the best answer.
   a. Teamwork and collaboration
   b. Safety
   c. Informatics
   d. Quality improvement

CHAPTER 15

Assessing

ASSESSING YOUR UNDERSTANDING

FILL IN THE BLANKS

1. The primary source of patient assessment data is the _____; two other sources of patient data are the patient's _____ people and the patient _____.

2. The nursing assessment that is performed during the nurse's first contact with the patient and collects data about all aspects of the patient's health is referred to as the _____ assessment.

3. When a nurse acts to keep assessment data free of error, bias, or misinterpretation, the nurse is engaging in _____.

4. The _____ is an assessment tool that incorporates social determinants of health and assesses a person's ability to manage their health through evaluation of patient complexity.

5. A nurse admitting patient to the telemetry unit for hypertensive emergency who now reports blurred will perform a(n) _____ assessment.

6. A patient is brought to the emergency department with loss of consciousness and tachycardia. The patient's wife states that the patient has diabetes. The nurse performs a(n) _____ assessment.

7. Most schools of nursing and health care institutions establish the specific information that must be collected from every patient in a structured assessment form. This information is known as a(n) _____ data set.

MATCHING EXERCISES

Matching Exercise 1

Match the term in Part A with the appropriate example in Part B.

PART A

a. Database

b. Interview

c. Health assessment

d. Nursing history

e. Physical assessment

f. Observation

PART B

_____ 1. Examination of a patient for objective data that may better define the patient's condition and help the nurse in planning care

_____ 2. Conscious and deliberate use of the five physical senses to gather information

_____ 3. Clearly identifies patient strengths and weaknesses, health risks, and potential and existing health problems

_____ 4. Planned communication to obtain patient data

_____ **5.** Includes all pertinent patient information collected by the nurse and other health care professionals, enabling a comprehensive and effective plan of care to be designed and implemented

_____ **6.** May be used by nurses to help patients identify potential and actual health risks and to explore the habits, behaviors, beliefs, attitudes, and values that influence their health

Matching Exercise 2

Write the letter "S" beside data that is subjective and the letter "O" beside data that is objective.

_____ **1.** Redness and swelling at an incision site

_____ **2.** Patient reports pain in their left arm

_____ **3.** Patient has a violent spell of coughing

_____ **4.** Patient is nauseated at the sight of food

_____ **5.** Patient worries about their child during their hospital stay

_____ **6.** Patient is fidgety and cannot focus

SHORT ANSWER

1. List the five sources of data for the nursing assessment.

a. _____

_____

b. _____

_____

c. _____

_____

d. _____

_____

e. _____

_____

2. Give two examples of when data need to be validated.

a. _____

_____

b. _____

_____

3. Give two examples of open-ended questions that could be used to elicit information from your patient who passed out at work and was diagnosed with diabetes. The patient has been admitted to the hospital for stabilization with insulin and IV fluids.

a. _____

_____

b. _____

_____

4. Briefly describe why the following characteristics of data are important when collecting and recording patient data.

a. Purposeful: _____

_____

b. Prioritized: _____

_____

c. Complete: _____

_____

d. Systematic: _____

_____

e. Accurate: _____

_____

f. Relevant: _____

_____

g. Recorded in a standard manner: _____

_____

5. Give an example of three observations nurses should make each time they encounter a patient.

a. _____

_____

b. _____

_____

c. _____

_____

6. Give an example of when immediate communication of data is indicated. Document your communication to the health care provider in the SBAR format.

   a. Example: _____

   _____

   b. S: _____

   _____

   c. B: _____

   _____

   d. A: _____

   _____

   e. R: _____

   _____

7. Explain how the following factors affect assessment priorities when collecting patient data.

   a. Patient's health orientation: _____

   _____

   b. Patient's developmental stage: _____

   _____

   c. Patient's culture: _____

   _____

   d. Patient's need for nursing: _____

   _____

APPLYING YOUR KNOWLEDGE

CRITICAL THINKING QUESTIONS

1. Role-play nursing interview with your classmates for a patient with diabetes and diabetic foot ulcers who was brought to the emergency room after she experienced a syncopal episode. Discuss which approaches and types of questions resulted in the best interviews.

2. Recall the last time you went to a health care provider's office or hospital for a problem. How did it feel to be a patient? Did you feel empowered or at the mercy of others? How will you incorporate this learning into your nursing practice?

REFLECTIVE PRACTICE: CULTIVATING QSEN COMPETENCIES

Use the following expanded scenario from Chapter 14 in your textbook to answer the questions below.

Scenario: Susan is a 34-year-old woman newly diagnosed with multiple sclerosis (MS). She says, "How am I going to tell my husband? We were just married last year and planned to do lots of hiking and outdoor sports. It's not fair for him to be tied down to me if I can't be the wife and partner that he thought he had married."

1. Patient-centered care/safety: How might the nurse facilitate Susan's ability to cope with disability?

   _____

   _____

   _____

2. Patient-centered care/safety: What would be a successful outcome for this patient?

   _____

   _____

   _____

3. Patient-centered care/evidence-based practice: What intellectual, interpersonal, and/or ethical/legal competencies are most likely to bring about the desired outcome?

   _____

   _____

   _____

4. Teamwork and collaboration: What resources might be helpful for Susan?

   _____

   _____

   _____

PRACTICING FOR NCLEX

MULTIPLE-CHOICE QUESTIONS

Circle the letter that corresponds to the best answer for each question.

1. A nurse is documenting findings gathered during a patient assessment. What will the nurse include under objective data?
   a. Reporting nausea
   b. Reporting feeling anxious
   c. Reporting dizziness
   d. Skin having a yellow tint

2. A nurse is performing an initial assessment on a patient who reports abdominal pain. What question is most appropriate to gather needed data?
   a. "You haven't eaten any spoiled food, have you?"
   b. "Do you think you might have appendicitis?"
   c. "Are you feeling poorly besides your stomachache?"
   d. "What do you believe contributed to this problem?"

3. A nurse is interviewing a hospitalized patient. What position will the nurse adopt to best facilitate exchange of information?
   a. When the patient is in bed, the nurse stands at the foot of the bed.
   b. The nurse and patient are seated with their chairs at right angles, 1 ft apart.
   c. For a patient in bed, the nurse places their chair at a 45-degree angle to the bed.
   d. If the patient is in bed, the nurse stands at the side of the bed.

4. A nurse in the short procedure unit is assessing a new patient prior to surgery. During the introductory phase of the interview, which action will the nurse perform first?
   a. Determining the patient's comfort and ability to participate
   b. Reviewing important points of the interview with the patient
   c. Ensuring the environment for the interview is quiet and private
   d. Gathering all necessary information to form the subjective database

5. A nurse is assessing a patient admitted to the hospital who reports left-sided weakness and difficulty speaking. What represents appropriate documentation of the findings?
   a. Neurologic examination reveals partial paralysis and aphasic speech.
   b. Brain scan shows evidence of a clot in the middle cerebral artery.
   c. Patient is unable to communicate basic needs or perform tasks with left hand.
   d. Left-sided weakness and speech deficit indicate probable stroke.

6. A clinic nurse is assessing an energetic older adult who reports difficulty urinating, bloody urine, and burning on urination. What best reflects the priority assessment for this patient?
   a. Performing a quick priority assessment of only the urinary system
   b. Focusing on altered patterns of elimination common in older adults
   c. Performing a detailed assessment of the patient's sexual history
   d. Performing a thorough systems review to validate data on the patient's record

7. A nurse notes a patient became very tired during the initial nursing assessment, but there are outstanding questions needed for planning care. Which action will the nurse take next?
   a. Asking the patient to wake up and try to answer the interview questions
   b. Asking the patient's husband to come in and answer the interview questions
   c. Waiting until the next day to obtain the answers to the interview questions
   d. Obtaining the patient's permission for their partner to answer the questions

8. A patient is admitted to the medical-surgical unit with a diagnosis of scleroderma. The nurse is unfamiliar with this condition. What is the nurse's best source of information?
   a. Consulting with the patient
   b. Consulting with the patient's primary care provider
   c. Reviewing the medical record
   d. Consulting a nursing reference

9. Prior to feeding a patient with dysphagia, a nurse reviews the speech pathologist's recommendations for preventing aspiration. Where in the electronic medical record will the nurse find this information?
   a. Laboratory testing
   b. History and physical
   c. Radiology reports
   d. Progress notes

10. The nurse in an inpatient psychiatric unit is validating a portion of the assessment. What is most appropriate to ask?
   a. "Have you been experiencing side effects of your prescription medications?"
   b. "When did the problem begin?"
   c. "Do you have family in the area?"
   d. "You say you're not hearing voices, but you seem to be listening to something?"

ALTERNATE-FORMAT QUESTIONS

Multiple-Response Questions

Circle the letters that correspond to the best answers for each question.

1. Nurses perform assessments routinely, and when indicated by a change in status. What accurately describes the unique focus of nursing assessments? Select all that apply.
   a. They validate medical assessments.
   b. They target data pointing to pathologic conditions.
   c. They focus on the patient's responses to health problems.
   d. Findings from a nursing assessment may contribute to the medical diagnosis.
   e. They focus on actual, not potential, health problems.
   f. Initial assessments establish a database for problem solving and care planning.

2. A nurse is organizing data obtained during the patient interview according to Gordon's functional health pattern model. Which statements reflect the focus of this model? Select all that apply.
   a. Data are clustered or organized according to a hierarchy of basic human needs.
   b. Data are collected regarding the health perception/health management of the patient.
   c. The perception of the major roles and responsibilities in the patient's life is explored.
   d. The major body systems are assessed, and data are collected.
   e. Data related to human response patterns are collected and organized.
   f. Elimination, activity, sleep, and sexuality are components of the assessment data.

3. Nurses collect objective and subjective data during the patient interview. Which data will the nurse document as subjective data? Select all that apply.
   a. Patient wringing her hands before signing consent for surgery
   b. Redness and swelling at an IV site
   c. Patient describing pain as an 8 on the pain assessment scale
   d. Patient reporting nausea after eating breakfast
   e. Blood pressure 152/90 following physical activity
   f. Patient reporting being cold and requesting an extra blanket

4. A nurse is performing a daily assessment on a patient who has pneumonia and a history of stroke. Which actions will the nurse include as part of an ongoing nursing assessment?
   a. Auscultation of lungs
   b. Questioning about pain
   c. Preparation of the meal tray
   d. Administration of daily insulin
   e. Observation of the pupils
   f. Evaluation of muscle strength

5. Nurses performing a physical examination (assessment) following the nursing history and interview. Which methods are used to collect these data?
   a. Auscultation
   b. Role-playing
   c. Inspection
   d. Palpation
   e. Teaching
   f. Percussion

Prioritization Questions

1. Place the following actions performed by a nurse during a patient interview in the order in which they would most likely occur. Keep in mind the four distinct phases of the interview process: preparatory phase, introduction, working phase, and termination.

   a. The nurse gathers all the information needed to form the subjective database.

   b. The nurse prepares to meet the patient by reading current and past records and reports.

   c. The nurse recapitulates the interview, highlighting the key points.

   d. The nurse initiates the interview by stating their name, identifying the purpose of the interview, and clarifying the roles of the nurse and patient.

   e. The nurse ensures that the environment in which the interview is to be conducted is private and relaxed.

   f. The nurse assesses the patient's comfort and ability to participate in the interview.

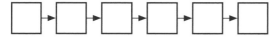

2. As the triage nurse in a pediatric practice, place the patients who need same-day appointments in order from first to last.

   a. School-aged child who fell off the bed and has a painful arm

   b. Adolescent needing a physical to play sports

   c. Infant with a fever and rash

   d. School-aged child who is wheezing

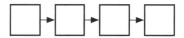

3. During the admission assessment, the patient develops a facial droop and garbled speech. Circle the letter of the action that takes priority at this time.

   a. Completing the health assessment and neurologic check

   b. Reporting change in status to the health care provider

   c. Documenting a focused neurologic assessment in the health record

   d. Developing the nursing diagnoses

CHAPTER 16

Diagnosis/Problem Identification

ASSESSING YOUR UNDERSTANDING

FILL IN THE BLANKS

1. Actual or potential health problems that can be prevented or resolved by independent nursing intervention are called nursing _____.

2. During the diagnosis phase of the nursing process, the nurse interprets and _____ the data.

3. A health _____ is a condition that necessitates intervention to prevent or resolve disease or illness or to promote coping and wellness.

4. When the nurse determines a potential health problem or risk for a problem is present, the nurse takes steps to _____ the problem.

5. When formatting a health problem, the nurse states the problem, the _____ and the _____ and _____.

6. When a nurse writes a patient outcome that requires a prescription for pain medication for goal achievement, the situation is a(n) _____ problem.

7. Patient reports of fever, chills, and nausea are considered significant data or _____.

8. When determining the significance of the results of a patient's urinalysis, the expected values to which the data can be compared are termed a(n) _____.

9. When a nurse groups patient cues that point to the existence of a patient health problem, the cues form what is known as a data _____.

10. A(n) _____ is a clinical judgment concerning a specific cluster of nursing diagnoses that occur together and are best addressed together and through similar interventions.

MATCHING EXERCISES

Match the appropriate step involved in the interpretation and analysis of data in Part A with the example in Part B. Answers may be used more than once.

PART A

a. Recognizing significant data
b. Recognizing patterns or clusters
c. Identifying strengths and problems
d. Reaching conclusions

PART B

___ 1. A nurse notes that a patient's refusal to stop smoking will adversely affect his recovery from cardiac surgery.

___ 2. A nurse compares a 15-month-old child's motor abilities with the norms for that age group.

___ 3. A nurse recognizes an unhealthy situation developing when a patient, recovering from a mastectomy, cries at night, refuses to eat, and sleeps all day.

____ 4. A nurse decides no further nursing response is indicated for a patient who recovered from gallbladder surgery according to schedule.

____ 5. A maternity nurse notices a newborn's skin tone is markedly different from that of the other babies and checks for jaundice.

____ 6. A nurse determines that a man with a history of diabetes is highly motivated to develop a healthy pattern of nutrition in response to his problem.

____ 7. A nurse notices that a patient with AIDS has an adverse reaction to a drug and consults the prescribing health care provider.

CORRECT THE FALSE STATEMENTS

Mark the statement "T" if true or "F" if false. If false, replace the underlined word or words to make the statement true.

____ 1. Actual or potential health problems that can be prevented or resolved by independent nursing intervention are termed <u>collaborative problems</u>. _____

____ 2. A <u>cue</u> is a generally accepted rule, measure, pattern, or model that can be used to compare data in the same class or category. _____

____ 3. A <u>data cluster</u> is a grouping of patient data or cues that points to the existence of a patient health problem. _____

____ 4. Nursing diagnoses should be derived from a <u>single cue</u>. _____

____ 5. The <u>problem</u> statement identifies the physiologic, psychological, sociologic, spiritual, and environmental factors believed to be related to the problem as either a cause or a contributing factor. _____

____ 6. The <u>etiology</u> of health problems and needs directs nursing intervention. _____

____ 7. A <u>possible</u> health problem is written when the nurse suspects that a health problem exists but needs to gather more data to confirm it. _____

____ 8. A <u>wellness health problem</u> is a clinical judgment about an individual, family, or community in transition from a specific level of wellness to a higher level of wellness. _____

____ 9. In the diagnosing step, the nurse <u>collects</u> patient data. _____

____ 10. A <u>possible health problem</u> is a clinical judgment that an individual, family, or community is more likely to develop the problem than others in the same or similar situation. _____

SHORT ANSWER

1. Place a check mark next to the health problems that are written correctly; state why the problem is incorrect on the lines that follow.

   a. Injury risk, etiology: absence of restraints and side rails _____

   _____

   b. Altered skin integrity, etiology: mobility deficit _____

   _____

   c. Grief, etiology: loss of breast _____

   _____

   d. Insomnia, etiology: inability to sleep _____

   _____

   e. Impaired mobility, etiology: lower extremity amputation _____

   _____

   f. Malnutrition risk, etiology: loss of appetite _____

   _____

   g. Situational low self-esteem, etiology: powerlessness _____

   _____

   h. Deficient knowledge, etiology: noncompliance with diet _____

   _____

   i. Needs assistance walking, etiology: immobility _____

   _____

   j. Constipation, etiology: colon cancer _____

   _____

   _____

2. What questions would you ask a patient to validate the following health problem?

   a. Urinary retention: _____

   _____

   b. Polypharmacy: _____

   _____

   c. Coping impairment: _____

   _____

   d. Insomnia: _____

   _____

3. In the following examples, explain how standards can be used to identify significant cues.

   a. Blood pressure: _____

   _____

   b. Growth and development: _____

   _____

   c. Diagnostic laboratory study: _____

   _____

4. List nine questions a nurse should consider when using critical thinking in diagnostic reasoning.

   a. _____
   b. _____
   c. _____
   d. _____
   e. _____
   f. _____
   g. _____
   h. _____
   i. _____

5. Review the following two- and three-part health problem statements and briefly discuss the benefits of using each.

   Lack of knowledge, etiology: medications, warfarin (anticoagulant).

   Lack of knowledge, etiology: medications, warfarin (anticoagulant). Signs and symptoms: PT/INR well above the therapeutic level, nosebleed, patient states "I don't remember if I take my medications or not."

   _____

   _____

6. Read the mini-cases that follow. In each one, underline the cues that form a data cluster indicating a health problem and write an appropriate health problem as a three-part statement.

   a. The home care nurse is visiting Mr. Klinetob, age 86, whose wife of 52 years died 6 months ago. He has degenerative joint disease and had spoken for years about having "a touch of arthritis," which never kept him from being up and about. His family reports he sits in his room and has no desire to engage in self-care activities. He tells the nurse he is "too stiff" in the morning to bathe, and "I just don't seem to have the energy." The nurse notices that his hair is matted and uncombed, his face has traces of previous meals, and he has a strong body odor.

   Health problem: _____

   Etiology: _____

   Signs and symptoms: _____

   b. Ms. Adams sustained a right-sided stroke that resulted in left hemiparesis (paralysis on the left side of the body) and left-sided "neglect." She ignores the left side of her body and actually denies its existence, stating it belongs to the patient in the next bed. This patient was previously quite active: she walked for 45 to 60 minutes four or five times a week and was an avid swimmer.

   Health problem: _____

   Etiology: _____

   Signs and symptoms: _____

APPLYING YOUR KNOWLEDGE

CRITICAL THINKING QUESTION

1. Identify health problems for the following patient. Be sure to include actual and potential health problems or needs. Then, compare your findings with those of another classmate and note similarities and differences. Decide which problems best suit the patient's situation.

An older adult presents to the emergency department with fever, tachypnea, and shortness of breath for 2 days. Her pulse oximetry reading is 89%, and she is quite pale. She tells you that she thought she had bronchitis but now fears she may have contracted COVID-19 from her daughter, who is a nurse.

Health problem: _____

Etiology: _____

Signs and symptoms: _____

REFLECTIVE PRACTICE: CULTIVATING QSEN COMPETENCIES

Use the following expanded scenario from Chapter 16 in your textbook to answer the questions below.

Scenario: Martin, a 46-year-old man, comes to the health clinic for a routine physical examination. During the assessment, he states, "I've had problems with constipation and have seen some blood when I wipe myself after a bowel movement. It's just hemorrhoids, right? Nothing to worry about?"

1. Patient-centered care: What health problem could the nurse consider appropriate for Martin? How might the nurse advocate for Martin to ensure that he gets tested for colon cancer?

   _____

   _____

   _____

2. Patient-centered care/safety: What would be a successful outcome for this patient?

   _____

   _____

   _____

3. Patient-centered care/evidence-based practice: What intellectual, interpersonal, and/or ethical/legal competencies are most likely to bring about the desired outcome?

   _____

   _____

   _____

4. Teamwork and collaboration: What resources might be helpful for Martin?

   _____

   _____

   _____

5. Informatics: In what way will the nurse use the electronic health record to document Martin's care?

   _____

   _____

   _____

PRACTICING FOR NCLEX

MULTIPLE-CHOICE QUESTIONS

Circle the letter that corresponds to the best answer for each question.

1. During post-conference, nursing students discuss formulating accurate health problems. Which statement should be included in the discussion?

   a. Health problems remain the same for as long as the disease is present.

   b. Nurses formulate health problems to identify diseases.

   c. Nurses write health problems to describe patient problems that nurses can treat.

   d. Health problems focus on identifying healthy responses to health and illness.

2. A nurse documents the following in the patient chart: Risk for electrolyte imbalance, etiology: prescribed loop diuretic and anorexia. This is an example of which aspect of patient care?

   a. Identification of health problem

   b. Nursing assessment

   c. Medical diagnosis

   d. Collaborative problem

3. A nurse is caring for a toddler who has been treated on two different occasions for lacerations and contusions from parents' lax supervision. What is an appropriate health problem for this patient and family?

a. Impulsivity, etiology: frequent falls

b. Injury risk, etiology: impaired home management

c. Child abuse, etiology: abusive parents

d. Knowledge deficiency, etiology: developmental abilities of toddlers

4. A nurse suspects that a patient has a self-care deficit but needs more data to confirm this health problem. What clarifying information will the nurse add when writing this health problem?

a. Actual

b. Potential

c. Possible

d. Apparent

5. A patient has a health problem of nonadherence to the treatment plan for a medical problem. Further assessment reveals the patient's partner died 2 weeks ago, and they "feel lost." Which action related to the health problem will the nurse take?

a. Maintain the current health problem in the medical record

b. Develop a new health problem of cognitive dysfunction

c. Update the care plan with a health problem of grief

d. Revise the health problem to impaired health maintenance

6. The admission care plan contains the health problem of dietary nonadherence for a patient with diabetes whose blood glucose continues to be elevated. Which statement reflects a need to modify the health problem to "denial"?

a. "I don't like to cook for myself."

b. "I just have a 'touch of sugar'; it's nothing."

c. "I really like potatoes."

d. "I'm trying to switch to whole-grain pastas."

7. The nurse has developed a health problem of "bleeding risk" for a patient who takes an anticoagulant and continues to consume alcohol. After formulating the health problem, which step will the nurse take?

a. Formulate the outcomes.

b. Admonish the patient for consuming alcohol.

c. Evaluate coagulation studies.

d. Observe for hematuria and bruising.

ALTERNATE-FORMAT QUESTIONS

Multiple-Response Questions

Circle the letters that correspond to the best answers for each question.

1. A nursing student is learning how to write a health problem for a patient. Which actions are accurate guidelines when formulating a three-part health problem? Select all that apply.

a. Including the medical health problem in the health problem

b. Ensuring the problem statement precedes the etiology

c. Writing the health problem in legally advisable terms

d. Phrasing the health problem as a patient need rather than alteration

e. Ensuring the problem statement indicates what is unhealthy about the patient

f. Making sure signs and symptoms (defining characteristics) follow the etiology

2. Prior to developing a health problem for nonadherence to a medication, the nurse validates which factors? Select all that apply.

a. Whether the patient is experiencing side effects

b. Whether the patient has taken an overdose

c. Whether the patient is experiencing a drug interaction

d. Whether there is a likely allergy or adverse reaction

e. Whether the patient's partner objects to the medication

3. Nursing students in an acute care hospital are invited to an in-service on the legal obligation to formulate accurate problem statements and care plans. Which statements do the students learn are legally inadvisable? Select all that apply.

   a. Persistent pain related to no return phone call from the health care provider

   b. Pressure injury related to infrequent turning by the home health aid

   c. Impaired myocardial tissue perfusion related to reduced myocardial oxygen supply and demand

   d. Potential for injury related to weakness and malnutrition

   e. Risk for altered growth and development related to being nonverbal at age 4

   f. Impaired cognition: expressive aphasia related to altered cerebral blood flow

4. A nurse is caring for a male patient who had an appendectomy earlier that day. The nurse notes that the patient is hesitant to move, guards the surgical area, and grimaces frequently. The dressing is dry and intact. Which cues lead to a data cluster that the nurse can use to formulate a health problem? Select all that apply.

   a. Male sex

   b. Guarding

   c. Grimacing

   d. Surgical site

   e. Dressing dry and intact

   f. Avoiding moving

Prioritization Questions

1. Place the parts of the three-step health problem in the order in which they should be stated.

   a. Signs and symptoms

   b. Actual or potential health problem

   c. Etiology

   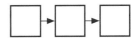

2. A nurse is caring for four patients with the following health problems. Based on Maslow's hierarchy of needs, which patients will the nurse assess first? Circle the letter that corresponds to the best answer.

   a. Hypotension, etiology: fever and diaphoresis

   b. Acute anxiety, etiology: unknown outcome of ovarian biopsy

   c. Constipation, etiology: post-anesthesia, use of opioid pain medication

   d. Infection risk, etiology: long-term immuno-suppressant medication

3. A nurse is caring for a group of patients. Based on their health problems, which patients will the nurse assess first? Circle the letter that corresponds to the best answer.

   a. Altered body image perception

   b. Ineffective airway clearance

   c. Aspiration risk

   d. Hypoglycemia risk

Outcome Identification and Planning

ASSESSING YOUR UNDERSTANDING

FILL IN THE BLANKS

1. A(n) _____ is the expected conclusion to a patient health problem or, in the event of a wellness diagnosis, an expected conclusion to a patient's health expectation.

2. While waiting in line for lunch, a nurse contemplates how to help a patient with cancer accept the loss of a limb. This nurse is using the process of _____ planning.

3. In acute care settings, the three stages of planning that are critical to comprehensive nursing care are _____, _____, and _____.

4. To develop patient-centered outcomes, the nurse bases the goals on what the _____ would like to achieve.

5. Follow-up documentation to the care plan in the electronic health record states, "Goal partially met; patient ate approximately one half of food offered for lunch." This reflects a(n) _____ statement of the nursing care plan.

6. *Healthy People 2030* established _____ national health objectives to guide efforts to improve health across the country.

7. When a nurse provides education on sodium reduction by encouraging patients to read food labels and avoid adding salt to food, the nurse is performing a(n) _____ intervention.

8. When a nurse administers health care provider–prescribed pain medication to a patient after surgery, they are performing a(n) _____ intervention.

9. A(n) _____ is a set of clinical rules or steps, typically embedded in a branching flowchart, that approximates the decision process of an expert clinician.

10. A clinical _____ guideline is a statement or a series of statements outlining appropriate practice for a clinical condition or procedure generally based on the latest, most comprehensive scientific evidence and expert analysis.

MATCHING EXERCISES

Matching Exercise 1

Match the type of care plan listed in Part A with the definition in Part B. Answers may be used more than once.

PART A

a. Initial care plan

b. Ongoing, problem-solving care plan

c. Discharge care plan

d. Standardized care plan

e. Clinical pathways

f. Concept map care plan

PART B

____ **1.** Diagram of patient problems and interventions, used to organize data, analyze data, and take a holistic view of the patient situation

____ **2.** Type of plan for leaving the institution is best prepared by the nurse who has worked most closely with the patient, in conjunction with a social worker familiar with the patient's community resources

____ **3.** Prepared plans of care that identify the nursing diagnoses, outcomes, and related nursing interventions common to a specific population or health problem

____ **4.** Emphasis is to clearly state expected patient outcomes and specific timeframes to achieve the outcomes

____ **5.** Benefits include ready access to an expanded knowledge base, improved record keeping and documentation, and decreased paperwork

____ **6.** Developed by the nurse who performs the admission nursing history and physical assessment

Matching Exercise 2

Match the type of goal in Part A with the appropriate example in Part B. Answers may be used more than once.

PART A

a. Cognitive

b. Psychomotor

c. Affective

PART B

____ **1.** Patient will demonstrate self-blood glucose monitoring by 12/22/25

____ **2.** Patient will state the normal blood glucose value by 12/20/25

____ **3.** Patient will state willingness to change the diet to regain health and maintain HbA_{1C} <7 by discharge

____ **4.** Patient will state the effects of simple carbohydrates on blood glucose prior to discharge

____ **5.** Patient will demonstrate self-administration of insulin by 12/23/25

Matching Exercise 3

Match the step of the nursing process in Part A with its appropriate example in Part B. Answers may be used more than once.

PART A

a. Assessment

b. Analysis/diagnosis

c. Planning/outcome

d. Implementation

e. Evaluation

PART B

____ **1.** Bowel sounds return; bowel movement within 24 hours

____ **2.** Constipation

____ **3.** Order salad, fruit, or vegetable with each meal; offer MOM

____ **4.** Ambulated twice; missed third time due to pain

____ **5.** Patient will ambulate three times daily

____ **6.** Postoperative day 4, no bowel movement for 6 days; feels bloated; diminished bowel sounds

SHORT ANSWER

1. Revise the nursing orders for the following patients to reflect a clear, individualized, and specific statement.

    a. Child with asthma who must be taught to use an inhaler: _____

    _____

    b. New mother who must ambulate after having a cesarean delivery:

    _____

    _____

    c. Overweight adolescent who would like to lose weight: _____

    _____

2. During care planning, from which part of the problem statement, "Pain, etiology: delayed surgical wound healing" would nursing interventions be derived?

_____

_____

3. Briefly define the following elements of planning. Explain why they are necessary to the planning step of the nursing process.

a. Setting priorities: _____

_____

b. Writing goals/outcomes that determine the evaluative strategy: _____

_____

c. Selecting appropriate evidence-based nursing interventions: _____

_____

d. Communicating the nursing care plan:

_____

_____

4. Explain why nursing students are often asked to support their care plan and nursing interventions with a scientific rationale.

_____

_____

5. Individualize the following standard plans to meet the patient's specific goals.

a. Manage pain for a terminally ill patient:

_____

_____

b. Explore support people for a patient with AIDS: _____

_____

c. Provide sensory stimulation for an older adult in a long-term care facility:

_____

_____

d. Teach a patient being discharged to their home after a stroke about safety:

_____

_____

6. Describe the following types of nursing care and give an example of each type.

a. Nursing care related to basic human needs: _____

_____

Example: _____

_____

b. Nursing care related to nursing diagnoses:

_____

Example: _____

c. Nursing care related to the medical and interdisciplinary plan of care:

_____

_____

Example: _____

_____

7. List four considerations a nurse should employ when planning nursing care for each day.

a. _____

_____

b. _____

_____

c. _____

_____

d. _____

_____

8. Place a check mark next to the patient goals that are written correctly; rewrite those that are incorrect on the lines that follow.

____ a. Teach Mrs. Myers one lesson per day on the nutritional value of foods.

_____

_____

____ b. Mrs. Gray will know the dangers of smoking after viewing a video on smoking. _____

_____

____ c. By the end of the shift, the patient ambulates in the hallway using crutches. _____

_____

____ d. By 2/7/25, the patient correctly demonstrates insulin self-injection.

_____

_____

____ e. By next visit, the patient will understand the benefits of psychotherapy.

_____

_____

_____ **f.** By 6/12/25, patient correctly demonstrates application of wet-to-dry dressing on leg ulcer. _____

_____

9. Identify a patient goal that shows a direct resolution of the health problem expressed in the problem statements below.

a. Dehydration related to decreased fluid intake during fever

Patient goal: _____

_____

b. Sexual dysfunction: Loss of desire related to change in body image and feelings of unattractiveness following mastectomy

Patient goal: _____

_____

c. Stress urinary incontinence related to age-related degenerative changes and weak pelvic muscles and structural supports

Patient goal: _____

_____

d. Acute pain related to fear of taking prescribed analgesics

Patient goal: _____

_____

10. List six measures nurses should consider to correctly plan health care for a patient.

a. _____

_____

b. _____

_____

c. _____

_____

d. _____

_____

e. _____

_____

f. _____

_____

11. Give four examples of questions a nurse should ask when thinking critically about setting priorities for a patient plan of care.

a. _____

_____

b. _____

_____

c. _____

_____

d. _____

_____

12. When developing outcomes, the nurse uses the memory jogger or acronym for SMART goals. Explain each element in this mnemonic.

a. S: _____

b. M: _____

c. A: _____

d. R: _____

e. T: _____

APPLYING YOUR KNOWLEDGE

CRITICAL THINKING QUESTIONS

1. Explain what type of outcomes would be appropriate in each of the three stages of planning (initial planning, ongoing planning, discharge planning) using the following patient data.

a. A mother brings her young school-aged child to the emergency room. She reports that the child has been running a low-grade fever and has had abdominal pain and headache. His skin is pale with bruising and purpura on the arms and legs. On examination, you note splenic enlargement and abdominal tenderness. Diagnostic testing confirms acute leukemia.

b. A middle-aged adult presents with low-grade fevers, weight loss, chronic fatigue, and night sweats. The patient has a productive cough with yellowish mucus and chest pain. A TB skin test comes back positive.

c. A 12-year-old girl presents with fatigue, weight loss, excessive thirst, and frequent urination. Laboratory tests confirm a diagnosis of diabetes mellitus.

2. Why is the identification of goals in each stage necessary for optimal care and outcomes?

REFLECTIVE PRACTICE: CULTIVATING QSEN COMPETENCIES

Use the following expanded scenario from Chapter 17 in your textbook to answer the questions below.

Scenario: Glenda, a 35-year-old woman, comes to the health center for a routine checkup. During the visit, she expresses a strong motivation and desire to become physically fit, lose weight, increase her muscle tone, and improve her cardiorespiratory capacity. "I know it will involve some major lifestyle changes, including diet. What's with all these diets and diet supplements now?" she asks.

1. Patient-centered care/evidence-based practice: How might the nurse respond to Glenda's questions regarding dietary supplements?

_____

_____

_____

2. Patient-centered care/evidence-based practice: What would be a successful outcome for this patient?

_____

_____

_____

3. Patient-centered care/evidence-based practice: What intellectual, technical, interpersonal, and/or ethical/legal competencies are most likely to bring about the desired outcome?

_____

_____

_____

4. Teamwork and collaboration: What resources might be helpful for Glenda?

_____

_____

_____

PRACTICING FOR NCLEX

MULTIPLE-CHOICE QUESTIONS

Circle the letter that corresponds to the best answer for each question.

1. A nurse is planning care for a patient who has just been diagnosed with type 2 diabetes. Which nursing action is performed during the planning step of the nursing process?
   a. Interpreting and analyzing the patient data
   b. Establishing a database for the patient
   c. Identifying patient strengths and weaknesses
   d. Selecting individualized interventions, including patient teaching

2. A nurse is writing outcomes for a patient who must ambulate following hip replacement surgery. What is a correctly written goal for this patient?
   a. Within 24 hours, the patient will walk 20 feet and back using a walker.
   b. The nurse will help the patient ambulate the length of the hallway once a day.
   c. Offer to help the patient walk the length of the hallway each day.
   d. Patient will become mobile within a 24-hour period.

3. A nurse is caring for a patient with a new colostomy. Which patient outcome is written correctly?
   a. Teach the patient proper care of the stoma by 3/29/25.
   b. Patient will know how to care for his stoma by 3/29/25.
   c. Patient will demonstrate proper care of stoma by 3/29/25.
   d. Patient will be able to care for stoma and cope with psychological loss by 3/29/25.

4. When planning nursing interventions, a nurse includes the etiology in the problem statement to direct outcomes and interventions. What best reflects the etiology portion of a diagnostic statement?
   a. Identifies the unhealthy response preventing desired change
   b. Identifies factors or barriers leading to undesirable response
   c. Suggests patient goals to promote desired change
   d. Identifies patient strengths

5. A nurse is engaging in discharge planning for an overweight, highly stressed executive who has undergone coronary bypass surgery. What is an effective goal for this patient?

   a. By 6/30/25, the patient will list three benefits of daily exercise.

   b. By 6/30/25, the patient will correctly demonstrate breathing techniques to reduce stress.

   c. By 6/30/25, the patient will value his health sufficiently to reduce the dietary cholesterol.

   d. By 6/30/25, the patient will be able to plan healthy weekly menus.

6. A primary nurse is updating the patient care plans, evaluating and revising nursing interventions. Which guideline is essential for the nurse to use when designing the plan of care?

   a. Making sure the nursing interventions are a separate entity from the original outcomes

   b. Dating the nursing interventions when written and when the plan of care is revised

   c. Ensuring nursing interventions are cosigned by the health care provider

   d. Being certain the nursing intervention does not describe the nursing action to be performed

ALTERNATE-FORMAT QUESTIONS

Multiple-Response Questions

Circle the letters that correspond to the best answers for each question.

1. A nurse is planning care for patients on a medical-surgical unit. Which actions will the nurse perform during this step of the nursing process? Select all that apply.

   a. Establishing and setting priorities

   b. Collecting and interpreting patient data

   c. Identifying expected patient outcomes

   d. Selecting evidence-based nursing interventions

   e. Recording patient outcomes

   f. Communicating the nursing care plan

2. A nurse is performing initial care planning for a hospitalized patient. Which actions occur during the initial planning of patient care? Select all that apply.

   a. The nurse who performs the admission nursing history and physical assessment makes the initial plan.

   b. After the initial plan is developed, the nurse prioritizes problem statements.

   c. The nurse identifies patient goals and the related nursing care in the initial plan.

   d. The nurse uses tailored plans as opposed to standardized care plans as a basis for the initial plan.

   e. The nurse collects new data and analyzes it to make the plan more specific and effective.

   f. The nurse making the initial plan focuses on using teaching and counseling skills to help the patient carry out necessary self-care behaviors at home.

3. A nurse is writing outcomes for patients in a rehabilitation facility. Which guidelines should the nurse consider? Select all that apply.

   a. Derive each set of outcomes from a combination of nursing diagnoses.

   b. At least one outcome should show a direct resolution of the problem statement.

   c. The nurse should not be concerned if patient and family do not value the outcomes if they support the plan of care.

   d. Outcomes should be brief, specific, and support the overall plan of care.

   e. The outcomes need not support the overall treatment plan if they specify a goal.

   f. Expected outcomes are not required to specify a timeline if they are linked with other outcomes.

4. Nurses write learning outcomes that are categorized by cognitive, psychomotor, or affective domains. What are outcomes in the cognitive domain? Select all that apply.

   a. Within 1 week of teaching, the patient will list three benefits of quitting smoking.

   b. By 6/8/25, the patient will correctly demonstrate injecting himself with insulin.

   c. Before discharge, the patient will verbalize valuing health sufficiently to follow reduce trans fat in the diet.

   d. By 6/8/25, the patient will describe a meal plan that is high in fiber.

   e. By 6/8/25, the patient will correctly demonstrate ambulating with a walker.

   f. After viewing a cardiac rehabilitation video, the patient will verbalize four benefits of daily exercise.

5. A nurse is writing a measurable outcome for a patient learning to ambulate with a new prosthesis. Which components must be included in the outcome? Select all that apply.

   a. Action the patient will perform

   b. Modifiers describing the end result

   c. Description in subjective terms of the expected patient behavior

   d. Circumstances in which the outcome is to be achieved

   e. Patient or some aspect of the patient's health

   f. Target time when the patient is expected to be able to achieve the outcome

6. A nurse is writing goals for patients being discharged from an acute care setting. Which goals are written correctly? Select all that apply.

   a. The nurse will demonstrate the correct use of crutches to the patient prior to discharge.

   b. The patient will know how to dress their wound after receiving a demonstration.

   c. After attending an infant care class, the patient will correctly demonstrate the procedure for bathing their newborn.

   d. By 4/5/25, the patient will demonstrate how to care for a colostomy.

   e. The patient will list the dangers of smoking and quit.

   f. After counseling, the patient will describe two coping measures to deal with stress.

7. Nurses in a large community hospital system use computerized nursing care plans. What are the beneficial attributes of this type of care plan? Select all that apply.

   a. Ready access to a large knowledge base

   b. Improved record keeping and quality assurance

   c. Printouts for the patient's record and for change-of-shift reports

   d. Less time spent on paperwork

   e. Less individualization of care

8. The nurse is carrying out the care plan for a sacral pressure injury requiring wet-to-dry dressings twice daily. The outcome is written as: "The sacral pressure wound will decrease from stage 2 to stage 1 within 2 weeks." Which planning steps will the nurse use prior to the intervention? Select all that apply.

   a. Document the length, width, depth, and quality of drainage of the wound

   b. Gather sterile water, 4 × 4 gauze pads, and clean gloves

   c. Bring extra pillow to turn the patient off the affected area

   d. Identify the patient's strength and ability to turn in bed

   e. Administer an analgesic every 4 hours, as needed for sacral pain

Prioritization Questions

1. Using Maslow's hierarchy of needs, place the care plan goals in the order in which the nurse will prioritize patient care.

   a. Patient will sit upright while demonstrating coughing and deep breathing every 2 hours.

   b. Parents of a newborn will bring an infant car seat to the hospital prior to discharge.

   c. Parents of a school-aged child will facilitate visits with siblings during prolonged hospitalization.

   d. Adolescent who sustained a spinal cord injury will verbalize the ability to complete high school using a wheelchair.

   e. Patient will value returning to work as a chef.

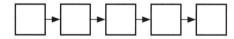

2. When planning care for a group of patients, a nurse uses Maslow's hierarchy of human needs to prioritize care. Which patient will the nurse assess first? Circle the letter that corresponds to the best answer.

   a. Patient who reports depression after having a myocardial infarction (MI)

   b. Adolescent patient with a spinal cord injury who wants friends to visit the hospital

   c. Adult with emphysema reports shortness of breath when walking to the bathroom

   d. Postmastectomy patient whose dressing is saturated with bright red blood

CHAPTER 18

Implementing

ASSESSING YOUR UNDERSTANDING

FILL IN THE BLANKS

1. _____ are written plans that detail the nursing activities to be executed in specific situations, such as might occur in the emergency department of a hospital.

2. _____ orders empower the nurse to initiate actions that ordinarily require prescription, order, or supervision of a health care provider.

3. _____ interventions are targeted to promote and preserve the health of populations.

4. A(n) _____ care intervention is a treatment performed away from the patient but on behalf of a patient or group of patients.

5. _____ interventions are developed by nurses and an interprofessional health care team.

6. An _____ reaction is an unwanted or harmful experience following the administration of a drug, diagnostic test, or therapeutic intervention under normal conditions of use.

7. When a nurse delegates care to another, such as to AP, the nurse transfers the responsibility for the performance of an activity to this person while retaining accountability for the _____.

8. A (care) _____ is a standard set of evidence-based practices, that, when performed together and applied consistently, have been proven to improve patient outcomes.

9. Administering medications using the electronic health record's medication administration record is an example of the QSEN competency _____.

MATCHING EXERCISES

Match the type of intervention in Part A with appropriate example of interventions in Part B. Answers may be used more than once.

PART A

a. Nurse-initiated, independent

b. Health care provider–initiated, dependent

c. Collaborative, interdependent

PART B

____ 1. A nurse notices that a patient is extremely anxious about surgery with general anesthesia and asks the nurse anesthetist to speak with the patient before surgery.

____ 2. A nurse administers the prescribed analgesic to a patient recovering from knee surgery.

____ 3. A nurse teaches the daughter of a patient who has leg ulcers how to change the dressings.

____ 4. A nurse meets with a patient's health care provider to discuss a patient's response to prescribed therapy.

_____ **5.** A nurse administers enemas and antibiotics prior to intestinal surgery.

_____ **6.** A nurse attends a care conference with the health care provider, social worker, and psychiatrist to discuss a patient's progress.

CORRECT THE FALSE STATEMENTS

Mark the statement "T" if true or "F" if false. If false, replace the underlined word or words to make the statement true.

_____ **1.** The <u>health care provider</u> is legally responsible for the assessments nurses make and for their nursing responses. _____

_____ **2.** <u>Nurse-initiated interventions</u> involve carrying out nurse-prescribed orders written on the nursing care plan. _____

_____ **3.** <u>Standing orders</u> are written plans that detail the nursing activities to be executed in specific situations. _____

_____ **4.** The <u>health care provider</u> acts as coordinator within the health care team. _____

_____ **5.** The <u>nursing team</u> carries out the nursing orders detailed in the nursing care plan. _____

_____ **6.** When working with patients to achieve the goals/outcomes specified in the care plan, it is important to remember that the <u>plan of care is fluid</u>. _____

_____ **7.** When choosing nursing interventions, it is important to consider the <u>patient's background</u>. _____

_____ **8.** Sincere motivation to benefit the patient and conscientious attempts to implement nursing orders are <u>sufficient</u> to protect a nurse from legal action due to negligence. _____

_____ **9.** When a patient fails to follow the care plan despite the nurse's best efforts, it is time to <u>change the patient's attitude toward their care</u>. _____

_____ **10.** All nursing actions for implementing the care plan must be <u>consistent with standards for practice</u>. _____

SHORT ANSWER

1. List three duties nurses perform when acting as coordinators for the health care team.
   a. _____
   b. _____
   c. _____

2. Give an example of a nurse variable, a patient variable, and a health care variable that might influence the implementation of the care plan.
   a. Nurse variable: _____
   b. Patient variable: _____
   c. Health care variable: _____

3. Explain why the following nursing actions are important to the continuity of nursing care.
   a. Promoting self-care: teaching, counseling, and advocacy: _____
   b. Assisting patients to meet health goals: _____

4. Mr. Franks, a new resident in a long-term care facility, is recovering from a minor surgery. He shows no interest in his condition and refuses to participate in self-care. You suspect an underlying problem of loneliness and boredom beginning with his admission to the facility. How would you reevaluate the nursing care plan and incorporate self-care for Mr. Franks, taking into consideration his mental state? _____

5. You suspect your pregnant patient living in a subsidized housing development is not receiving proper nutrition. She has two other children and states that there is not enough money to put three square meals a day on the table. How would you reevaluate the nursing care plan for this patient to include options for proper nutrition? _____

6. Give an example of the following types of interventions defined by the *Nursing Intervention Classification* report.

  a. Direct care intervention: _____

  _____

  b. Indirect care intervention: _____

  _____

  c. Community (or public health) intervention:

  _____

  _____

7. State the five rights of delegation.

  a. _____
  b. _____
  c. _____
  d. _____
  e. _____

APPLYING YOUR KNOWLEDGE

CRITICAL THINKING QUESTIONS

1. List factors (nurse, health care team, patient/ family, health care setting, resources, and so on) that might interfere or facilitate the nurse's ability to implement a care plan for the following patients. Think about how you can use this knowledge.

  a. A 5-year-old girl with cystic fibrosis is being discharged into the care of her family, which consists of a single working mother and two older brothers.

  b. A 17-year-old single mother who is living with her parents is being sent home with her newborn son. She is having difficulty nursing the baby, and the baby is being treated for jaundice.

2. Observe nurses as they care for patients. Consider whether the nursing actions you observe involved the use of the nurse's cognitive skills, interpersonal skills, technical skills, ethical/legal skills, or a blend of these skills. Rate your own skills in these areas and note in which areas you feel confident and in which areas you need improvement. What actions will help you improve these skills?

REFLECTIVE PRACTICE: CULTIVATING QSEN COMPETENCIES

Use the following expanded scenario from Chapter 18 in your textbook to answer the questions below.

Scenario: Antoinette, a toddler, is brought to the well-child community clinic by her grandmother. The health history reveals recurrent nausea, vomiting, and diarrhea. Her physical examination reveals a negligible gain in height and weight, lethargy, and a delay in achieving developmental milestones.

1. Patient-centered care: What might be the nurse's response when advocating for Antoinette and her family?

  _____

  _____

  _____

2. Patient-centered care, evidence-based practice: What would be a successful outcome for this patient?

  _____

  _____

  _____

3. Patient-centered care: What intellectual, technical, interpersonal, and ethical/legal competencies are most likely to bring about the desired outcome?

  _____

  _____

  _____

4. Teamwork and collaboration: What resources might be helpful for this family?

  _____

  _____

  _____

PRACTICING FOR NCLEX

MULTIPLE-CHOICE QUESTIONS

Circle the letter that corresponds to the best answer for each question.

1. The Joint Commission (TJC) encourages patients to become active, involved, and informed participants of the health care team. Which nursing action is consistent with their recommendations for improving patient safety by encouraging patients to speak up?
   a. Explaining each procedure twice to prevent patient questions from wasting time
   b. Encouraging the patient to participate in all treatment decisions as the center of the health care team
   c. Encouraging patients to advocate for themselves instead of choosing a trusted family member or friend
   d. Assuring the patient who questions a medication that it is the right medication prescribed for him and administers the medicine

2. Nurses perform many independent nursing actions when caring for patients. Which action is considered an independent, nurse-initiated action?
   a. Inserting an indwelling catheter
   b. Participating in interprofessional rounds to discuss patient care
   c. Helping to allay a patient's anxiety about an upcoming surgery
   d. Administering oral medication to a patient

3. A nurse follows set guidelines to titrate intravenous anticoagulation for patients based on their weight and diagnostic test results. Through which mechanism does the nurse have the legal authority to initiate actions normally requiring a prescription?
   a. Protocols
   b. Nursing interventions
   c. Collaborative orders
   d. Standing orders

4. A nursing student asks why the nurse assesses a patient's skin integrity, ability to respond to simple directions, and their muscle tone during bathing. What is the nurse's best response?
   a. "It is difficult to collect complete data in the initial assessment."
   b. "It is the most efficient use of the nurse's time."
   c. "It enables the nurse to revise the care plan appropriately."
   d. "It meets current standards of care."

5. A patient with high blood pressure is put on a low-sodium diet and instructed to quit smoking. The nurse finds the patient in the bathroom with the door locked and the smell of cigarette smoke coming from under the bathroom door. The patient tells the nurse there is no way they will quit smoking. What is the nurse's focus when implementing care for this patient?
   a. Explaining the effects of sodium and smoking on blood pressure
   b. Identifying barriers that interfere with the patient following the treatment plan
   c. Collaborating with other health care professionals about the patient's treatment
   d. Revising the nursing care plan

6. A nurse is administering medications to a patient who refuses to take them. To provide patient-centered care, what response by the nurse is most appropriate?
   a. "Your health care provider has written prescriptions for these medications; I'll show you."
   b. "I only have a few more minutes to discuss this; others need their medications."
   c. "Let me ask the health care provider to come speak with you."
   d. "Could you explain your concern about these medications?"

7. Which collaborative action best reflects safe, evidence-based practice?
   a. Using a bundle when assisting with insertion of a central venous catheter
   b. Crushing medications for a patient who has difficulty swallowing pills
   c. Using an infusion pump when administering maintenance intravenous fluids
   d. Documenting the outcome of nursing care in the electronic health record

8. When implementing the plan of care, a nurse enters the patient's room to administer a prescribed ointment to a skin lesion. What will the nurse do first?

    a. Clean away any ointment previously prescribed.

    b. Explain the purpose of the medication to the patient.

    c. Revise the nursing diagnosis.

    d. Assess the patient's skin to determine the appearance of the lesion.

ALTERNATE-FORMAT QUESTIONS

Multiple-Response Questions

Circle the letters that correspond to the best answers for each question.

1. A nurse is writing interventions for their assigned patient's care plans. Which activities are typically be carried out during the implementation step of the nursing process? Select all that apply.

    a. Collecting additional patient data

    b. Modifying the patient care plan

    c. Performing an initial assessment of the patient

    d. Developing patient outcomes and goals

    e. Measuring how well the patient has achieved patient goals

    f. Collecting a database to enable an effective care plan

2. Nurses use the *Nursing Interventions Classification* (NIC) report of research when choosing nursing interventions for patients. What are advantages of having standard NICs? Select all that apply.

    a. Limiting the amount of reimbursement allowed for nursing services

    b. Teaching decision making

    c. Allocating nursing resources

    d. Allowing the use of multiple systems of nomenclature

    e. Developing information systems

    f. Communicating nursing to non-nurses

Prioritization Question

1. A nurse is caring for a group of patients on a medical-surgical unit. Which intervention will the nurse prioritize? Circle the letter that corresponds to the best answer.

    a. Discussing the impact of mastectomy with a patient who is crying

    b. Suctioning the airway of a patient with copious secretions and weak cough

    c. Providing range of motion to a patient who sustained a spinal cord injury

    d. Administering an antibiotic to a patient with pneumonia

CHAPTER 19

Evaluating

ASSESSING YOUR UNDERSTANDING

FILL IN THE BLANKS

1. When evaluating the patient's response to the care plan, the nurse makes a determination to _____, _____, or _____ the care plan.

2. Nurses are involved in many types of evaluation, but the _____ is always the nurse's primary focus.

3. The most important act of evaluation performed by nurses is evaluating _____ achievement with the patient.

4. The nurse evaluates a patient's outcome by measuring the skills and knowledge that the patient has achieved. These measurable qualities, attributes, or characteristics are called _____.

5. The nurse evaluates four types of outcomes: cognitive, _____, affective, and _____.

6. When documenting the outcome of care, the nurse uses a two-part evaluative statement including whether the outcomes were met, partially met, or not met and nursing _____ that supports the evaluation decision.

7. _____ are the levels of performance accepted by and expected of the nursing staff or other health care team members established by authority, custom, or consent.

8. _____ practice guidelines are recommendations for how care should be managed in specific diseases, problems, or situations.

9. The nurse manager of a hospital unit sets up a program to help promote teamwork. This type of program that promotes excellence in nursing is referred to as a _____ improvement program.

10. A person who evaluates nursing care by using post discharge questionnaires, patient interviews (by telephone or face to face), or chart review (nursing audit) to collect data is conducting a(n) _____ evaluation.

MATCHING EXERCISES

Matching Exercise 1

Match the type of evaluation listed in Part A with its definition in Part B.

PART A

a. Concurrent

b. Retrospective

c. Outcome

d. Process

e. Structure

PART B

____ 1. Focuses on the environment in which care is provided

____ 2. Focuses on measurable changes in the health status of the patient

____ 3. Focuses on nursing care and patient goals while the patient is receiving the care

_____ **4.** Focuses on the nature and sequence of activities carried out by the nurse implementing the nursing process

_____ **5.** Collects data after discharge usually by using post discharge interviews and questionnaires and chart review

Matching Exercise 2

Match the measurement tool in Part A with its appropriate example in Part B. Answers may be used more than once.

PART A

a. Criterion

b. Standard

PART B

_____ **1.** Patient will walk the length of the hall by 5/15/25.

_____ **2.** Nurses will complete the admission database on all patients within 24 hours of admission.

_____ **3.** All patients in active labor will have continuous external fetal heart monitoring.

_____ **4.** Upon completion of an ECG course, the nurse will recognize common arrhythmias appearing on a heart monitor.

_____ **5.** The student will name and describe steps of the nursing procedure by the end of the semester.

_____ **6.** Nurses will complete the Braden skin assessment for each patient daily.

SHORT ANSWER

1. Explain how you would evaluate whether a patient has achieved the following outcomes.

a. Cognitive: _____

b. Psychomotor: _____

c. Affective: _____

2. Explain how the following elements of evaluation help to determine whether goals/outcomes have been met.

a. Identifying evaluative criteria: _____

b. Determining whether these criteria and standards are met: _____

c. Terminating, continuing, or modifying the plan: _____

3. Give an example of a variable that may influence goal/outcome achievement in the following areas.

a. Patient: _____

b. Nurse: _____

c. Health care system: _____

4. When the outcome for the plan of care is not achieved, the nurse modifies the plan in what four ways?

a. _____

b. _____

c. _____

d. _____

5. Mr. Bogash, a 28-year-old man with leukemia, recently had a bone marrow transplantation. His medical condition has improved, but he is unable to meet his goal of being up and alert during the daytime hours. What would be the appropriate step to take after evaluating Mr. Bogash? How would you document Mr. Bogash's failure to progress? How would you revise his care plan?

_____

_____

_____

6. Explain the following three essential components of quality care and how nursing care is evaluated in each area.

a. Structure: _____

b. Process: _____

c. Outcome: _____

7. Explain why the following revisions may be made to a care plan.

a. Delete or modify the nursing diagnosis: _____

b. Make the goal statement more realistic: ___

_____

c. Adjust the time criteria in the goal statement: _____

_____

d. Change nursing interventions: _____

_____

8. Would you rather work in an environment that ensures the quality of the profession using quality by inspection or quality as opportunity? Explain your answer.

_____

_____

9. Give four examples of the type of evaluations nurses are involved in as members of the health care team.

a. _____

b. _____

c. _____

d. _____

10. Briefly state the purpose of the publicly reported Hospital Consumer Assessment of Healthcare Providers and Systems (HCAHPS), the Centers for Medicare and Medicaid Services' patient satisfaction program. What is your role in helping your hospital achieve positive ratings?

_____

_____

APPLYING YOUR KNOWLEDGE

CRITICAL THINKING QUESTIONS

1. Give an example of each of the following "Seven Crucial Conversations in Health Care" and provide a recommendation for solving the problems.

a. Broken rules: _____

_____

b. Mistakes: _____

_____

c. Lack of support: _____

_____

d. Incompetence: _____

_____

e. Poor teamwork: _____

_____

f. Disrespect: _____

_____

g. Micromanagement: _____

_____

2. Reflect on the role that evaluation plays in promoting your scholastic achievement. Has it been positive or negative? Think of specific ways nurses can use evaluation to motivate patients to achieve healthy goals.

_____

_____

REFLECTIVE PRACTICE: CULTIVATING QSEN COMPETENCIES

Use the following expanded scenario from Chapter 19 in your textbook to answer the questions below.

Scenario: Ms. Otsuki, an older adult female with a history of heart failure being treated with diuretics, is receiving home care. Questioned about her prescribed drug-therapy regimen, Ms. Otsuki states, "I take this one labeled 'furosemide' every day in the morning along with this other one labeled 'Lasix'."

1. Patient-centered care/safety: What should be the focus of an evaluation of Ms. Otsuki's nursing care plan conducted by the home health care nurse?

_____

_____

_____

2. Patient-centered care/safety: What would be a successful outcome for this patient?

_____

_____

_____

3. Patient-centered care/evidence-based practice: What intellectual, technical, interpersonal, and ethical/legal competencies are most likely to bring about the desired outcome?

_____

_____

_____

4. Teamwork and collaboration: What resources might be helpful for Ms. Otsuki?

_____

_____

_____

PRACTICING FOR NCLEX

MULTIPLE-CHOICE QUESTIONS

Circle the letter that corresponds to the best answer for each question.

1. A nurse evaluates patients prior to discharge from a hospital setting. What is the focus of the evaluation?
   a. Patient's goal/outcome achievement
   b. Interventions on the care plan
   c. Competence of nurses on the unit
   d. Types of health care services available to the patient

2. A nurse observes a colleague applying restraints on an agitated and uncooperative patient without a health care provider's prescription. Which action will the nurse take next?
   a. Reporting the nurse applying the restraints to the supervisor
   b. Completing an event/incident report and having the second nurse sign it
   c. Discussing the need for the restraints and a prescription with the colleague
   d. Contacting the health care provider for an order for the restraints.

3. Nurses formulate different types of goals for patients when planning patient care. What is considered a psychomotor patient goal?
   a. By 8/18/25, patient will value his health sufficiently to quit smoking.
   b. By 8/18/25, patient will demonstrate lifting the left arm overhead.
   c. By 8/18/25, patient will list three foods that are low in sodium.
   d. By 8/18/25, patient will demonstrate three leg strengthening exercises.

4. A nurse is evaluating nursing care and patient outcomes by using a retrospective evaluation. Which action would the nurse perform in this approach?
   a. Directly observing the nursing care being provided
   b. Reviewing the patient chart while the patient is being cared for
   c. Interviewing the patient while they are receiving the care
   d. Devising a post discharge questionnaire to evaluate patient satisfaction

5. What action should the nurse take when patient data indicate that the stated goals have not been achieved?
   a. Collect more data for the database.
   b. Review each preceding step of the nursing process.
   c. Implement a standardized care plan.
   d. Change the nursing orders.

6. The long-term goal for a patient with motor deficits is that they will be able to dress themselves after 6 weeks of physical and occupational therapy. What is the best timing for evaluating the patient's progress toward this goal?
   a. When the patient is discharged
   b. At the end of the 6-week therapy
   c. When the patient shows progress
   d. With each patient contact

7. The quality assurance model of the ANA identifies three essential components of quality care. Which component does the nurse use when determining whether a patient has met the goals stated on the care plan?
   a. Structure
   b. Process
   c. Retrospect
   d. Outcome

8. Which action is appropriate when evaluating a patient's responses to a care plan?

   a. Reinforcing the care plan when each expected outcome is achieved

   b. Terminating the plan if there are difficulties achieving the goals/outcomes

   c. Terminating the care plan upon patient discharge

   d. Continuing the care plan if more time is needed to achieve the goals/outcomes

9. A nurse is evaluating the care plan for a surgical patient whose family members are at the bedside. Which action will best evaluate pain relief in this patient?

   a. Observing the patient for signs of distress, grimacing, and protecting the surgical area

   b. Asking the family members if the patient appears comfortable to them

   c. Asking the patient to rate their pain on a scale of 1 to 10

   d. Documenting that the patient is comfortable after assisting them to the commode

10. A nurse is overheard stating that plans of care are busywork. As their colleague, you recognize that plans of care lacking corresponding interventions recorded in the electronic health record may result in what negative outcome?

   a. Poor patient satisfaction scores

   b. Legal grounds to state care was not provided

   c. Understanding that nurses were busy yet administered care

   d. Shift report providing updates to the oncoming nurses

ALTERNATE-FORMAT QUESTIONS

Multiple-Response Questions

Circle the letters that correspond to the best answers for each question.

1. Nurses formulate physiologic goals for patients when providing patient care. Which are examples of physiologic goals? Select all that apply.

   a. By 4/6/25, the infant will demonstrate adequate sleep–wakefulness patterns.

   b. Before discharge, the parents of a newborn will verbalize decreased anxiety about taking care of their infant.

   c. By 4/6/25, the parents will list appropriate resources in case questions arise after discharge.

   d. By 4/6/25, the infant will show an adequate comfort level indicating satisfactory parenting.

   e. Before discharge, the infant will have reached a target weight gain of 8 lb (birth weight: 7 lb, 6 oz).

   f. Before discharge, the parents will demonstrate correctly bathing and feeding their infant.

2. A nurse is documenting evaluation of the care provided for an infant born with Down syndrome. Which nursing actions exemplify the appropriate documentation process? Select all that apply.

   a. After assessment data have been collected to determine outcome achievement, the nurse writes an evaluative statement to summarize the findings.

   b. The nurse writes an evaluative statement that includes how well the outcome was met and patient data that support the decision.

   c. The nurse selects one of the three options to describe how goals have been met.

   d. The nurse determines whether a patient goal has been met or not met, then the goal is discontinued.

   e. The nurse does not increase the complexity of a goal after it has been achieved to prevent patient anxiety and distrust.

   f. If a nurse writes a properly written goal, it is not affected by patient, nurse, or health care variables.

3. A nurse is following the rules recommended by the Institute of Medicine's Committee on Quality of Health Care in America to help redesign and improve patient care. Which nursing actions are based on these rules? Select all that apply.

   a. Basing patient care on established nursing needs and values

   b. Becoming the source of control for patient care

   c. Basing care on evidence-based decision making

   d. Customizing care based on availability of resources

e. Promoting shared knowledge and the free flow of information

f. Acknowledging that continuous decrease in waste improves patient care

4. A nurse manager and nursing staff engage in a performance improvement project to improve the triage process in the hospital's emergency department. Which steps will the nurses take? Select all that apply.

a. Discovering a problem exists with the triage system in place

b. Calling a meeting of the emergency department interdisciplinary team to affect change in the triage process

c. Organizing a task force to implement change in the triage process

d. Meeting with the emergency department staff to assess changes made to the triage process

e. Discontinuing efforts to force change if the goal of changing the triage process is not met

f. Involving the administration to force the changes when met with resistance to change from the staff

Prioritization Question

1. A nurse caring for a group of patients is evaluating each patient's progress toward the expected outcomes as stated on their care plans. Which patient evaluation data requires immediate follow-up?

a. Blood pressure 212/108

b. Dry cough

c. No adventitious breath sounds noted

d. Pain scaled 2/10; patient reports it is tolerable

CHAPTER 20

Documenting and Reporting

ASSESSING YOUR UNDERSTANDING

FILL IN THE BLANKS

1. The _____ health record is the permanent document detailing the nurse's interactions with the patient and includes patient assessments, nursing diagnoses or patient needs, nursing interventions, and patient outcomes.

2. Nursing documentation reflecting unexpected events, the cause of the event, actions taken in response to the event, and discharge planning, if appropriate, is termed _____ charting.

3. A nurse in a Medicare-approved long-term care facility documents care for nursing, medical, psychological, and social problems by using _____ data sets, a core set of screening, clinical, and functional status elements that forms the foundation of the comprehensive assessment.

4. The adult home care nurse uses _____ (give acronym) to document core items of a comprehensive assessment and form the basis for measuring patient outcomes for purposes of outcome-based quality improvement.

5. Nurses document care in long-term care settings as specified by the resident assessment _____, which helps the staff gather definitive information on a resident's strengths and needs and develop an individualized care plan.

6. The _____ report refers to the communication of a summary of the patient condition by the primary nurse to their replacement in oral, written, or audiotaped format.

7. A nurse uses the _____ report, a risk management tool, to document unexpected events that result in, or have the potential to result in harm to a patient, person, or damage property.

8. Nurses on a medical-surgical unit request an interprofessional nursing care _____ to discuss discharge planning for a patient with complex needs.

9. Documenting and reporting are two methods nurses use for _____.

10. The electronic health record's computer provider order entry (CPOE) is associated with a 13% to 99% reduction in _____ errors.

11. Members of the health care team would expect to find patient information such as pulse, respiratory rate, weight, and intake and output in the _____ record.

12. To ensure safety, communication using the situation, _____, _____, and recommendation format is often used.

13. The process of sending or guiding the patient to another source for assistance is called a _____.

MATCHING EXERCISES

Match the types of formats of nursing documentation listed in Part A with their appropriate examples in Part B.

PART A

a. Critical/collaborative pathways
b. Graphic record
c. (Electronic) Medication administration records (e)MAR
d. Discharge and transfer summary
e. PIE format nursing note
f. Nursing care plan

PART B

____ 1. The nurse documents a patient's nursing diagnosis, specific nursing interventions, and outcomes of care.

____ 2. The nurse documents administration of ciprofloxacin IV, 400 mg every 12 hours.

____ 3. The nurse uses this form to record a patient's body temperature, pulse, respiratory rate, blood pressure, and bowel movements.

____ 4. This is an interprofessional, collaborative master list of patient problems, documenting patient progress.

____ 5. The nurse summarizes a patient's reason for treatment, significant findings, procedure performed, treatment rendered, and any specific instructions for the patient/family.

____ 6. The nurse documents the case management plan for a patient population with a designated diagnosis that includes expected outcomes, interventions, and the sequence and timing of these interventions.

SHORT ANSWER

1. List four areas of nursing care data that, according to the Joint Commission, must be permanently integrated into the patient record.

a. _____
b. _____
c. _____
d. _____

2. Briefly describe the nurse's role in the following methods of reporting patient data.

a. Change-of-shift/hand-off reports: _____

b. Telephone orders: _____

c. Transfer and discharge reports: _____

d. Reports to family members and significant others: _____

e. Incident reports: _____

f. Conferring about care: _____

g. Consultations and referrals: _____

h. Nursing and interdisciplinary team care conference: _____

i. Nursing care rounds: _____

3. Briefly explain the following purposes of the patient record.

a. Communication: _____

b. Care planning: _____

c. Quality process and performance improvement: _____

d. Research: _____

e. Decision analysis: _____

f. Education: _____

g. Credentialing, regulation, and legislation: _____

h. Legal documentation: _____

    i. Reimbursement: _____

_____

    j. Historical document: _____

_____

4. List five guidelines nurses should follow when reporting a significant change in a patient's condition to other health care professionals by telephone.

    a. _____

    b. _____

    c. _____

    d. _____

    e. _____

5. Complete the chart below listing the purpose (description), advantages, and disadvantages of the various methods of documentation.

6. Describe the procedure for correcting an error in documentation in the written and electronic medical record.

_____

_____

APPLYING YOUR KNOWLEDGE

CRITICAL THINKING QUESTIONS

1. Consider the following patient: A 79-year-old female with Alzheimer's disease is admitted to a long-term care unit. She no longer recognizes her daughter, who was taking care of her. She has a history of falls and hip fracture. The daughter insists that the nurses physically restrain her mother to prevent falls.

Documentation Method	Description/Advantages/Disadvantages
SOURCE-ORIENTED RECORD	Description: Advantages: Disadvantages:
PROBLEM-ORIENTED MEDICAL RECORDS	Description: Advantages: Disadvantages:
PIE—PROBLEM, INTERVENTION, EVALUATION	Description: Advantages: Disadvantages:
FOCUS CHARTING	Description: Advantages: Disadvantages:
CHARTING BY EXCEPTION	Description: Advantages: Disadvantages:
CASE MANAGEMENT MODEL	Description: Advantages: Disadvantages:
OCCURRENCE OR VARIANCE CHARTING	Description: Advantages: Disadvantages:
ELECTRONIC HEALTH RECORDS	Description: Advantages: Disadvantages:

Consider the information the team will need to provide safe, quality care for this patient. What types of data should the admitting nurse record, and what system of documentation is most likely to bring the information to the attention of everyone who needs it?

2. How would you go about scheduling a consultation for an amputee who needs physical therapy? Write a brief summary of the patient's condition and how you would present his case to the physical therapy department or PT.

3. Make an appointment to interview a nurse risk manager of a health care system. Find out how important the documentation of patient care is to the patient, nurse, and health facility when legal questions arise. How can this knowledge help to safeguard your practice?

REFLECTIVE PRACTICE: CULTIVATING QSEN COMPETENCIES

Use the following expanded scenario from Chapter 20 in your textbook to answer the questions below.

Scenario: Phillippe is a 52-year-old man being discharged from the outpatient surgery department after undergoing a colonoscopy for removal of three polyps. He will be going home with his wife, who is a nurse, and they both require discharge teaching.

1. Patient-centered care/safety: What should be the focus of discharge teaching for Phillippe and his wife?

_____

_____

_____

2. Patient-centered care/safety: What would be a successful outcome for this patient?

_____

_____

_____

3. Patient-centered care/evidence-based practice: What intellectual, interpersonal, and ethical/legal competencies are most likely to bring about the desired outcome?

_____

_____

_____

4. Teamwork and collaboration/informatics: What resources might be helpful for this patient?

_____

_____

_____

PRACTICING FOR NCLEX

MULTIPLE-CHOICE QUESTIONS

Circle the letter that corresponds to the best answer for each question.

1. A patient post hip replacement surgery accuses a nurse of negligence after he trips while ambulating for the first time. Which action by the nurse reflects the best defense against allegations of negligence?
   a. Notifying the nursing team of the patient condition
   b. Documenting patient data on the flow sheet
   c. Keeping an accurate medication record
   d. Accurately documenting patient care on the patient record

2. Which nursing action is an example of properly handling the patient record?
   a. Sharing the patient record with a close family member
   b. Not sharing the patient record with interprofessional team members
   c. Not allowing a patient to update his health record
   d. Allowing a patient to see and copy their own health record

3. A nurse documents the following patient data in the patient record according to the SOAP format:
   S. Patient complains of unrelieved pain
   O. Patient is seen clutching his side and grimacing
   A. Patient's pain currently 8/10
   P. Call in to primary care provider to adjust analgesic prescription.
   What charting method does this represent?
   a. Source-oriented
   b. PIE
   c. Problem-oriented
   d. Focus

4. A nurse helps a patient who has cystic fibrosis prepare a tethered personal health record. Which statement by the nurse best explains this type of information?

   a. "You can fill in information from your own records and store it on your computer or the Internet."

   b. "You can link your record to a specific health care organization's electronic health record system."

   c. "Your health care provider is obligated to read your personal health record and share it with your insurance provider."

   d. "Your entire health care team may access and securely share your vital medical information electronically."

5. A nurse is finding it difficult to plan and implement care for a patient and requests a nursing care conference. Which action would the nurse take to facilitate this process?

   a. Consulting with someone in order to exchange ideas or seek information, advice, or instructions

   b. Meeting with nurses or other health care professionals to discuss some aspect of patient care

   c. Visiting patients with similar problems individually at each patient's bedside in order to plan nursing care

   d. Directing someone to take action in a specific nursing care problem

6. A nurse is documenting the effectiveness of a patient's pain management on the electronic health record. What reflects accurate documentation?

   a. Patient is receiving sufficient relief from pain medication.

   b. Patient appears comfortable and is resting adequately.

   c. Patient reports that on a scale of 1 to 10, the pain they are experiencing is a 3.

   d. Patient appears to have a low pain tolerance and complains frequently about intense pain.

7. A nurse is arranging for home care for older adult patients and reviews the Medicare reimbursement requirements. Which patient meets these requirements?

   a. Homebound and needs skilled nursing care

   b. Poor rehabilitation potential

   c. Complete stabilized status

   d. Not making progress toward expected outcomes

8. A nurse takes a patient's pulse, respiratory rate, blood pressure, and body temperature. Where in the electronic health record will the nurse document the results?

   a. Progress note

   b. Flow sheet

   c. Graphic record

   d. Medical record

9. A nurse has a two-way video communication with the specialist involved in the care of a patient in a long-term care facility. What nursing informatics technology does this represent?

   a. Patient engagement

   b. Data aggregation

   c. Telemedicine

   d. Population health management

ALTERNATE-FORMAT QUESTIONS

Multiple-Response Questions

Circle the letters that correspond to the best answers for each question.

1. A nurse is documenting care for an older adult patient recovering from a stroke. Which documentation entries meet recommended guidelines for communicating and documenting patient information? Select all that apply.

   a. The patient rates their headache as 2 compared to a 7 yesterday.

   b. The patient seems comfortable today.

   c. The patient drank an average amount of fluids.

   d. Vital signs returned to normal.

   e. The patient appears anxious about having another stroke.

   f. Radial pulse is 72, +2, and regular.

2. A nurse manager of a health care provider's office is responsible for obtaining signed authorizations for releasing patient information to third parties. In which situations will the nurse not need an authorization from the patient? Select all that apply.

   a. Reporting the incidence of an infectious disease to the Centers for Disease Control and Prevention

b. Releasing a medical record requested by the court for a lawsuit

c. Sharing information regarding home care with a patient's spouse

d. Submitting charges for nursing services

e. Facilitating organ donation of a deceased patient

f. Providing statistics related to the use of a dangerous piece of equipment

3. A nurse preceptor is reviewing a new graduate nurse's documentation of patient care in a hospital setting. For which documentation entries will the preceptor provide guidance and assist the new nurse to correct? Select all that apply.

a. The content reflects patient needs.

b. The content includes descriptions of situations that are out of the ordinary.

c. The notes criticize another health care professional.

d. There are blank lines between the entries.

e. The documentation is not signed.

f. Dates are present, but times of entries are omitted.

4. HIPAA allows incidental disclosure of patient health information if it cannot reasonably be prevented, is limited in nature, and occurs as a byproduct of an otherwise permitted use or disclosure of PHI. What actions reflect a breach in PHI disclosure? Select all that apply.

a. The nurse uses sign-in sheets that contain information about the reason for the patient visit.

b. A visitor hears a confidential conversation between two nurses in surroundings that are appropriate and with voices that are kept low.

c. The nurse uses white boards on an unlimited basis.

d. The nurse uses x-ray light boards that can be seen by passersby; however, patient x-rays are not left unattended on them.

e. The nurse calls out names in the waiting room but does not disclose the reason for the patient visit.

f. The nurse leaves a detailed appointment reminder message on a patient's voice mail.

5. A nurse is using the ISBARR format to report a surgical patient's deteriorating condition to a health care provider. Which actions will the nurse take when using this format? Select all that apply.

a. Asking the health care provider to describe the admitting diagnosis of the patient

b. After introductions, stating the patient's name, room number, and problem

c. Asking the health care provider to estimate the discharge date for the patient

d. Asking the health care provider to comment on the present situation before giving recommendations

e. Stating that the patient's condition "could be life threatening"

f. Reading back the health care provider's new orders at the conclusion of the call

6. First-year nursing students are learning about confidential patient information. What will the students correctly identify as confidential, protected information? Select all that apply.

a. Patient name

b. Patient address

c. Reason for admission

d. Tests performed

e. Past health conditions

f. Dietary preferences

Ordered Response

1. Place the components of the SOAP note in order

a. Pedal pulse +1, toes cold and dusky but able to wiggle

b. Patient lying stiff in bed, unwilling to move

c. "My leg and ankle are killing me under this cast"

d. Requested health care provider assess cast and pain

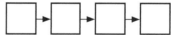

Prioritization Question

1. A nurse notes a blood pressure of 182/100 in a patient who is 5 months' pregnant. After reassessing the blood pressure and fetal heart sounds, which action will the nurse take next? Circle the letter that corresponds to the best answer.

a. Complete documentation of the visit.

b. Report the findings to the health care provider using the SBAR format.

c. Schedule the patient's next prenatal visit.

d. Teach the patient about normal blood pressure at this stage of pregnancy.

CHAPTER 21

Informatics and Health Care Technologies

ASSESSING YOUR UNDERSTANDING

FILL IN THE BLANKS

1. A(n) _____ is a computer-based system designed for collecting, storing, manipulating, and making clinical information available for the health care delivery process.

2. A digital version of a patient's chart or medical history is called a(n) _____.

3. A nurse who integrates nursing science with multiple information management and analytical sciences into her nursing practice is using the QSEN competency of nursing _____.

4. An informatics nurse who helps other nurses to implement the use of an electronic health record (EHR) in their practice may become a(n) _____, or a system expert who can navigate the EHR with ease.

5. The extent to which an informatics product can be used by specified users to achieve specified goals with effectiveness, efficiency, and satisfaction in a specified context of use is termed _____.

6. A patient may use a computer or electronic device to access a patient _____ to review lab results, request prescription refills, or make an appointment.

7. The ability of analysts to present analytics graphically in order to identify new patterns or see difficult concepts is termed _____.

8. _____ data comprises the accumulation of health care–related data from various sources, combined with new technologies that allow for the transformation of data to information, to knowledge, and ultimately to wisdom.

9. When the informatics nurse posts a video on safely disposing of internal radiation devices (brachytherapy), the nurse is meeting the informatics standard of _____ health.

10. A group of nurse informaticists invite a representative group of nurses to provide feedback on whether an electronic health record's screens contain the needed information or if anything was left out. This occurs in the technology phase of _____ testing.

MATCHING EXERCISES
Matching Exercise 1
Match the standard of practice area for nursing informatics listed in Part A with the appropriate example listed in Part B.

PART A
a. Resource utilization
b. Education
c. Evidence-based practice and research
d. Quality of practice
e. Leadership
f. Collaboration

PART B

____ **1.** A nurse coordinates health care provision based on availability of operational resources.

____ **2.** A nurse teaches colleagues nursing informatics practices and helps to put them to use.

____ **3.** A nurse schedules a teleconference with a patient's primary care provider and nutritionist.

____ **4.** A nurse analyzes data to improve nursing and informatics outcomes in the facility.

____ **5.** A nurse attends an in-service on new informatics techniques to advance his practice.

____ **6.** A nurse uses available informatics resources to research evidence-based practices.

Matching Exercise 2

Match the standard of practice area for nursing informatics listed in Part A with the appropriate example listed in Part B.

PART A

a. Assessment

b. Diagnosis, problem, and issue identification

c. Outcome identification

d. Planning

e. Implementation

f. Evaluation

PART B

____ **1.** Provides leadership in the coordination of the information technology and health care activities for integrated delivery of efficient and cost-effective health care services

____ **2.** Uses workflow analysis to examine current practice, workflow, and the potential impact of an informatics solution on that workflow

____ **3.** Defines expected outcomes in terms of the health care consumer, health care worker, and other stakeholders, and their values, ethical considerations, and environmental, organizational, or situational considerations

____ **4.** Uses standardized clinical terminologies, taxonomies, and decision support tools

to identify problems, needs, issues, and opportunities for improvement

____ **5.** Develops a customized plan considering clinical and business characteristics of the environment and situation

____ **6.** Conducts a systematic, ongoing, and criterion-based appraisal of the outcomes in relation to the structures and processes prescribed by the project plan and indicated timeline

SHORT ANSWER

1. List four meaningful uses of certified EHR technology as defined by HealthIT.gov.

a. _____
b. _____
c. _____
d. _____

2. List five positive results of the meaningful use compliance of certified EHR technology.

a. _____
b. _____
c. _____
d. _____
e. _____

3. Describe the Informatics Scope and Standards Definitions (DIKW) listed below:

a. Data: _____
_____

b. Information: _____
_____

c. Knowledge: _____
_____

d. Wisdom: _____
_____

4. Nurses who use a clinical information system should be involved in all phases of a system development lifecycle (SDLC) to ensure the best chance that the system will meet its intended need. Consider the scenario of an organization converting to a different information system and EHR, and give an example of a nursing responsibility related to the following areas of focus of an SDLC.

a. Analyze and plan: _____
_____

b. Design: _____

_____

c. Test: _____

_____

d. Train: _____

_____

e. Implement: _____

_____

f. Maintain: _____

_____

g. Evaluate: _____

_____

5. Briefly define the following informatics concepts and state how they affect the implementation and maintenance of clinical information systems.

a. Usability: _____

_____

b. Optimization: _____

_____

c. Standard terminologies: _____

_____

d. Interoperability: _____

_____

e. Security and privacy: _____

_____

6. List five benefits of using a patient portal in a medical practice.

a. _____
b. _____
c. _____
d. _____
e. _____

7. Give two examples of the following types of mobile technologies:

a. Telehealth: _____

_____

b. Telecare: _____

_____

c. Telemedicine: _____

_____

APPLYING YOUR KNOWLEDGE

CRITICAL THINKING QUESTIONS

1. Nurses handle sensitive patient information daily when using clinical information systems. Interview an informatics nurse specialist to discuss how to keep this information safe.

2. Consider your response if your colleague placed a sticky note on a computer with their password written on it.

3. Nurses use analytics and big data to support population health. Consider the types of patient conditions that best respond to this type of analysis and what data can be retrieved from information systems to positively affect patient outcomes. Give an example of a risk a nurse could identify and provide interventions leading to improve patient care.

REFLECTIVE PRACTICE: CULTIVATING QSEN COMPETENCIES

Use the following expanded scenario from Chapter 21 in your textbook to answer the questions below.

Scenario: Frank is a 72-year-old patient who has chronic obstructive pulmonary disease. His wife, who has been his primary caretaker since his diagnosis 5 years ago, died last year, and he now lives alone in their original two-level family home. He has been sleeping on the couch in the living room because he can no longer go upstairs. He has a daughter who lives across country who tries to get home once a month to be sure he has food and medications. Not surprisingly, Frank has had four hospital readmissions in the past year.

1. Patient-centered care/safety: What should be the focus of an evaluation of Frank's nursing care plan. How can informatics be of help in this case?

_____

_____

_____

2. Patient-centered care/safety: What would be a successful outcome for this patient?

_____

_____

_____

3. Patient-centered care/evidence-based practice: What intellectual, technical, and interpersonal competencies are most likely to bring about the desired outcome?

_____

_____

_____

4. Teamwork and collaboration/informatics: What resources might be helpful for Frank?

_____

_____

_____

PRACTICING FOR NCLEX

MULTIPLE-CHOICE QUESTIONS

Circle the letter that corresponds to the best answer for each question.

1. A patient asks why the health care provider is planning to prescribe medications based on pharmacogenomics. What does the nurse teach the patient about the basis for this practice?
   a. Each drug works essentially the same for everyone with the same ethnicity.
   b. The health care provider includes patient preference in the drug choice.
   c. Choices of medications are based on the patient's economics or ability to pay.
   d. The effect of genetic makeup on the medication's effectiveness is assessed.

2. A nurse using the facility's information system's EHR for patients must reset their password. What reflects the best practice guideline for setting a password to protect patient information?
   a. Never use a password manager for EHR access.
   b. Use at least six characters for your password.
   c. Consider using multifactor authentication.
   d. Use the same password for all electronic needs to prevent password resetting.

3. A nurse is using the SDLC to implement the placement of new computers in the workplace. In which stage of this process would the nurse most likely consult with coworkers for their input in creating the new workstations?
   a. Analyze and plan
   b. Design
   c. Test
   d. Implement

4. A nurse meets with coworkers to discuss and make improvements to a new EHR reporting system being used in their office. What is the technical term for this core concept?
   a. Usability
   b. Optimization
   c. Interoperability
   d. Standard terminologies

5. A nurse is able to share patient data stored on an EHR with a specialist in another country. What is the term for this advantage of informatics use?
   a. Interoperability
   b. Data visualization
   c. Big data
   d. System usability

6. A nurse is reviewing data from EHRs that has been transformed into pie charts. What is the term for this presentation of analytics?
   a. Data visualization
   b. Big data
   c. Graphic picture
   d. Predictive analytics

7. A nurse in a hospital with a new information system is having difficulty documenting a preoperative assessment. What individual will the nurse contact?
   a. Surgeon
   b. Nurse manager
   c. System superuser
   d. Unit educator

8. A nurse informaticist is performing monthly maintenance of the hospital's information system. Which activities will the nurse do in this phase?
   a. Update the system with new medication and clinical alerts
   b. Obtain superusers to assist in training
   c. Perform a literature search to determine if the system is well designed
   d. Determine if patient care and safety have improved

9. Nurses on multiple hospital units express concern that descriptive terms for patient assessment are limited in the information system's dropdown menus. How does the nurse informaticist explain this?

   a. Standard terminology allows for sharing data nationally.

   b. It promotes safety in decision making.

   c. Dropdown boxes are limited as they are costly.

   d. Less options promote enhanced security.

10. Students in a nursing informatics class are concurrently studying about polypharmacy. What information can be obtained using health care analytics?

    a. Most popular pharmacies patients in the health care system use

    b. Number of patients older than age 65 who take more than five medications

    c. Pie chart demonstrating the most commonly prescribed medications

    d. Who is at risk for hospital readmission

ALTERNATE-FORMAT QUESTIONS

Multiple-Response Questions

Circle the letters that correspond to the best answers for each question.

1. A nurse is using a dropdown menu to enter patient activity level on an EHR. Which entries are most likely to be presented? Select all that apply.

   a. Walks without assistance

   b. Nonambulatory

   c. Walks with a cane

   d. Able to walk short distances

   e. Requires an assistive device

   f. Sometimes uses a walker

2. A nurse is using technology testing phases to evaluate the use of a new patient reporting system. Which actions would the nurse perform during integration testing? Select all that apply.

   a. Using test scripts to validate one particular function of the system

   b. Ensuring that all systems are properly functioning and communicating

   c. Testing whether the new system can handle high volumes of information

   d. Using test scripts to validate that multiple components of the system are working

   e. Test driving the system to ensure all components are working as designed

3. A nurse in a health care provider's office suggests patients use the portal to increase their engagement in their care. What functions will the nurse teach the patient are available through the portal? Select all that apply.

   a. Requesting prescription delivery

   b. Communicating privately with the health care provider

   c. Paying a bill

   d. Receiving lab and diagnostic test results

   e. Receiving a reminder for influenza vaccine

   f. Ordering medical equipment

Sequencing Questions

1. Place the following steps in informatics evaluation in the order in which they would occur.

   a. Conducting a literature search

   b. Determining the question

   c. Determining the study type

   d. Collecting, analyzing, and displaying data

   e. Determining what will be evaluated

   f. Determining the needed data

   g. Documenting the outcome evaluation

   h. Determining the data collection method and sample size

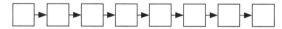

2. Place the following testing technology testing phases in the order in which they should be performed.

   a. Function testing

   b. Performance testing

   c. User acceptance testing

   d. Unit testing

   e. Integration testing

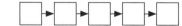

CHAPTER 22

Developmental Concepts

ASSESSING YOUR UNDERSTANDING

FILL IN THE BLANKS

1. A nurse in a pediatric setting notes that infants' and children's growth progresses from gross motor movements, such as lifting the head, to fine motor movements, such as holding a toy. This trend in growth development is known as _____ development.

2. A nurse is counseling a 16-year-old female who is seeking contraception at a local health clinic. According to developmental theorist Sigmund Freud, this patient is in the _____ stage.

3. A 6-year-old child says bedtime prayers together with his parents at night. According to the developmental theorist Fowler, this child is in stage _____ of spiritual development also called the intuitive-projective _____.

4. According to Erik Erikson, during the middle _____ years, a person desires to make a contribution to the world, and, if this is not accomplished, stagnation may occur.

5. _____ studies how genetic variation affects a person's response to drugs, helping to determine whether patient is likely to have a strong therapeutic response or develop adverse effects to a drug.

6. According to Piaget, a child who enters pre-school and integrates the experience into existing schemata is using the _____ process of restructuring knowledge.

7. A 13-year-old female is using deductive reasoning to test beliefs regarding her sexuality. This female is in the formal _____ stage of Piaget's theory of cognitive development.

8. Levinson and associates based their theory of human development on the organizing concept of "individual life structure." This theory centered on the belief that the pattern of life at any point in time is formed by the interaction of three components: the _____, the social and cultural aspects of one's life, and the particular set of _____ in which a person participates.

9. The characteristics inherited from each parent are carried in gene pairs on the 23 pairs of _____, which carry the genetic information that determines the person's cellular differentiation, growth, and function.

10. Failure to _____, a condition of early infancy, has been linked to both nutritional and emotional deprivation.

MATCHING EXERCISES

Matching Exercise 1

Match Erikson's stages of development listed in Part A with the appropriate example listed in Part B. May use an answer more than once; not all answers will be used.

PART A

a. Trust versus mistrust

b. Autonomy versus shame and doubt

c. Initiative versus guilt

d. Industry versus inferiority

e. Identity versus role confusion

f. Intimacy versus isolation
g. Generativity versus stagnation
h. Ego integrity versus despair

PART B

____ **1.** A toddler wants to dress themself.

____ **2.** A middle-aged adult meets a goal of guiding their two children into rewarding careers.

____ **3.** An adolescent fights with their parent about appropriate attire for religious services.

____ **4.** An older adult reflects positively on their past life experiences.

____ **5.** An adult volunteers Saturday mornings to work with the homeless.

____ **6.** An infant believes that his parents will provide food.

Matching Exercise 2

Match the stages of faith development listed in Part A with the appropriate definition listed in Part B.

PART A

a. Stage 1: Intuitive–projective faith
b. Stage 2: Mythical–literal faith
c. Stage 3: Synthetic–conventional faith
d. Stage 4: Individuative–reflective faith
e. Stage 5: Conjunctive faith
f. Stage 6: Universalizing faith

PART B

____ **1.** This is the characteristic stage for many adolescents. An ideology has emerged, but it has not been closely examined until now; attempts to stabilize own identity.

____ **2.** This stage involves making tangible the values of absolute love and justice for humankind; total trust in principle of being and existence of future.

____ **3.** In this stage, children imitate religious gestures and behaviors of others; they follow parental attitudes toward religious or moral beliefs without a thorough understanding of them.

____ **4.** This stage is critical for older adolescents and young adults because the responsibility for their commitments, beliefs, and attitudes becomes their own.

____ **5.** This stage predominates in the school-aged child with increased social interaction. Stories represent religious and moral beliefs, and the existence of a deity is accepted.

____ **6.** This stage integrates other viewpoints about faith into one's understanding of truth.

CORRECT THE FALSE STATEMENTS

Mark the item "T" for true or "F" for false. If false, correct the underlined word or words to make the statement true in the space provided.

____ **1.** The human processes of growth and development result from two interrelated factors: heredity and environment.
_____

____ **2.** Growth and development follow irregular and unpredictable trends. _____

____ **3.** Different aspects of growth and development occur at the same stages and rates in all people. _____

____ **4.** In the third level of Carol Gilligan's theory of moral development, nonviolence governs all moral judgments and actions.
_____

____ **5.** According to Freud, the ego is the part of the psyche concerned with self-gratification by the easiest and quickest available means. _____

____ **6.** In Freud's phallic stage, the child has increased interest in biologic sex differences, curiosity about the genitals, and masturbation increases. _____

____ **7.** According to Havighurst, developing a conscience, morality, and a scale of values should occur in middle childhood.
_____

____ **8.** In Kohlberg's preconventional level, stage 2, instrumental relativist orientation, the motivation for choices of action is fear of physical consequences or authority's disapproval. _____

____ **9.** According to Gould, between ages 22 and 28 years, self-acceptance increases as the person's need to prove their competence disappears. _____

_____ **10.** According to Havighurst, living and growing are based on <u>learning</u>. _____

_____ **11.** The <u>superego</u> is the part of the mind commonly called the conscience. It develops from the ego during the first year of life, as the child learns praise versus punishment for actions.

_____

_____ **12.** Alcohol and drug abuse is more prevalent in teenagers who have poor family relationships, low self-esteem, and <u>poor social skills</u>. _____

SHORT ANSWER

1. Complete the following chart, using the first theorist (Sigmund Freud) as an example.

2. Describe Lawrence Kohlberg's three levels of moral development and give an example of behavior that would typify each level.

a. Preconventional level: _____

_____

Example: _____

_____

b. Conventional level: _____

_____

Example: _____

_____

c. Postconventional level: _____

_____

Example: _____

_____

Theorist and Theory	Basic Concepts of Theory	Stages of Development
Sigmund Freud Psychoanalytic theory	Stressed the impact of instinctual human drives on determining behavior: unconscious mind, the id, the ego, the superego, stages of development based on sexual motivation	Oral stage Anal stage Phallic stage Latent stage Genital stage
Erik Erikson		
Robert J. Havighurst		
Roger Gould		
Daniel Levinson		
Jean Piaget		
James Fowler		

3. What is a major difference between Kohlberg's and Gilligan's moral development theory.

_____

_____

4. A 6-year-old girl with leukemia is admitted to the hospital for her first session of chemotherapy. What insight into this patient's needs could be gained from the following theorists?

a. Freud: _____

_____

b. Erikson: _____

_____

c. Havighurst: _____

_____

d. Piaget: _____

_____

e. Kohlberg: _____

_____

f. Gilligan: _____

_____

g. Fowler: _____

_____

5. Identify the stage of the patient as explained by the theorists noted below. The statements below were made by a 15-year-old boy admitted to the hospital following an ATV accident. He has multiple fractures and several deep cuts in his face that require stitches.

a. Freud: _____ "My dad told me not to ride that thing. I should have listened to him, and this never would have happened."

b. Erikson: _____ "I'm going to be so ugly with these scars on my face. No girl will ever look at me again."

c. Piaget: _____ "What's the best way to be sure I don't lose strength in my muscles? If I do those exercises you taught me, will I be able to play basketball next year."

d. Fowler: _____ "I don't believe in God. If there were a God, He never would have let this happen to me."

6. What role does the family play in health promotion and illness prevention? How has your family affected your attitudes toward health and illness?

_____

_____

_____

APPLYING YOUR KNOWLEDGE

CRITICAL THINKING QUESTIONS

1. Reflect on the nursing plan you would develop for a 3-year-old, a 10-year-old, and a 16-year-old undergoing heart surgery. How would you provide developmentally appropriate explanations of the surgery to each child? Support your teaching with a rationale from at least two different developmental theories for each age group.

Toddler: _____

_____

School-aged child: _____

_____

Adolescent: _____

_____

2. Observe children in different settings and find an example of each stage of development. Talk with classmates about how these findings would influence your nursing practice.

REFLECTIVE PRACTICE: CULTIVATING QSEN COMPETENCIES

Use the following expanded scenario from Chapter 22 in your textbook to answer the questions below.

Scenario: Joseph, an older adult, who fell and fractured his hip while repairing the exterior of his home, states, "Go away and leave me alone. I'm a grown man, I can take care of myself … and get rid of this tray. I'm not hungry." Further investigation reveals that the patient has been the traditional head of his household and is now troubled by needing others, including his wife, to care for him.

1. Patient-centered care/safety: What developmental considerations may affect care planning for Joseph?

_____

_____

_____

2. Patient-centered care/safety: What would be a successful outcome for this patient?

_____

_____

_____

3. Patient-centered care/evidence-based practice: What intellectual, technical, interpersonal, and/or ethical/legal competencies are most likely to bring about the desired outcome?

_____

_____

_____

4. Teamwork and collaboration: What resources might be helpful for Joseph and his family?

_____

_____

_____

PRACTICING FOR NCLEX

MULTIPLE-CHOICE QUESTIONS

Circle the letter that corresponds to the best answer for each question.

1. A nurse is caring for a school-aged child hospitalized after sustaining femur fractures in a motor vehicle accident (MVA). Based on Havighurst's developmental tasks, the nurse suggests which diversional activity for this patient?
   a. Reading a book
   b. Playing video games
   c. Watching television
   d. Speaking to friends on the phone

2. A nurse is assessing the psychosocial development of children in an afterschool program. Which child would the nurse expect to be experiencing the most intense period of speech development?
   a. Young toddler
   b. Preschool child
   c. Young school-aged child
   d. Preteen

3. A nurse is teaching parents of preschoolers about growth and development. Which teaching point is important for the nurse to include?
   a. "The pace of growth and development is specific for each child."
   b. "Growth and development occur at similar stages and rates for each age group."
   c. "Aspects of growth and development cannot be modified."
   d. "Growth and development do not follow regular predictable trends."

4. A nurse is caring for a hospitalized preschool child having surgery for a cleft palate repair. The parents tell the nurse that the child was previously potty-trained and has begun to wet their pants. What is the nurse's best response?
   a. "We can have a child psychologist assess your child."
   b. "It's best to put a diaper on your child while they are in the hospital."
   c. "Children often regress during difficult periods or crises."
   d. "Try offering a reward for not wetting her pants or bed."

5. A nurse is caring for older adults in a long-term care facility. The nurse will include interventions to aid patients with which appropriate developmental task?
   a. Developing a conscious and morality
   b. Adjusting to decreasing physical status and health
   c. Becoming financially independent
   d. Depending on family for psychosocial needs

6. A child is learning to sit quietly during story hour in kindergarten, thereby integrating this new experience into their existing schema. What behavior does this reflect?

    a. Accommodation

    b. Dissemination

    c. Assimilation

    d. Orientation

7. A nurse is caring for a child who states, "I don't like the taste of this medicine, but my parents told me it will help me get better, so I'll take it." This exemplifies which stage of Piaget's cognitive development theory?

    a. Sensorimotor stage

    b. Preoperational stage

    c. Concrete operational stage

    d. Formal operational stage

8. A nurse observes a hospitalized adolescent refuse his meal tray and state, "I usually eat pizza at home. I can't eat the food here." This type of rebellious behavior is characteristic of which of Erik Erikson's stages of psychosocial development?

    a. Autonomy versus shame and doubt

    b. Initiative versus guilt

    c. Industry versus inferiority

    d. Identity versus role confusion

9. A nurse is counseling a woman who states, "I'm never going to find a husband, every time I start dating, I end up getting hurt. I'm not even going to try anymore." This woman is in what stage of Carol Gilligan's theory of moral development?

    a. Level 1—selfishness

    b. Level 2—goodness

    c. Level 3—nonviolence

    d. Level 3—ethic of care

10. A parent brings their newborn for their first pediatric checkup and tells the nurse, "my friends tell me not to hold the baby so much and let them cry more." The nurse explains to the parent that according to which stage of Erikson's theory of development, the parent is showing the baby their needs will be met?

    a. Phallic

    b. Industry versus inferiority

    c. Trust versus mistrust

    d. Ego integrity versus despair

11. A nurse on your unit has been terminated for diverting controlled substances. Which of Kohlberg's stages of development is this nurse likely in?

    a. Punishment and obedience

    b. Instrumental relativist

    c. Law and order

    d. Social contract

ALTERNATE-FORMAT QUESTIONS

Multiple-Response Questions

Circle the letters that correspond to the best answers for each question.

1. A nurse assesses the effect of the environment and nutrition on patients visiting a walk-in clinic in a low-income community. Which statements accurately describe these effects? Select all that apply.

    a. Infants who are malnourished in utero develop the same amount of brain cells as infants who had adequate prenatal nutrition.

    b. Substance abuse during pregnancy increases the risk for congenital anomalies in her developing fetus.

    c. Failure to thrive cannot be linked to emotional deprivation.

    d. Drug and alcohol abuse is more prevalent in teenagers who have poor family relationships.

    e. An increased incidence of teenage pregnancy can be linked to substance abuse by adolescents.

    f. Child abuse can lead to deficits in physical development, but psychosocial development is not affected.

2. A nurse is using Freud's theory of psychoanalytic development to assess the development of children in the phallic stage of this theory. Which developmental milestones would the nurse expect in this age group? Select all that apply.

    a. The child becomes toilet trained.

    b. The child shows increased interest in biologic sex differences.

    c. The child is possessive of the opposite-sex parent.

    d. The child is curious about genitals and masturbation increases.

    e. The child prepares for adult roles and relationships.

    f. The child experiences sexual pressures and conflicts.

3. A school nurse is using Havighurst's developmental theory to teach parents of adolescents what to expect at this developmental stage. Which behaviors are typical of adolescents? Select all that apply.

   a. Learning physical skills necessary for games

   b. Accepting their body and using it effectively

   c. Learning to get along with peers

   d. Achieving emotional independence from parents

   e. Acquiring an ethical system as a guide to behavior

   f. Achieving social and civic responsibility

4. A nurse is assessing children using Kohlberg's theory of moral development. What are examples of milestones achieved in the preconventional level of this theory? Select all that apply.

   a. Learning to follow parent's rules

   b. Identifying with family members and conforming to their expectations

   c. Being motivated by punishment for not conforming to rules

   d. Striving for approval in an attempt to be viewed as "good"

   e. Developing moral judgment that is rational and internalized into self

   f. Developing a perception of goodness or badness

Sequencing Questions

1. Place the examples of stages of Sigmund Freud's theory of psychoanalytic development in the order in which they occur.

   a. The child has increased interest in biologic sex differences and their own biologic sex.

   b. The child increases sex-role identification with the parent of the same sex.

   c. The child uses their mouth as a major source of gratification and exploration.

   d. The child begins overt sexual relationships with others.

   e. The child develops neuromuscular control necessary for toilet training.

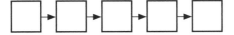

2. Place the stages of Havighurst's theory of development (developmental tasks) in the order in which they occur.

   a. Achieving biologic sex–specific social role; achieving independence; acquiring a set of values and ethical system to guide behavior

   b. Learning sex differences; forming concepts; getting ready to read

   c. Learning to walk; learning to talk; learning to control body waste elimination

   d. Achieving social and civic responsibility; accepting and adjusting to physical changes

   e. Learning physical skills; learning to get along with others; developing conscience and morality

   f. Adjusting to decreasing physical status and health; adjusting to retirement

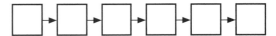

Prioritization Question

1. The nurse in a family practice is assessing a group of patients. Who will the nurse prioritize as needing further assessment? Circle the letter corresponding to the best answer.

   a. 10-week-old who does not lift their head

   b. Toddler who is slender and a picky eater

   c. Adolescent whose parents state they are defiant

   d. Newborn who awakens to eat every 2 hours

CHAPTER 23

Conception Through Young Adulthood

ASSESSING YOUR UNDERSTANDING

FILL IN THE BLANKS

1. The nurse explains to a class of pregnant persons that the _____ layer of the zygote will eventually become the respiratory system, the digestive system, the liver, and the pancreas.

2. The nurse is assessing a pregnant person who is 6 weeks pregnant. This fetus is in the _____ stage of the development in which there is initiation of rapid growth and differentiation of the cell layers.

3. The nurse assesses the neonate using the _____ rating scale at 1 and 5 minutes after birth.

4. A nurse encourages a new mother to cuddle and talk to her newborn to stimulate _____, the mother's emotional link to her newborn.

5. A nurse documents inadequate growth in height and weight resulting from the infant's inability to obtain or use calories needed for growth. The term for this condition is _____ to _____.

6. A nurse uses the Denver _____ Screening Test to determine quickly and inexpensively atypical developmental patterns in infants and children.

7. Parents of _____ should childproof their home.

8. Young children who are overweight are more likely to be overweight adults with chronic health problems such as high blood pressure or _____, among others.

9. _____ from puberty to about age 18 years.

MATCHING EXERCISES

Matching Exercise 1

Match the stage of development listed Part A with the risk factor in Part B.

PART A

a. Neonate

b. Infant

c. Toddler

d. Preschooler

e. School-aged

f. Adolescent and young adult

PART B

____ 1. Hormonal changes cause physical responses.

____ 2. Communicable diseases and respiratory tract infections begin to develop in this stage.

____ 3. Congenital disorders, such as hypospadias, inguinal hernias, and cardiac anomalies, require surgery at this stage.

____ 4. The suicide rate is highest for this group.

____ 5. A mother who smokes cigarettes, drinks alcohol, or uses drugs may cause developmental deficits in this stage.

_____ 6. Scabies, impetigo, and head lice are more prevalent in this stage.

_____ 7. Accidents, poisonings, burns, drowning, aspiration, and falls remain the major causes of death in this stage.

SHORT ANSWER

1. Indicate the age group in which the following physiologic characteristics and behaviors are commonly developed. Use *N* for neonate, *I* for infant, *T* for toddler, *P* for preschooler, *S* for school-aged, and *A* for adolescent/young adult.

   a. _____ Motor abilities include skipping, throwing and catching, copying figures, and printing letters and numbers

   b. _____ Puberty begins

   c. _____ Brain grows to about half the adult size

   d. _____ Reflexes include sucking, swallowing, blinking, sneezing, and yawning

   e. _____ Temperature control responds quickly to environmental temperatures

   f. _____ Walks forward and backward, runs, kicks, climbs, and rides tricycle

   g. _____ Drinks from a cup and uses a spoon

   h. _____ Sebaceous and axillary sweat glands become active

   i. _____ Height increases 2 to 3 inches and weight increases 3 to 6 lb a year

   j. _____ Feet, hands, and long bones grow rapidly, and muscle mass increases

2. Indicate the age group in which the following psychosocial characteristics and behaviors commonly develop. Use *N* for neonate, *I* for infant, *T* for toddler, *P* for preschooler, *S* for school-aged, and *A* for adolescent/young adult.

   a. _____ Is in oral stage (Freud); strives for immediate gratification of needs; strong sucking need

   b. _____ Developmental task of learning appropriate sex's social role

   c. _____ Self-concept is being stabilized, with peer group as greatest influence

   d. _____ Achieves personal independence; develops conscience, morality, and scale of value

   e. _____ Develops skill in reading, writing, and calculating, as well as concepts for everyday living

   f. _____ More mature relationships with both males and females of same age

   g. _____ Personal appearance accepted; set of values internalized

   h. _____ Developmental tasks of learning to control elimination; begins to learn sex differences, concepts, language, and right from wrong

   i. _____ Developmental tasks of learning sex differences and modesty

3. Briefly describe the prenatal growth and development in the following stages.

   a. Pre-embryonic stage: _____

   _____

   b. Embryonic stage: _____

   _____

   c. Fetal stage: _____

   _____

4. List the four critical areas of development that are assessed by the Denver Developmental Screening Test.

   a. _____

   b. _____

   c. _____

   d. _____

5. After observing infants in a neonatal unit, describe the physical symptoms of the following temperaments:

   a. "Easy": _____

   b. "Slow to warm": _____

   c. "Difficult": _____

6. Define the following infant health problems and teaching and nursing interventions used for each.

   a. Colic: _____

   _____

   b. Failure to thrive: _____

   _____

   c. Sudden infant death syndrome and sudden unexpected infant death syndrome:

   _____

   _____

d. Child maltreatment and adverse child-hood experiences: _____

_____

e. Choking: _____

_____

7. Describe age-appropriate methods for preparing the following age groups for eye surgery; explain why you have chosen this method.
   a. Toddler: _____

   _____

   _____

   b. Preschooler: _____

   _____

   _____

   c. School-aged child: _____

   _____

   _____

   d. Adolescent and young adult: _____

   _____

   _____

8. The nurse plays an important role in health care for each stage of development. Explain how you would tailor your care plan for the various age groups listed below.
   a. Infant: _____

   _____

   b. Toddler: _____

   _____

   c. Preschooler: _____

   _____

   d. School-aged child: _____

   _____

   e. Adolescent and young adult: _____

   _____

9. Briefly describe the following stages of puberty.
   a. Prepubescence: _____

   _____

   b. Pubescence: _____

   _____

c. Postpubescence: _____

_____

10. Describe three immunizations preteens and adolescents should receive.
    a. _____

    _____

    b. _____

    _____

    c. _____

    _____

APPLYING YOUR KNOWLEDGE

REFLECTIVE PRACTICE: CULTIVATING QSEN COMPETENCIES

Use the following expanded scenario from Chapter 23 in your textbook to answer the questions below.

Scenario: Darlene, a pregnant 14-year-old in her third trimester, comes to the prenatal clinic for the first time. Her history reveals sexual activity with multiple partners, smoking two packs of cigarettes per day, beer "4 or 5 nights a week," and eating mostly "fast foods." She has received no prenatal care and hasn't been taking any prenatal vitamins. She is experiencing homelessness but occasionally stays with an older girlfriend since her parents "threw me out of the house."

1. Patient-centered care/evidence-based practice: What should be the focus of the nursing care plan developed for Darlene?

   _____

   _____

   _____

2. Patient-centered care/evidence-based practice: What would be a successful outcome for this patient?

   _____

   _____

   _____

3. Patient-centered care/evidence-based practice: What intellectual, technical, interpersonal, and ethical/legal competencies are most likely to bring about the desired outcome?

_____

_____

_____

4. Teamwork and collaboration: What resources might be helpful for this patient?

_____

_____

_____

PRACTICING FOR NCLEX

MULTIPLE-CHOICE QUESTIONS

Circle the letter that corresponds to the best answer for each question.

1. A nurse records an Apgar score of 3 for a newborn taken 1 minute after birth. What is the nurse's next action?
   a. No intervention is needed, this is a normal score.
   b. Provide respiratory support.
   c. Provide immediate life-saving support.
   d. Report the Apgar score to the primary care provider.

2. During assessment of a female adolescent, a nurse notes the following data: presence of breast tissue, growth spurt in height and weight, appearance of axillary hair, and onset of menarche. Which stage of sexual development does this data confirm?
   a. Prepubescence
   b. Pubescence
   c. Postpubescence
   d. Precocious puberty

3. The nurse observes a hospitalized preschooler who clings excessively to their parents and uses infantile speech patterns. How does the nurse explain this behavior to the parents?
   a. Regression
   b. Separation anxiety
   c. Negativism
   d. Self-expression

4. A nurse in a pediatrician's office teaches parents about age-related health problems for children. Which problem would be most appropriate for a school-aged child?
   a. Suicide
   b. Infections
   c. Failure to thrive
   d. Substance abuse

5. A nurse on the postpartum unit is teaching class for parents of newborns. What is the priority teaching point for this developmental age?
   a. Place the infant on the side or stomach when sleeping.
   b. Line the crib with bumpers to protect the infant's head.
   c. If choking occurs, give back blows, chest thrusts, or CPR.
   d. Wean the infant from the breast or bottle when 9 months old.

6. A nurse in a children's hospital observes for separation anxiety. Which child does the nurse identify would be at highest risk for separation anxiety?
   a. Infant who was abandoned by his parents
   b. Newly hospitalized toddler
   c. Preschooler who is in an isolation room
   d. School-aged child who has low self-esteem

7. A school nurse is implementing a sex education program for adolescents. Which information will the nurse prioritize?
   a. Early sexual activity can lead to loss of self-esteem.
   b. Become familiar with your breast and testicles.
   c. Practice saying "no" to pressures to have sex.
   d. Secondary sex characteristics are fully developed.

8. When assessing the health of a neonate, the nurse bases priorities of care on which of these developmental responses by the baby?
   a. Reflexes that allow sucking, swallowing, or blinking are not yet developed.
   b. Labile temperature control that responds slowly to environmental temperatures is likely.
   c. The neonate is alert to the environment but cannot distinguish color and form.
   d. Hearing and turning toward sound and ability to smell and taste is present.

9. A school nurse is teaching parents of adolescents about the development of self-concept. The nurse teaches that self-concept is stabilized with which group acting as the greatest influence?

   a. Parents

   b. Siblings

   c. Peers

   d. Teachers

10. A nurse is providing education on health maintenance and promotion for the mother and fetus. What information will the nurse include?

   a. If you eat a varied diet, vitamins are unnecessary.

   b. Cut down on smoking.

   c. Avoid cleaning a cat's litter box.

   d. Enjoy only one alcoholic beverage daily.

ALTERNATE-FORMAT QUESTIONS

Multiple-Response Questions

Circle the letters that correspond to the best answers for each question.

1. A nurse is assessing neonates in a hospital nursery. Which are the expected behaviors? Select all that apply.

   a. Displays the Moro and stepping reflex

   b. Body temperature responds slowly to environmental temperature

   c. Senses are not developed enough to feel pain from a heel-stick

   d. Eliminates urine and stool

   e. Exhibits both an active crying state and a quiet alert state

   f. Inherits a transient immunity from infections from the mother

2. A nurse in a pediatric practice is assessing infants during scheduled office visits. Which findings reflect normal physical characteristics of an infant? Select all that apply.

   a. Brain grows to about one third the adult size.

   b. Body temperature stabilizes.

   c. Eyes begin to focus and fixate.

   d. Heart triples in weight.

   e. Heart rate slows and blood pressure rises.

   f. Birth weight usually doubles by 1 year.

3. A nurse is assessing toddlers in a community health care clinic. Which toddlers would the nurse refer for follow-up care? Select all that apply

   a. 2-year-old whose birth weight quadrupled

   b. 2-year-old who cannot kick a ball

   c. 3-year-old who is drawing stick figures

   d. 1½-year-old whose arms and legs are not increasing in length

   e. 1-year-old who does not pick up small objects with fingers

   f. 1-year-old who does not have bladder control during the day

4. A nurse is teaching parents of preschoolers about normal development for this age group. Which teaching points would the nurse include? Select all that apply.

   a. Their head is close to adult size.

   b. Their body is less chubby and more coordinated.

   c. They still have baby teeth.

   d. The average weight of a preschooler is 60 lb.

   e. They are able to skip, jump, and throw a ball.

   f. They are more egocentric than the toddler.

5. A school nurse is assessing school-aged children for achievement of developmental milestones. Which findings require follow up by the nurse? Select all that apply.

   a. 8-year-old who cannot write with a pencil

   b. 10-year-old who has not begun puberty

   c. 12-year-old who still has baby teeth

   d. 9-year-old who has not developed a set of values

   e. 8-year-old whose height remained the same since preschool

   f. 11-year-old who is not developing skills for physical games

6. A nurse is counseling adolescents in a group home setting. Which statements accurately describe the cognitive and psychosocial development of this age group? Select all that apply.

   a. The concept of time and its passage enables the adolescent to set long-term goals.

b. According to Piaget, adolescence is the stage when the cognitive development of formal operations is developed.

c. In the adolescent, egocentrism diminishes and is replaced by an awareness of the needs of others.

d. Based on Erikson's theory, the adolescent tries out different roles and personal choices and beliefs in the stage called generativity versus stagnation.

e. The parents act as the greatest influence on the adolescent.

f. According to Havighurst, more mature relationships with boys and girls are achieved by the adolescent.

Chart/Exhibit Questions

Use the chart below to determine the 5-minute Apgar score of the following neonates:

1. A neonate has a pink skin tone on the body with blue extremities, displays minimum resistance to having extremities extended, has a hearty cry, and has a heart rate of 105 beats/min. Score _____

2. A neonate has a pale skin tone, heart rate of 96 beats/min, respiratory rate of 20 breaths/min, a weak cry, and no response to being slapped on the sole. Score _____

3. A neonate has a pink skin color, cries vigorously, clenches fists and flexes knees, and has a heart rate of 130 beats/min. Score _____

Apgar Scoring Chart			
Category[a]	0	1	2
Heart rate	Absent	Slow (less than 100 beats/min)	More than 100 beats/min
Respiratory effort	Absent	Slow, irregular	Good, crying
Muscle tone	Flaccid	Some flexion of extremities	Active motion
Reflex irritability	No response	Weak cry or grimace	Vigorous cry
Color	Blue, pale	Body pink, extremities blue	Completely pink

[a]Each category is rated as 0, 1, or 2. The rating for each category is then totaled to a maximum score of 10. Normal neonates score between 7 and 10. Neonates who score between 4 and 6 require special assistance; those who score below 4 are in need of immediate life-saving support.

Middle and Older Adulthood

ASSESSING YOUR UNDERSTANDING

FILL IN THE BLANKS

1. According to the _____ theory of aging, a chemical reaction produces damage to the DNA and cell death interfering with normal cell function.

2. A nurse in the medical clinic is assessing a 50-year-old patient. This patient's age category is termed _____ adult.

3. A nurse is examining a middle-aged adult who cares for their grandson and disabled mother. The term generation _____ describes the middle adult who is involved in relationships with their own children and aging family members.

4. The older adult period is often further divided into the young-old, ages _____ to _____; the middle-old, ages _____ to _____; and the old-old, ages _____ and older.

5. A nurse who believes that all older adults take more time to answer interview questions due to slowed mental processes is displaying a form of stereotyping known as _____.

6. The _____ and _____ theory of aging suggests organisms wear out from increased metabolic functioning, and cells become exhausted from the constant energy depletion that occurs from continual adaptation to stressors.

7. When an older adult residing in a long-term care facility tells the nurse about his successes on the golf course, he is engaging in what is termed life _____ or _____.

8. _____ disease is the most common degenerative neurologic illness and the most common cause of cognitive impairment.

9. _____ is the scientific and behavioral study of all aspects of aging and its consequences.

10. The nurse uses the SPICES acronym to identify common problems in older adults. The letters in the acronym stand for: _____ disorders, problems with _____, _____, confusion, evidence of _____, and skin _____.

CORRECT THE FALSE STATEMENTS

Mark the item "T" for true or "F" for false. If false, correct the underlined word or words to make the statement true in the space provided.

____ 1. Most older adults <u>use technology</u>. _____

____ 2. Older adults' enjoyment of sexual activity lasts into their <u>50s</u>. _____

____ 3. Older men often develop prostate <u>cancer</u>. _____

____ 4. The older adults develop decreased <u>depth</u> perception. _____

_____ **5.** The older adult sleeps <u>more</u> at night. _____

_____ **6.** Wrinkles develop due to decreased <u>pigmentation</u> of the skin. _____

_____ **7.** Adults over <u>70</u> years should not receive colon cancer screenings. _____

_____ **8.** Hearing tends to be lost in the <u>higher pitch</u> range. _____

_____ **9.** A previous fall in the older adult <u>doubles</u> the chances of another fall. _____

_____ **10.** <u>Delirium</u> is a progressive cognitive disorder. _____

SHORT ANSWER

1. Briefly describe the following characteristics of middle and older adulthood.

   a. Middle adulthood

   Physiologic development: _____

   Psychosocial development: _____

   Cognitive, moral, and spiritual development: _____

   b. Older adulthood

   Physiologic development: _____

   Psychosocial development: _____

   Cognitive, moral, and spiritual development: _____

2. List five health-promotion activities recommended for all older adults.

   a. _____
   b. _____
   c. _____
   d. _____
   e. _____

3. Briefly define the following theories on aging.

   a. Genetic theory: _____

   b. Immunity theory: _____

   c. Free radical theory: _____

   d. Disengagement theory: _____

   e. Activity theory: _____

4. The family of a patient with Alzheimer's disease (AD) who is mildly forgetful asks the nurse what to expect as the disease progresses. Describe what physical and psychological changes they can expect to develop over time.

_____

5. Give an example of expected changes in the following body systems.

   a. Integumentary: _____

   b. Musculoskeletal: _____

   c. Neurologic: _____

   d. Cardiopulmonary: _____

   e. Gastrointestinal: _____

   f. Genitourinary: _____

APPLYING YOUR KNOWLEDGE

CRITICAL THINKING QUESTIONS

1. Due to advances in medical technology and the increased awareness of proper nutrition and exercise, there has been a dramatic increase in the number of active older adults. Discuss nursing strategies that would enhance the cognitive development and overall functioning (physiologic, social, emotional, spiritual) in this age group.

2. Discuss how the home care nurse would educate about and promote safety for older adults?

3. After attending a senior center or observing older adults you know, discuss what can you learn from this healthy group that will enable you to help others?

REFLECTIVE PRACTICE: CULTIVATING QSEN COMPETENCIES

Use the following expanded scenario from Chapter 24 in your textbook to answer the questions below.

Scenario: Larry, a 67-year-old man with diabetes, states, "Everything's gone downhill since I retired 5 months ago." He reports being "bored out of my mind" and drinking more alcohol simply because "there's nothing else to do!"

1. Patient-centered care/safety: How might the nurse use blended nursing skills to provide holistic, developmentally sensitive care for Larry?

2. Patient-centered care/safety: What would be a successful outcome for this patient?

3. Patient-centered care/safety: What intellectual, technical, interpersonal, and ethical/legal competencies are most likely to bring about the desired outcome?

4. Teamwork and collaboration: What resources might be helpful for this patient?

PRACTICING FOR NCLEX

MULTIPLE-CHOICE QUESTIONS

Circle the letter that corresponds to the best answer for each question.

1. A parish nurse is assessing middle adults living in their area. What behavior would the nurse expect to find in the middle adult?
   a. Establishing a sense of self but fearing being pulled back into the family
   b. Substituting new roles for old roles and perhaps continuing formal roles in a new context
   c. Looking inward; accepting life as finite; and having special interest in spouse, friends, and community
   d. Looking forward but also looking back and beginning to reflect on their lives

2. A nurse encourages residents of a long-term care facility to continue a similar pattern of behavior and activity that existed in their middle adulthood years to ensure healthy aging. This intervention is based on which aging theory?
   a. Identity-continuity
   b. Disengagement
   c. Activity
   d. Life review

3. Based on an understanding of the cognitive changes that normally occur with aging, the nurse plans assessments and care based on which of these expected behaviors of the older adult?
   a. Speaking rapidly and being frequently confused
   b. Withdrawing from strangers
   c. Interrupting frequently with questions
   d. Needing a longer time to respond and react

4. A nurse is admitting the older adult to a medical-surgical unit. What nursing action would the nurse prioritize to help maintain safety?
   a. Treating each patient as a unique person
   b. Orienting the patient to new surroundings
   c. Encouraging independence
   d. Providing planned rest and activity times

5. The nurse in a long-term care facility integrates Erikson's theory of ego integrity versus despair and disgust. Which intervention would the nurse use to best foster older adults' ego integrity?

   a. Distracting the patient

   b. Praising the patient

   c. Encouraging life review

   d. Promoting independent living

6. Based on Havighurst's theory of human development, which nursing intervention would best facilitate the accomplishment of a developmental task of older adulthood?

   a. Assisting a patient move independently using a walker

   b. Suggesting a patient move in with their daughter

   c. Helping a patient cope with living alone after the death of a spouse

   d. Recommending services as a patient becomes established in the community

7. Gould viewed the middle years as a time when adults increase their feelings of self-satisfaction, value their spouse as a companion, and become more concerned with health. Which nursing action best facilitates this process?

   a. Counseling a patient who complains of being depressed

   b. Providing diversional activities for a patient on bed rest

   c. Arranging for social services to assist with meals for a homebound patient

   d. Encouraging a patient to have regular checkups

8. A nurse is caring for a middle adult who is being treated for depression following the death of their spouse. Which action best facilitates the accomplishment of a developmental task of this middle adult?

   a. Encouraging the patient to start dating again to find a life partner

   b. Helping them to see the value of guiding his children to become responsible adults

   c. Helping them to establish a social network within the community

   d. Encouraging the formation of a personal philosophical and ethical structure

9. A nurse caring for older adults in a long-term care facility is precepting a new graduate nurse. The preceptor corrects the graduate nurse when they state that which statement reflects ageism?

   a. "Old age begins at age 65."

   b. "Personality is not changed by chronologic aging."

   c. "Most older adults are ill and institutionalized."

   d. "Intelligence declines with age."

10. Nursing students who attend clinical in a long-term care facility plan to use reminiscence or life review with their older adult residents. Which actions would the students use to enhance reminiscence?

    a. Bringing a birthday card for a resident's birthday

    b. Determining the residents' favorite foods

    c. Asking what music they listened to in their 20s

    d. Determining if they've had visitors recently

11. A nurse working in a gerontology practice assesses patients for risk for injury. Which of these statements by the patient requires the nurse to follow up?

    a. "I received my flu shot last week."

    b. "A new produce store just opened around the corner from me."

    c. "My daughter took my walker and said I don't need it."

    d. "I take the bus to the senior center once a week."

ALTERNATE-FORMAT QUESTIONS

Multiple-Response Questions

Circle the letters that correspond to the best answers for each question.

1. A nurse and nursing student are assessing a middle-adult patient. The nurse recognizes the student understands normal physical changes in this population when they make which statement? Select all that apply.

   a. "Skin moisture increases."

   b. "Hormone production increases."

   c. "Hearing acuity diminishes."

   d. "Cognitive ability diminishes."

   e. "Cardiac output begins to decrease."

   f. "Bones lose calcium."

2. A nurse working in a community clinic assists middle-adult patients to follow guidelines for health-related screenings and immunizations. What preventive measures would the nurse recommend for this population? Select all that apply.

   a. Have a physical exam every year from age 40 onward

   b. Have a clinical skin examination every 3 years

   c. Report any breast changes to the health care provider

   d. Have a pelvic examination and Pap exam at least every 5 years (females)

   e. Have a prostate-specific antigen (PSA) test every 5 years (males)

   f. Get the Zoster vaccine (adults 50 years and older)

3. A nurse is screening for Alzheimer's disease (AD) in patients in a long-term care facility. Which facts regarding AD are accurate? Select all that apply.

   a. AD accounts for about one third of the cases of dementia in the United States.

   b. AD primarily affects young to middle adults.

   c. Scientists estimate that more than 5 million people have AD.

   d. Nearly half of 85-year-old adults have AD.

   e. AD affects brain cells and is characterized by the formation of amyloid plaques and tangles of tau proteins.

   f. AD is a progressively serious but not a life-threatening disease.

4. When caring for older adults, nurses must be aware of common conditions found in this population. Which statements accurately describe these conditions? Select all that apply

   a. Sundowning syndrome is a condition in which an older adult habitually becomes confused, restless, and agitated after dark.

   b. Delirium is a permanent state of confusion occurring in older adulthood.

   c. Depression is a prolonged or extreme state of sadness occurring in many older adults.

   d. Researchers have shown no link between delirium and hospitalization of the older adult.

   e. Polypharmacy is a term that is used to describe the habit of older adults to use many pharmacies to obtain their prescription drugs.

   f. A significant percentage of older adults limit their activities because of fear of falling that might result in serious health consequences.

Prioritization Question

1. The nurse on a surgical unit is receiving report on a group of patients. Which patient will the nurse assess first? Circle the letter that corresponds to the best answer.

   a. Middle adult who will need an influenza vaccine before discharge

   b. Older adult who needs liquids thickened before eating

   c. Older adult whose Jackson–Pratt drain requires emptying

   d. Middle adult with an acute change in mental status

CHAPTER 25

Asepsis and Infection Control

ASSESSING YOUR UNDERSTANDING

FILL IN THE BLANKS

1. The _____ and _____ Education for _____ (QSEN) initiative has identified safety, including effective infection control practices, as one of the leading issues in health care.

2. The _____ for Disease _____ and _____ (CDC) is the U.S. government agency responsible for investigating, preventing, and controlling disease.

3. Bacteria that require oxygen to live and grow are _____; those that can live without oxygen are _____.

4. Bacteria that stain violet with Gram stain are gram _____; those not taking up the stain are gram _____.

5. Microorganisms that commonly inhabit various body sites and are part of the body's natural defense system are referred to as normal _____.

6. The natural habitats of organisms, such as humans, animals, soil, and food and water, are examples of _____, which can support organisms that are pathogenic to humans.

7. Failing to properly sterilize equipment exposes patients to infection by introducing microorganisms at the _____ of _____, or the point at which organisms enter a new host.

8. During the immune response to an invading organism, the body responds by producing a(n) _____; the foreign material is called the _____.

9. A _____ is not present on admission but develops during the course of treatment for other conditions.

10. A(n) _____ infection results from a treatment or diagnostic procedure.

11. A nurse assessing patients for athlete's foot, ringworm, and yeast infections recognizes these problems are caused by organisms known as _____.

12. The nurse uses _____ asepsis by practicing hand hygiene and wearing clean gloves; _____ asepsis refers to processes to keep objects and areas free from microorganisms.

MATCHING EXERCISES

Matching Exercise 1

Match the term in Part A with its definition in Part B.

PART A

a. Fungi

b. Virus

c. Parasite

d. Normal flora

e. Opportunist

f. Fomite

PART B

_____ **1.** Normal flora that becomes potentially harmful by taking advantage of a susceptible host

_____ **2.** Plant-like organisms, present in air, soil, and water, that can cause infection

_____ **3.** Microorganisms that commonly inhabit various body sites and are part of the body's natural defense system

_____ **4.** Organisms that live on or in a host and rely on it for nourishment

_____ **5.** Smallest of all microorganisms, visible only with an electron microscope

_____ **6.** Inanimate objects, such as equipment or countertops, that can transmit organisms

Matching Exercise 2

Match the term in Part A with its definition in Part B.

PART A

a. Exogenous

b. Endogenous

c. Colonized/colonization

d. Surgical asepsis

e. Medical asepsis

f. Contact tracing

PART B

_____ **1.** Infection in which the causative organism is normally harbored within the patient

_____ **2.** Infection caused by an organism acquired from other people

_____ **3.** Clean technique that uses procedures and practices to reduce the number and transfer of pathogens

_____ **4.** Organism present in the body but not causing symptoms; the patient remains healthy and uninfected

_____ **5.** Sterile technique and practices used to render and keep objects and areas free from microorganisms

_____ **6.** Identifies people with an infectious disease and locates their direct contacts to interrupt transmission

CORRECT THE FALSE STATEMENTS

Mark the item "T" for true or "F" for false. If false, correct the underlined word or words to make the statement true in the space provided at the end of the line.

_____ **1.** The purpose of using <u>Gram stain on bacteria</u> is to inform prescribers in selecting appropriate antibiotic therapy.

_____

_____ **2.** Methicillin-resistant *Staphylococcus aureus* (MRSA) and vancomycin-resistant enterococci (VRE) are most often transmitted by <u>the hands of health care providers</u>.

_____

_____ **3.** <u>Wearing gloves</u> is the most effective way to help prevent the spread of organisms.

_____

_____ **4.** <u>Resident bacteria</u>, normally picked up by the hands in the course of usual activities of daily living, are relatively few on clean and exposed areas of the skin.

_____

_____ **5.** <u>Nonantimicrobial agents</u> are considered adequate for routine mechanical cleansing of the hands and removal of most transient microorganisms.

_____

_____ **6.** <u>Sterilization</u> is the process by which all microorganisms, including spores, are destroyed. _____

_____ **7.** In a home environment, contaminated items may be disinfected by placing them in boiling water for <u>10 minutes</u>.

_____

_____ **8.** When observing <u>medical asepsis</u>, areas are considered contaminated if they are touched by any object that is not sterile.

_____

_____ **9.** Using <u>body substance isolation precautions</u> eliminates the need for category-specific or disease-specific systems, except for certain airborne diseases that require special precautions.

_____

SHORT ANSWER

1. List four factors that influence an organism's potential to produce disease.

a. _____

b. _____

c. _____

d. _____

2. Give an example of a disease that is transmitted by organisms from the following reservoirs.

a. Other humans: _____

b. Animals: _____

c. Soil: _____

3. List three portals of exit of microorganisms from the human body.

a. _____

b. _____

c. _____

4. Give an example of the following means of transmission.

a. Direct contact: _____

b. Indirect contact: _____

c. Vectors: _____

d. Fomite: _____

e. Airborne: _____

5. Briefly describe the following body defenses against infection.

a. Inflammatory response: _____

b. Immune response: _____

6. List four factors that influence the susceptibility of a host.

a. _____

b. _____

c. _____

d. _____

7. Use the steps of the nursing process to briefly describe the nurse's role in controlling or treating infection.

a. _____
_____
_____

b. _____
_____
_____

c. _____
_____
_____

d. _____
_____
_____

e. _____
_____
_____

8. Give two examples of how you would teach the patient to practice medical asepsis in the following areas.

a. Patient's home: _____
_____

b. Public facilities: _____
_____

c. Community: _____
_____

d. Health care facility: _____
_____

9. List three measures that health care agencies have found to be successful in reducing the incidence of hospital-acquired infections.

a. _____

b. _____

c. _____

10. Explain why the following factors should be considered when selecting sterilization and disinfection methods.

a. Nature of organisms present: _____
_____

b. Number of organisms present: _____
_____

c. Type of equipment: _____
_____

d. Intended use of equipment: _____
_____

e. Available means for sterilization and disinfection: _____
_____

f. Time: _____
_____

11. Describe the role of the infection control nurse in the following situations.

   a. Hospital: _____

   _____

   b. Home care setting: _____

   _____

12. You are caring for a patient who sustained third-degree burns on his upper body. Describe how you can help to control or prevent infection for this patient.

   _____

   _____

13. In the emergency department, a patient you are treating for lacerations tells you that he was recently diagnosed with tuberculosis (TB). Discuss the infection control precautions for this patient compared to others in the emergency department patient?

   _____

   _____

APPLYING YOUR KNOWLEDGE

CRITICAL THINKING QUESTIONS

1. The nurse uses aseptic techniques to halt the spread of microorganisms and minimize the threat of infection. During a breach of asepsis, the patient may develop an infection or sepsis. What symptoms and outcome of this process would you anticipate?

2. Imagine what it must feel like to be in strict isolation, then interview a patient whose medical condition necessitated the use of isolation precautions. Elicit their feelings of being isolated and, perhaps feared by health care workers. What was done to help alleviate the loneliness and meet the patient's basic needs of love and belonging? Briefly discuss what you will apply when caring for patients in isolation.

3. A nurse is obligated to provide care to all patients regardless of race, creed, religion, etc. Should nurses be able to choose whether to take care of a patient who has a communicable disease? Should there be consequences for medical personnel who refuse to take care of these patients? Do you believe the precautions being taken with these

patients offer adequate protection for the health care provider? Consider employees of the COVID 19 pandemic as part of your response.

Share your responses with your classmates and see if you agree.

REFLECTIVE PRACTICE: CULTIVATING QSEN COMPETENCIES

Use the following expanded scenario from Chapter 25 in your textbook to answer the questions below.

Scenario: Giselle, a 38-year-old woman undergoing chemotherapy treatment for leukemia, states: "I know that my risk for infection is really high because of my poor immune status. But how do I respond to my Sunday school students, who are used to greeting me with a big hug? I want to be safe, but I know that I need these hugs too!"

1. Patient-centered care/safety: How might the nurse respond to Giselle in a holistic manner that respects her human dignity, while at the same time maintaining a safe environment for her?

   _____

2. Patient-centered care/safety: What would be a successful outcome for Giselle?

   _____

3. Patient-centered care/evidence-based practice: What intellectual, technical, interpersonal, and ethical/legal competencies are most likely to bring about the desired outcome?

   _____

4. Teamwork and collaboration: What resources might be helpful for this patient?

   _____

PRACTICING FOR NCLEX

MULTIPLE-CHOICE QUESTIONS

Circle the letter that corresponds to the best answer for each question.

1. An infection control nurse is rounding on a surgical unit to study whether nurses use proper hand hygiene during patient care. Which action represents the appropriate use of hand hygiene?

   a. Using gloves in place of hand hygiene

   b. Keeping fingernails less than ¼ inches long

   c. Replacing gloves with hand hygiene when touching blood

   d. Avoiding hand moisturizer following hand hygiene

2. A nurse is caring for a patient who is diagnosed with active tuberculosis. Which nursing intervention best promotes infection control?

   a. Admitting the patient to a private room

   b. Using droplet precautions when providing care for the patient

   c. Having visitors maintain a 3-ft distance from the infected person

   d. Placing the patient in a private room with negative air pressure

3. A nursing student performs hand hygiene after providing patient care, using soap and water. Which nursing action is performed correctly according to the procedure?

   a. Using soap and cold water to wash hands

   b. Using about 2 teaspoons of liquid soap to wash hands

   c. Washing at least 1 inch above the area of contamination if present

   d. Rinsing thoroughly with water flowing away from the fingertips

4. The mother of four children asks the nurse in a pediatric practice why everyone in the household got sick with a viral illness so quickly. What information does the nurse convey?

   a. "During the incubation period, the individual is asymptomatic and most likely to shed the most virus."

   b. "Once the patient enters the prodromal stage, with signs of the illness, the virus is no longer transmitted."

   c. "In the acute full stage of illness, family members become immune to the virus."

   d. "While convalescing, only the adults will transmit the virus."

5. A nurse prefers to use an alcohol-based handrub when providing care for patients. In which instance will the infection control nurse correct the nurse?

   a. While providing care to a patient with *Clostridioides difficile*

   b. While performing routine care and moving from one patient to another.

   c. After cleaning a patient's bedside table

   d. While completing patient care where hands are not visibly soiled

6. A nurse is setting up a sterile field to insert a urinary catheter when the patient touches the end of the sterile field. What reflects the nurse's most appropriate action?

   a. Changing the sterile field but reusing the sterile equipment

   b. Proceeding with the procedure since it was only touched by the patient

   c. Discarding the sterile field and the supplies and start over

   d. Calling for assistance

7. A nurse is inserting an intravenous catheter in preparation for administration of IV fluids. Which infection control precaution is followed during this procedure?

   a. Surgical aseptic technique

   b. Medical aseptic technique

   c. Droplet precautions

   d. Strict reverse isolation

8. A nursing student prepares to care for a patient whose infection was likely spread by fomites. Which intervention will the student use to prevent disseminating the infection?

   a. Washing hands with a dilute bleach solution

   b. Decontaminating surfaces in the patient room

   c. Wearing an N95 respirator mask

   d. Placing a mask on the patient when they leave their room

9. A nurse caring for patients in a hospital setting institutes CDC recommendations for standard precautions for which patients?

   a. Patients with diagnosed infections
   b. Patients with visible blood, body fluids, or sweat
   c. Patients with nonintact skin
   d. Every patient receiving care in hospitals

ALTERNATE-FORMAT QUESTIONS

Multiple-Response Questions

Circle the letter that corresponds to the best answer for each question.

1. A nurse is following medical asepsis when caring for patients in a critical care unit. Which nursing actions follow these principles? Select all that apply.

   a. Carrying soiled items away from the body
   b. Placing soiled bed linen on the floor
   c. Moving soiled equipment away from the body when cleaning it
   d. Opening a window and dusts the room in the direction of the window
   e. Cleaning least soiled areas first and then moving to more soiled ones
   f. Pouring discarded liquids into a basin then into the drain

2. A nurse is setting up a sterile field in preparation for a biopsy. Which actions follow recommended guidelines for this procedure? Select all that apply.

   a. Considering the outer 1-inch edge of the sterile field to be contaminated
   b. Placing the cap of an opened solution on the table with edges down
   c. Discarding a sterile field when a portion of it becomes contaminated
   d. Calling for help when realizing a supply is missing
   e. Dropping a sterile item on a sterile field from the height of 12 inches
   f. Holding a facility-wrapped item with top flap opening toward the body

3. An operating room nurse is putting on sterile gloves to assist with surgery. Which actions are performed correctly in this procedure? Select all that apply.

   a. Placing the sterile gloves on a clean dry surface at or below waist level

   b. Opening the outside wrapper by peeling the top layer back
   c. Placing the inner package on the work surface with the side labeled "cuff end" furthest from body
   d. Opening the inner package by folding open the top flap, then the bottom and sides
   e. Lifting and holding the glove up and off the inner package with fingers down and inserting hand palm up into the glove
   f. Touching only the inner surface of the package and the gloves

4. A nurse is removing soiled gloves after assisting with a sterile procedure. Which actions follow recommended guidelines for this procedure? Select all that apply.

   a. Using the dominant hand to grasp the opposite glove near cuff end on the outside exposed area
   b. Removing the glove by pulling it off, inverting it as it is pulled, and keeping the contaminated area on the inside
   c. Sliding the fingers of the ungloved hand between the remaining glove and the wrist
   d. Removing the second glove by pulling the cuff up, inverting it as it is pulled, and keeping the contaminated area on the outside
   e. Securing the second glove inside the first glove while keeping the contaminated area on the outside
   f. Discarding the gloves in appropriate container, removing additional PPE, and performing hand hygiene

5. Nurses wear PPE to protect themselves and patients from infectious materials. Which examples accurately represent the proper use of PPE in a health care facility? Select all that apply.

   a. Applying clean gloves only when performing or assisting with invasive patient procedures
   b. Possibly needing to change gloves more than once when caring for a patient
   c. Using a waterproof gown more than once
   d. Removing PPE, except for the respirator, at the doorway or in an anteroom
   e. When removing a gown, unfastening the ties, if at the neck and back, and allowing the gown to fall away from shoulders
   f. Lowering a mask around the neck when not being worn and bringing it back over the mouth and nose for reuse

6. Nursing students are discussing which patients require the nurse to use droplet precautions. Which patients will the students correctly include in the discussion? Select all that apply.

a. Patient with rubella

b. Patient with tuberculosis

c. Patient with SARS

d. Patient with mumps

e. Patient with MRSA

f. Patient with diphtheria

7. A community health nurse is discussing basic principles of medical asepsis that can be used to prevent infections at home. What will the nurse include in the discussion?

a. "Wash your hands before preparing food and before eating."

b. "Wash your hands after using the bathroom."

c. "Wash cutting boards and utensils with hot, soapy water before and after handling raw poultry and meat."

d. "Consume natural, unpasteurized milk and fruit juices."

e. "Wash raw fruits and vegetables before serving them."

f. "Boil toddlers' plates, cups, and utensils for 10 minutes."

Sequencing Questions

1. Place the steps the nurse will take when removing PPE in the order in which they should occur.

a. Remove gown

b. Remove mask/respirator

c. Remove gloves

d. Remove goggles/face shield

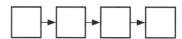

2. Place the steps of the infection cycle in order.

a. Portal of exit

b. Infectious agent

c. Means of transmission

d. Reservoir

e. Portal of entry

f. Susceptible host

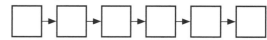

3. Place the following phases of an infection in the order it occurs.

a. Prodromal stage

b. Full (acute) stage

c. Convalescent period

d. Onset stage

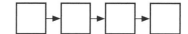

CHAPTER 26

Vital Signs

ASSESSING YOUR UNDERSTANDING

FILL IN THE BLANKS

1. Vital signs assess _____ function; they include _____, _____, _____ and _____. _____ and _____ may also be assessed.

2. The nurse is choosing a bladder width and length to measure the blood pressure of an older child with an arm circumference of 20 cm. The bladder width and length (in centimeters) that would typically be used for this child is: width: _____ and length: _____.

3. A nurse is palpating peripheral pulses and notes the radial pulse is weak. The nurse will document the amplitude or strength of this pulse as _____.

4. A nurse measures a patient's oral temperature at 101°F; therefore, the axillary temperature likely correlates to a temperature of _____.

5. A nurse converts a patient's temperature of 39°C to _____°F.

6. A nurse converts a patient's temperature of 99.5°F to _____°C.

7. _____ is referred to as a "silent killer" due to its few symptoms.

8. Orthostatic hypotension, especially in the older adult, can predispose the patient to _____.

9. The nurse auscultates the appearance and disappearance of _____ sounds to determine the blood pressure.

10. If the patient's blood pressure is inaudible, the nurse may obtain the systolic blood pressure using a _____ device.

DEVELOPING YOUR KNOWLEDGE BASE

IDENTIFICATION

1. Identify the areas for assessment of pulses by placing your answers on the lines provided.

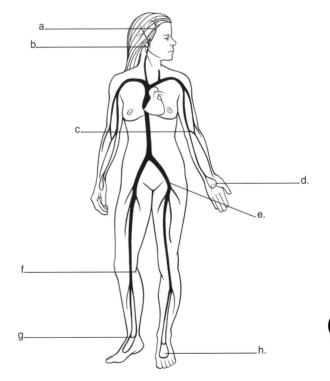

a._____
b._____
c._____
d._____
e._____
f._____
g._____
h._____

MATCHING EXERCISES

Matching Exercise 1

Match the term in Part A with its definition in Part B.

PART A

a. Tachycardia

b. Palpitation

c. Bradycardia

d. Pulse amplitude

e. Arrhythmia

f. Pulse deficit

PART B

____ **1.** Patient is aware of own rapid heartbeat without having to feel their pulse

____ **2.** Irregular pattern of heartbeats

____ **3.** Heart rate <60 beats/min in an adult

____ **4.** Difference between apical and radial pulse rates

____ **5.** Pulse rate >100 beats/min in an adult

____ **6.** Quality of pulse in terms of fullness; reflects strength of left ventricular contraction

Matching Exercise 2

Match the term in Part A with definition in Part B.

PART A

a. Apnea

b. Dyspnea

c. Orthopnea

d. Tachypnea

e. Ventilation

f. Respiration

PART B

____ **1.** Movement of gases in and out of the lungs

____ **2.** Difficult or labored breathing

____ **3.** Ability to breathe more easily in an upright position

____ **4.** Periods of no breathing

____ **5.** Respiratory rate >20 breaths/min

____ **6.** Involves ventilation, diffusion, and perfusion

Matching Exercise 3

Match the term in Part A with its definition in Part B.

PART A

a. Pyrexia

b. Febrile

c. Afebrile

d. Hyperpyrexia

e. Hypothermia

f. Hyperthermia

g. Ineffective thermoregulation

PART B

____ **1.** High fever, typically >106°F

____ **2.** Body temperature below limit of normal

____ **3.** Hyperthermia

____ **4.** Person with normal body temperature

____ **5.** Fever caused by extreme heat exposure

____ **6.** State in which temperature fluctuates between above-normal and below-normal ranges

SHORT ANSWER

1. Briefly describe how the following factors affect body temperature.

a. Circadian rhythms: _____

_____

_____

b. Age: _____

_____

_____

c. Biologic sex: _____

_____

_____

d. Stress: _____

_____

_____

e. Environmental temperature: _____

_____

_____

2. Complete the table below describing the types of thermometers used to assess body temperature.

Type of Thermometer	Brief Description	Contraindication	Normal Reading
A. ELECTRONIC AND DIGITAL			
B. TYMPANIC MEMBRANE			
C. DISPOSABLE SINGLE USE			
D. TEMPORAL ARTERY			
E. AUTOMATED MONITORING DEVICE			

3. List three methods that can be used to assess the pulses.

_____

_____

_____

4. Briefly describe how the following variables may affect a patient's blood pressure.

a. Pumping action of the heart: _____

_____

b. Blood volume: _____

_____

c. Blood viscosity: _____

_____

d. Elasticity of vessel walls: _____

5. Briefly explain how the following problems cause alterations in pulse and blood pressure.

a. Decrease in peripheral tissue perfusion: ____

_____

b. Loss of fluid volume: _____

_____

c. Excess fluid volume: _____

_____

d. Reduced cardiac output: _____

_____

e. Anxiety: _____

_____

6. After taking vital signs, a nurse documents the findings as T = 98.6°F, P = 66, R = 18, BP = 124/82. Which of these numbers represents the systolic blood pressure?

_____

7. Complete the table with the correct age-related value for vital signs.

Age	Temperature °C °F	Pulse beats/min	Respirations breaths/min	Blood Pressure mm Hg
Newborns	°C °F	95–170	30–60	60–70/40
Infants	35.6–37.6°C 96–99.7°F		30–50	85/37
Toddler	35.6–37.2°C 96–99°F	70–150	20–40	
Child	35.6–37.2°C 96–99°F		15–25	95/57
Adolescent	35.8–37.5°C 96.4–99.5°F		12–20	
Adult	°C °F			

APPLYING YOUR KNOWLEDGE

CRITICAL THINKING QUESTIONS

1. Using a partner, locate the nine sites for pulse assessment. Practice the technique for obtaining radial and apical pulses, measuring respirations, and assessing blood pressure. Why is it important to be proficient in assessing vital signs with various equipment and reporting deviations from normal measurements? If you were unsure of one of your vital sign assessments, what would you do?

2. An obese woman in the clinic needs a large blood pressure cuff, but one is not available. The resident tells you, "Just use the cuff you have." How do you respond, and why?

REFLECTIVE PRACTICE: CULTIVATING QSEN COMPETENCIES

Use the following expanded scenario from Chapter 26 in your textbook to answer the questions below.

Scenario: Noah, a 2-year-old, is brought to the emergency department by his mother who reports he has had a high fever and has refused food and fluids for 24 hours. When you attempt to obtain a tympanic temperature, he begins to scream uncontrollably, crying and pushing the device away from his ear.

1. Patient-centered care/evidence-based practice: What might be causing Noah's reaction to the nurse's attempt to assess a tympanic temperature?

_____

_____

_____

2. Patient-centered care: What would be a successful outcome for Noah?

_____

_____

_____

3. Patient-centered care: What intellectual, technical, and interpersonal competencies are most likely to bring about the desired outcome?

Intellectual: _____

_____

Technical: _____

_____

Interpersonal: _____

_____

4. Teamwork and collaboration: What resources might be helpful for the nurse caring for Noah?

_____

_____

_____

PRACTICING FOR NCLEX

MULTIPLE-CHOICE QUESTIONS

Circle the letter that corresponds to the best answer for each question.

1. A nurse documents the following assessment for an infant: temperature 98.2°F, pulse 90 beats/min, respirations 32 breaths/min, and blood pressure 73/55. Which nursing action is appropriate based on these assessments?
   a. Reporting the pyrexia
   b. Reporting tachycardia and bradypnea
   c. Reporting hypotension and tachypnea
   d. No action is needed; these are normal results

2. A nurse is taking the vital signs of a 9-year-old child who is anxious about the procedures. Which action would be appropriate when assessing this child?
   a. Making sure the child does not touch the assessment equipment.
   b. Performing as many tasks as possible with the child lying on the examining table.
   c. Performing the blood pressure measurement last.
   d. Performing the assessments quickly while maintaining a serious demeanor.

3. A nurse has delegated morning vital signs to an AP. Which action requires the nurse to intervene?
   a. Assessing blood pressure of a patient with a left A-V fistula in their right arm
   b. Taking a radial pulse by placing three fingers over the radial artery
   c. Taking the blood pressure of a patient with bilateral mastectomy and lymph node removal on the arm
   d. Assessing an axillary temperature on a patient who is experiencing vomiting and diarrhea

4. A nurse is assessing an adult who has an irregular pulse rate of 130 beats/min. Which action will the nurse take next?
   a. Assess the apical pulse
   b. Initiate CPR
   c. Document this in the health record
   d. Place the patient flat in bed

5. A nurse is taking a rectal temperature on a patient who reports feeling lightheaded during the procedure. What is the nurse's priority action in this situation?
   a. Leaving the thermometer in and notifying the health care provider
   b. Removing the thermometer and assessing blood pressure and heart rate
   c. Removing the thermometer and assessing the temperature via another method
   d. Calling for assistance and anticipating the need for CPR

6. A nurse is assessing a patient's apical pulse. Which action will the nurse perform after placing the diaphragm over the apex of the heart?
   a. Listen for extra heart sounds
   b. Count the heart rate for 2 minutes
   c. Count each "lub-dub" as 1 beat
   d. Palpate the space between the fifth and sixth ribs

7. A nurse is assessing the respirations of a patient and finds that the patient is breathing so shallowly that the respirations cannot be counted. What would be the appropriate initial nursing intervention in this situation?
   a. Notifying the primary care provider
   b. Performing a pain assessment
   c. Administering oxygen
   d. Auscultating the lung sounds and count respirations

8. Which patient would the nurse consider at risk for low blood pressure?
   a. Patient with high blood viscosity
   b. Patient with decreased blood volume
   c. Patient with decreased elasticity of arteriole walls
   d. Patient with strong pumping action of blood into the arteries

9. A nurse has delegated taking VS to an AP for a patient admitted with new-onset seizures. Which action by the AP will require intervention by the nurse?

   a. Measuring the blood pressure via the brachial artery

   b. Counting the patient's respirations while holding the wrist

   c. Taking the patient's temperature by the oral route

   d. Measuring oxygen saturation on the dominant hand

ALTERNATE-FORMAT QUESTIONS

Multiple-Response Questions

Circle the letters that correspond to the best answers for each question.

1. A nurse is assessing a patient's blood pressure and obtains a low pressure reading, inconsistent with previous results. Which actions might have contributed to this false reading? Select all that apply.

   a. Performing the assessment in a noisy environment

   b. Placing the bell beyond the direct area of the artery

   c. Using a non-facility issued manometer that was not calibrated

   d. Viewing the meniscus from below eye level

   e. Failing to pump the cuff 20 to 30 mm Hg above disappearing pulse

   f. Applying a cuff that is too narrow

2. A nurse is assessing a patient for orthostatic hypotension. When the patient stands, what additional signs and symptoms will the nurse assess? Select all that apply.

   a. Dizziness

   b. Bradycardia

   c. Erythema

   d. Fever

   e. Lightheadedness

   f. Pallor

3. A nurse is assessing vital signs for a group of patients in the Emergency Department. Which reflects proper technique when assessing body temperature by various methods? Select all that apply.

   a. When assessing tympanic membrane temperature, wipe the tympanic probe cover

with alcohol before inserting it snugly into the ear.

   b. When assessing an oral temperature with an electronic thermometer, place the probe beneath the patient's tongue in the posterior sublingual pocket.

   c. When assessing rectal temperature with an electronic thermometer, lubricate about 1 in of the probe with a water-soluble lubricant.

   d. When assessing axillary temperature, place the tip in the center of the axilla and bring the patient's arm down close to the body. Leave the thermometer in place for 6 minutes.

   e. When assessing temperature with an electronic thermometer, hold the thermometer in place in the assessment site until a beep is heard.

   f. Note the site used because axillary temperatures are generally about 1° higher than oral temperatures and rectal temperatures are generally about 1° lower than oral temperatures.

4. A nurse is providing discharge teaching for a patient diagnosed with hypertension. Which teaching points about monitoring blood pressure should the nurse include in the plan? Select all that apply.

   a. Using the blood pressure devices in public places to measure BP whenever possible

   b. Using manual cuffs over digital BP monitoring equipment

   c. Taking the blood pressure every day at the same time

   d. Recommending a cuff size appropriate for the patient's limb size

   e. Recommending the use of lower extremities when monitoring BP

   f. Telling the patient to keep their wrist at heart level when using a wrist monitor

5. A nursing student is assessing a patient's blood pressure using the brachial artery. Which nursing actions will the primary nurse correct? Select all that apply.

   a. Centering the bladder of the cuff over the brachial artery about midway on the arm

   b. Placing the cuff over the patient's clothing and fastens it snugly

   c. Recording the point on the gauge at which the first faint but clear sound appears and increases in intensity as the diastolic pressure

d. Having the patient lying or sitting down with the forearm supported at the level of the heart and the palm of the hand upward

e. Wrapping the cuff around the arm smoothly and snugly and fastening it

f. Repeating any suspicious reading before 1 minute has passed since the last reading

6. A nurse is assessing the blood pressure of a hospitalized patient using a Doppler ultrasound device. Which actions are performed correctly? Select all that apply.

a. Placing the patient in a comfortable lying or sitting position

b. Centering the bladder of the cuff over the artery lining

c. Wrapping the cuff around the limb smoothly and snugly and fastening it

d. Checking that the needle on the aneroid gauge is within the zero mark

e. Checking to see that the manometer is in the horizontal position

f. Opening the valve to the sphygmomanometer once the pulse is found

Sequencing Question

Place the following descriptions of the phases of Korotkoff sounds in order from phase I to phase V.

a. Characterized by muffled or swishing sounds that may temporarily disappear; also known as the auscultatory gap

b. Characterized by distinct, loud sounds as the blood flows relatively freely through an increasingly open artery

c. The last sound heard before a period of continuous silence, known as the second diastolic pressure

d. Characterized by the first appearance of faint but clear tapping sounds that gradually increase in intensity; known as the systolic pressure

e. Characterized by a distinct, abrupt, muffling sound with a soft, blowing quality; considered to be the first diastolic pressure

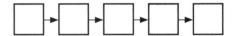

CHAPTER 27

Health Assessment

ASSESSING YOUR UNDERSTANDING

FILL IN THE BLANK

1. A health _____ is a collection of subjective information that provides information about the patient's health status, while the _____ assessment is a collection of objective data that provides information about the patient's body systems.

2. Accurate health assessment provides the foundation for _____ nursing care.

3. _____ and respect are primary concerns when conducting a health assessment.

4. The Full Outline of UnResponsiveness (FOUR) Coma Scale includes assessment of eye response, motor response, brainstem response, and _____.

5. When conducting a drug screen, in some locations, informed _____ is required.

6. The patient's reason for seeking health care is best documented using direct _____ rather than paraphrasing.

7. During auscultation, the nurse uses the _____ of the stethoscope to detect low-pitched sounds and the _____ to detect high-pitched sounds.

8. During vision screening, the nurse uses the _____ eye chart to assess visual acuity.

9. When using the technique of inspection, the nurse notes size, color, shape, position, movement, and _____.

10. _____ assessment can be considered a fifth vital sign.

CORRECT THE FALSE STATEMENTS

Mark the item "T" for true or "F" for false. If false, correct the underlined word or words to make the statement true in the space provided.

____ 1. During auscultation of the heart, the first heart sound heard is the lub or <u>S1</u> of "lub-dub." _____

____ 2. The first heart sound occurs when the <u>aortic</u> and mitral valves close. _____

____ 3. The lub or S1 is heard best in the <u>aortic</u> area. _____

____ 4. The second heart sound, S2 or <u>dub</u>, represents the closure of the aortic and pulmonic valves. _____

IDENTIFICATION QUESTIONS:
ANATOMY REVIEW

1. Locate the organs listed below that are found in the anterior section of the abdominal cavity. Place your answers on the lines provided in the illustration below.

Sigmoid colon

Small intestine

Stomach

Appendix

Bladder

Spleen

Transverse colon

Ascending colon

Cecum

Liver

Descending colon

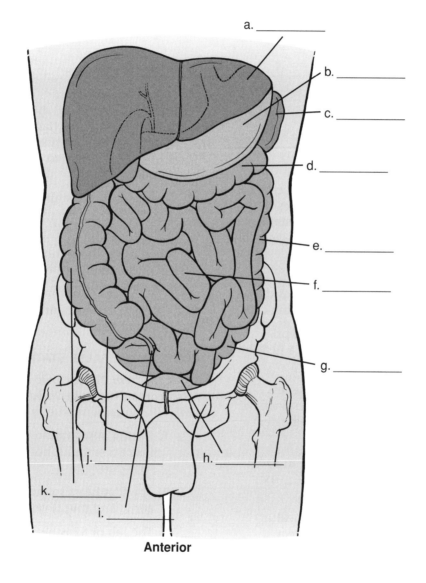

a. _____

b. _____

c. _____

d. _____

e. _____

f. _____

g. _____

j. _____

h. _____

k. _____

i. _____

Anterior

2. Locate the following list of internal structures of the ear and place your answers on the lines provided on the illustration below.

Incus
Facial nerve
Cochlea
Semicircular canals

Malleus
Tympanic membrane
Stapes and footplate
Cochlear and vestibular branch
Oval window
Eustachian tube
Round window

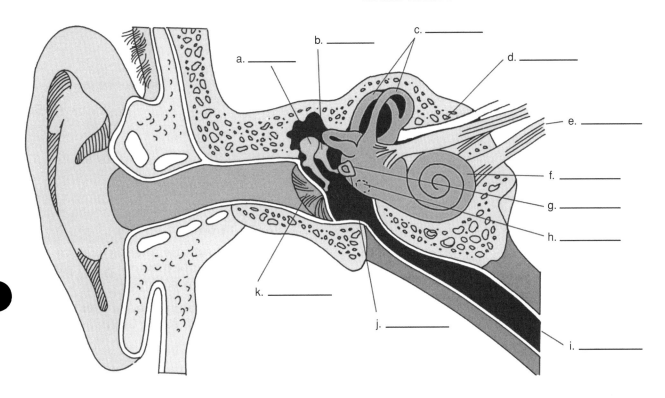

MATCHING EXERCISES

Matching Exercise 1

Match the location listed in Part A with the organ listed in Part B. Answers may be used more than once.

PART A

a. Right upper quadrant
b. Left upper quadrant
c. Right lower quadrant
d. Left lower quadrant
e. Midline

PART B

____ **1.** Liver

____ **2.** Stomach

____ **3.** Gallbladder

____ **4.** Sigmoid colon

____ **5.** Cecum

____ **6.** Spleen

____ **7.** Urinary bladder

____ **8.** Appendix

____ **9.** Body of pancreas

____ **10.** Left ovary and fallopian tube

Matching Exercise 2

Match the terms in Part A with the correct definitions for findings during skin assessment in Part B.

PART A

a. Cyanosis
b. Jaundice
c. Pallor
d. Ecchymosis
e. Petechiae
f. Lesion

PART B

____ **1.** Very small hemorrhagic spots

____ **2.** Dusky, blue color

____ **3.** Yellow tint to the skin

____ **4.** Paleness

____ **5.** Diseased or injured tissue

____ **6.** Purplish discoloration

Matching Exercise 3

Match the assessment findings in Part A with their description and function listed in Part B.

PART A

a. S3/third heart sound

b. Bruit

c. Bronchial breath sound

d. Vesicular breath sound

e. Bronchovesicular breath sound

f. Adventitious breath sound

PART B

____ **1.** High-pitched, harsh "blowing" sounds, heard over the larynx and trachea; sound on expiration is longer than inspiration

____ **2.** Moderate blowing sounds, with inspiration equal to expiration, heard over the mainstem bronchus

____ **3.** Soft, low-pitched, whispering sounds, heard over most of the lung fields, with sound on inspiration being longer than expiration

____ **4.** Extra, abnormal sounds, not normally heard in the lungs

____ **5.** Abnormal "swooshing or blowing" sounds heard over a blood vessel, caused by blood that is swirling in the vessel

____ **6.** Extracardiac sound, best heard with the bell; considered normal in children

Matching Exercise 4

Match the adventitious breath sound listed in Part A with its description in Part B.

PART A

a. Wheeze

b. Crackles

c. Rhonchi

d. Friction rub

PART B

____ **1.** Musical, squeaking, high pitched, and continuous; inspiratory and expiratory

____ **2.** Discrete, discontinuous, bubbling, crackling, popping; air passing through fluid in the airways

____ **3.** Sonorous or coarse; snoring quality; inspiratory and expiratory sound partially cleared by coughing

____ **4.** Rubbing or grating, loudest over the anterior surface during inspiration and expiration

COMPLETE THE CHART

1. Complete the chart below filling in missing information on name, function, or method of assessment.

Cranial Nerve	Name	Function	Method of Assessment
II	Optic	Visual acuity	Snellen eye chart
II, III, VI			Movement of eyes and lids, PERLA
V	Trochlear		
VII		Sensorimotor nerve that innervates the muscles of the face and functions to provide the taste sensation of the anterior two thirds of the tongue	
VIII	Acoustic		
IX			Motor nerve; ask patient to open the mouth and say "aaah"; observing the upward movement of the soft palate
XII			

2. Complete the chart below listing the four assessment techniques; give a brief description of each technique and the types of assessments made.

Technique	Definition	Assessment/Observation
a. Inspection:		
b. Palpation:		
c. Percussion:		
d. Auscultation:		

SHORT ANSWER

1. Identify five purposes of performing a health assessment.

    a. _____

    b. _____

    c. _____

    d. _____

    e. _____

2. Write the name of the instrument used during the health assessment.

    a. Lighted instrument used to visualize interior structures of the eyes: _____

    _____

    b. Lighted instrument used to visualize interior structures of the ears: _____

    _____

    c. Allows visualization of lower and middle turbinates of the nose: _____

    _____

    d. Two-bladed instrument used to examine the vaginal canal and cervix:

    _____

    _____

    e. Two-pronged metal instrument used to test auditory function and vibratory perception:

    _____

    _____

    f. Instrument with a rubber head for testing reflexes and tissue density: _____

    _____

3. List four factors that should be considered when deciding on a position for the physical assessment of a patient.

    a. _____

    b. _____

    c. _____

    d. _____

4. Describe how you would prepare a patient and the environment for a physical assessment.

    a. Patient: _____

    _____

    b. Environment: _____

    _____

5. List and describe the four characteristics of sound assessed by auscultation.

    a. _____

    b. _____

    c. _____

    d. _____

6. Briefly describe how you would assess a patient for the following conditions.

    a. Edema: _____

    _____

    b. Fluid loss: _____

    _____

    c. Assess difficulty with balance: _____

    _____

7. Describe the procedure for assessing the pupils of a patient for the following.

   a. Pupillary reaction: _____

   _____

   b. Accommodation: _____

   _____

   c. Convergence: _____

   _____

8. Give an example of a question you may ask to assess a patient's mental status in the following areas.

   a. Orientation: _____

   _____

   b. Immediate memory: _____

   _____

   c. Past memory: _____

   _____

   d. Abstract reasoning: _____

   _____

   e. Language: _____

   _____

9. Give an example of an interview question you would ask a patient to elicit the following eight components of the health history.

   a. Biographical data: _____

   _____

   b. Reason for seeking health care: _____

   _____

   c. Present health history: _____

   _____

   d. Past health history: _____

   _____

   e. Family history: _____

   _____

   f. Functional health: _____

   _____

   g. Psychosocial and lifestyle factors:

   _____

   _____

   h. Review of systems: _____

   _____

APPLYING YOUR KNOWLEDGE

CRITICAL THINKING QUESTIONS

1. Being prepared is a key factor in conducting a competent health assessment. The nurse must display well-developed cognitive, interpersonal, technical, and ethical skills. Describe what you would do to prepare the patient, the room, and the environment for an examination. How and why would you modify these preparations for the following patients?

   a. Patient who is comatose

   b. Patient who is uncooperative

   c. Patient who does not understand your language

   d. Young child

2. Rate yourself on your technical ability to use assessment instruments and the techniques for assessment. Practice using the instruments on a partner until you feel confident. Reflect on:

   a. How confident you need to be before you can assess a patient independently?

   b. When is it appropriate to practice assessment skills on a patient?

REFLECTIVE PRACTICE: CULTIVATING QSEN COMPETENCIES

Use the following expanded scenario from Chapter 27 in your textbook to answer the questions below.

Scenario: Billy, a 9-year-old boy with a history of allergies, including an allergy to insect stings, is spending a week at summer camp. He reports to the camp counselor that he was just stung by a bee.

1. Patient-centered care/safety: What type of health assessments would the nurse caring for Billy conduct?

   _____

   _____

   _____

2. Patient-centered care/safety: What would be a successful outcome for Billy and his family?

   _____

   _____

   _____

3. Safety/evidence-based practice: What intellectual, interpersonal, and ethical/legal competencies are most likely to bring about the desired outcome?

_____

_____

_____

4. Teamwork and collaboration/safety: What resources might be helpful to Billy, camp personnel and his family?

_____

_____

_____

PRACTICING FOR NCLEX

MULTIPLE-CHOICE QUESTIONS

Circle the letter that corresponds to the best answer for each question.

1. A nurse is performing eye assessments at a community clinic. Which assessment would the nurse document as normal?
   a. One eye moves toward midline when the nurse moves a finger toward the patient's nose.
   b. The patient's pupils are black, equal in size, and round and smooth.
   c. An older adult's pupils are pale and cloudy.
   d. Pupils dilate when looking at a near object and constrict when looking at a distant object.

2. The heath care provider documents a mass in the patient's right lung based on which assessment technique?
   a. Inspection
   b. Palpation
   c. Auscultation
   d. Percussion

3. A nurse is performing an abdominal assessment on a patient reporting RLQ pain. Which area will the nurse assess last?
   a. RLQ
   b. RUQ
   c. LUP
   d. LLQ

4. A nurse is caring for a group of patients. Patients with which integumentary assessment findings will the nurse assess first?
   a. Redness in the facial area
   b. Yellow tint to the skin
   c. Dusky, blue skin
   d. Pale skin

5. A nurse is assisting with assessment of the internal eye structures of patients in an ophthalmologist's office. What will the nurse document as a normal finding?
   a. Uniform yellow reflex
   b. Clear, reddish optic nerve disc
   c. Dark-red arteries and light-red veins
   d. Reddish retina

6. A nurse is assessing the lungs of a patient and auscultates soft, low-pitched sounds over the base of the lungs during inspiration. What will be the nurse's next action?
   a. Suspect an inflammation of the pleura.
   b. Document normal breath sounds.
   c. Recommend testing for infection.
   d. Assess for asthma.

7. A nurse is palpating the skin of a patient and documents that when picked up in a fold, the skinfold slowly returns to normal. What will be the nurse's next action?
   a. Document a normal skin finding on the patient chart.
   b. Assess the patient for oxygenation disorders.
   c. Report the finding as a positive sign for edema.
   d. Further assess the patient for fluid loss.

8. A nurse is assessing the ear canal and tympanic membrane of a patient using an otoscope. What finding will the nurse document as normal?
   a. The tympanic membrane is translucent, shiny, and gray.
   b. The ear canal is rough and pinkish.
   c. The tympanic membrane is reddish.
   d. The ear canal is smooth and white.

9. A nurse is assessing the bowel sounds of a patient who has Crohn's disease. Which assessment technique will the nurse use?
   a. Auscultation
   b. Palpation
   c. Percussion
   d. Inspection

10. A nurse is weighing a patient with a bed scale, when they become agitated as the sling rises in the air. What is the priority nursing intervention?
    a. Reassuring the patient that the procedure will only take a few minutes
    b. Stop lifting the patient and reassessing and reassuring them
    c. Administering a sedative to the patient and trying again when the sedative takes effect
    d. Enlisting the help of another nurse to hold the patient steady during the procedure

11. A nurse is assessing a patient in the emergency department with suspected stroke. When the nurse asks the patient to raise their eyebrows, smile, and puff out their cheeks, what is the nurse assessing?
    a. Facial cranial nerve VII
    b. Problems with swallowing
    c. Thyroid size
    d. Sensory function of the face

12. A nurse is testing the function of the spinal cord of a patient who presents in the emergency department following a motorcycle accident. What is the focus of this assessment?
    a. Motor ability
    b. Balance and gait
    c. Reflexes
    d. Sensory abilities

13. A nurse in the emergency department is assessing a patient who is not responsive to verbal and tactile stimuli. Which assessment tool will the nurse use to rapidly evaluate the patient's neurologic status?
    a. Palpation
    b. Stethoscope
    c. Glasgow Coma Scale (GCS)
    d. Snellen Chart

14. After receiving a patient from the OR, a nurse palpates a rapid, weak, thready pulse. Which action will the nurse take?
    a. Recommend a fluid restriction.
    b. Discuss possible blood loss with the provider.
    c. Document the patient has impaired circulation.
    d. Assess for postoperative pain.

15. A nurse in the pediatric clinic plans to measure head circumference in which patient?
    a. Preschool-aged children
    b. Children aged 0 to 2 years
    c. Newborns
    d. Children aged 6 to 18 months

ALTERNATE-FORMAT QUESTIONS

Multiple Response Questions

Circle the letters that correspond to the best answers for each question.

1. A nurse at a local clinic assesses breath sounds for patients presenting with dyspnea. Which sounds will the nurse document as normal? Select all that apply.
   a. Musical or squeaking sounds or high-pitched continuous sounds auscultated during inspiration and expiration
   b. Sonorous or coarse sounds with a snoring quality auscultated during inspiration and expiration
   c. Soft, low-pitched, whispering sounds heard over most of the lung fields
   d. Medium-pitched, medium-intensity, blowing sounds heard over the first and second interspaces anteriorly
   e. Blowing, hollow sounds; auscultated over the larynx and trachea

2. The nurse is testing a patient's peripheral vision. Which actions are recommended guidelines for this test? Select all that apply.
   a. Having the patient stand or sit about 12 inches away
   b. Having the patient cover one eye with a hand or index card
   c. Asking the patient to look directly at a predetermined spot on the wall behind you
   d. Covering your own eye opposite the patient's closed eye

e. Holding one arm outstretched to one side equidistant from you and the patient, and moving your fingers into the visual fields from various peripheral points

f. Asking the patient to tell you when the fingers are first seen (you should see the fingers before the patient)

3. The nurse asks the patient to focus on a finger from 2 ft away and moves the patient's eyes through the six cardinal positions of gaze. Which cranial nerves is this nurse testing? Select all that apply.

   a. II: Optic

   b. III: Oculomotor

   c. IV: Trochlear

   d. V: Trigeminal

   e. VI: Abducens

   f. VII: Facial

4. A nurse is assessing the thorax and lungs of patients visiting a health care provider's office. Which findings would the nurse document as normal, age-related thorax and lung variations? Select all that apply.

   a. Softer auscultated breath sounds found in newborns and children

   b. Children younger than age 10 years having a slower respiratory rate than an adult

   c. Newborns and children using abdominal muscles during respirations

   d. Older adults having an increased antero-posterior chest diameter

   e. Older adults having an increase in the dorsal spinal curve (kyphosis)

   f. Older adults having increased thoracic expansion

Hot Spot Question

Place an X on the figure below to mark the spot where the nurse would auscultate to best hear the S1 heart sound.

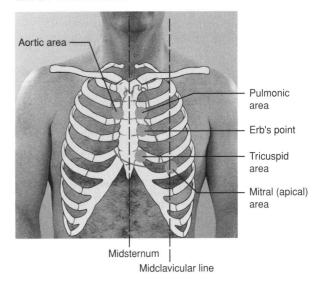

Aortic area

Pulmonic area

Erb's point

Tricuspid area

Mitral (apical) area

Midsternum

Midclavicular line

Prioritization Questions

1. Which assessment finding in an older adult will require immediate follow-up with the health care provider? Circle the letter that corresponds to the best answer.

   a. Poor skin turgor in an older adult

   b. Decreased peripheral vision

   c. Circumoral cyanosis

   d. Kyphosis

2. The nurse prioritizes assessment of the thorax in which individual? Circle the letter that corresponds to the best answer.

   a. Accountant

   b. Asbestos worker

   c. Caterer

   d. Gym teacher

Sequencing Question

1. Place the techniques of abdominal assessment in the proper order it is performed.

   a. Auscultation

   b. Inspection

   c. Palpation

   d. Percussion

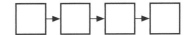

Safety, Security, and Emergency Preparedness

ASSESSING YOUR UNDERSTANDING

FILL IN THE BLANKS

1. Children younger than age _____ should not sit in the front seat of a motor vehicle.

2. Nurses educate adults that items that fit through a standard toilet paper roll can pose a _____ risk to young children under age 3.

3. Newborns of mothers who _____ have low birth weight.

4. If a child has swallowed a family member's medication, the nurse teaches the parents to first call the _____ control center (PCC).

5. Motor vehicle accidents are the number one cause of death for _____.

6. In children aged 1 to 17, death from _____ is the second leading cause of injury-related deaths.

7. Teaching individuals who are victims of intimate partner violence include removing _____ from the home and keeping their phone accessible at all times.

8. Evidence shows that self-reported history of falls is a significant predictor of future _____ and risk of fracture.

9. A strategy to prevent medication-related poisonings caused by polypharmacy is to fill all prescriptions at the _____ pharmacy.

10. The Centers for Medicare and Medicaid Services (CMS) has identified falls as a never _____ and includes falls and trauma on its list of Hospital-Acquired Conditions (HAC) for which reimbursement will be limited.

11. A _____ cause analysis is a tool used to study health care–related (actual) adverse events and close calls. The process supports the development of a culture of safety and is designed to prevent it from happening again.

12. Side rails on beds that prevent a patient from voluntarily getting out of bed are considered a _____ to be avoided.

13. To promote a culture of safety, The Joint Commission publishes an annual list of National Patient Safety _____.

14. After a patient falls, the nurse completes an _____ event report, which is included in the patient's health record.

15. A _____ is broadly defined as a tragic event of great magnitude that requires the response of people outside the involved community.

16. _____ involves the deliberate spread of pathogenic organisms into a community to cause widespread illness, fear, and panic.

MATCHING EXERCISES

Matching Exercise 1

Match the type of poisonous agent in Part A with its description in Part B.

PART A

a. Biotoxins

b. Vesicant

c. Toxic alcohols

d. Nerve agent

e. Organic solvents

f. Caustics (acids)

PART B

____ **1.** Agents that may cause damage to the heart, kidneys, and nervous system

____ **2.** Chemicals that severely burn the eyes, respiratory tract, and skin on contact

____ **3.** Highly poisonous chemicals that work by preventing the nervous system from working properly

____ **4.** Agents that damage the tissues of living things by dissolving fats and oils

____ **5.** Poisons from plants or animals that can cause harm to body systems

____ **6.** Chemicals that burn or corrode people's skin, eyes, and mucous membranes on contact

Matching Exercise 2

Match the age group in Part A with the safety precaution listed in Part B. Answers may be used more than once.

PART A

a. Fetus

b. Infant

c. Toddler and preschooler

d. School-aged child

e. Adolescent

f. Older adult

PART B

____ **1.** A young woman needs reinforcement about the risks associated with alcohol consumption, smoking, drug use, and exposure to dangers in the environment during pregnancy.

____ **2.** Safety care for this group entails never leaving them unattended, using crib rails, and monitoring objects that may be placed in the mouth and swallowed.

____ **3.** Education for this group must focus on safe driving skills, the dangers of drug and alcohol use, and creation of a healthy lifestyle as a way to respond to the stress of daily living.

____ **4.** This age group needs assistance to evaluate activities that are potentially dangerous and to discuss specific interventions that provide for safety at home, at school, and in the neighborhood.

____ **5.** Falls, fires, and motor vehicle crashes are significant hazards for this age group, and safety measures should be directed toward preventing these injuries.

____ **6.** Vigilant supervision by parents and guardians is required to anticipate hazards and provide protection for this group, with precautionary devices.

CORRECT THE FALSE STATEMENTS

Mark the item "T" for true or "F" for false. If false, correct the underlined word or words to make the statement true in the space provided.

____ **1.** An example of a modifiable intrinsic fall risk factor is postural hypotension. _____

____ **2.** In the older adult population, one out of five falls causes a serious injury such as broken bones or a head injury, with falls being the most common cause of traumatic brain injuries. _____

____ **3.** Dosing errors comprise 5% of medication poisoning cases and involve giving the medication twice by mistake, giving the medication doses too close together, giving the incorrect dose, confusing the units of measurement, and using the dispensing cup incorrectly. _____

____ **4.** Most exposures to toxic fumes occur in the workplace. _____

____ **5.** Asphyxiation may occur in any age group, but the incidence is greatest among <u>older adults</u>. _____

____ **6.** Keeping a gun in the home <u>increases</u> the risk for domestic homicide. _____

____ **7.** For the <u>school-aged child</u>, the focus of parental responsibility is on childproofing the environment. _____

____ **8.** As the primary reason for applying restraints, nurses consistently cite the risk for injury to patients and health care workers from <u>irrational behavior</u>. _____

____ **9.** Approximately one in five people who die from drowning are children aged <u>5 and younger</u>. _____

____ **10.** The number of deaths from accidental poisoning has <u>decreased</u> over the years. _____

____ **11.** Physical restraints <u>decrease</u> the possibility of serious injury due to a fall. _____

____ **12.** <u>Older adults</u> need education about ways to handle the stresses of daily life (e.g., raising a family, handling a demanding career) without relying on drugs and alcohol. _____

SHORT ANSWER

1. Identify two safety risks for each of the following age groups.

   a. Neonates and infants: _____

   _____

   b. Toddler and preschooler: _____

   _____

   c. School-aged child: _____

   _____

   d. Adolescent: _____

   _____

   e. Adult: _____

   _____

   f. Older adult: _____

   _____

2. List two examples of how the following factors can affect safety.

   a. Developmental considerations: _____

   _____

   b. Lifestyle: _____

   _____

   c. Limitation in mobility: _____

   _____

   d. Limitation in sensory perception: _____

   _____

   e. Limitation in knowledge: _____

   _____

   f. Limitation in ability to communicate:

   _____

   _____

   g. Limitation in health status: _____

   _____

   h. Limitation in psychosocial state: _____

   _____

   _____

3. Briefly explain why the following information is necessary when assessing the patient's safety.

   a. Nursing history: _____

   _____

   b. Physical assessment: _____

   _____

   c. Accident-prone behavior: _____

   _____

   d. Environment: _____

   _____

4. An older adult residing in a nursing home fell when getting out of bed to use the bathroom. List four characteristics the nurse should assess to determine whether this patient is at a greater risk for falls.

   a. _____

   b. _____

   c. _____

   d. _____

5. A home health nurse is visiting a home-bound older adult who lives with her daughter and toddler. The nurse observes the toddler pull a bottle of disinfectant out from under the sink. What education does the nurse provide about childproofing the home?

_____

_____

_____

6. List three questions you could ask a patient to assess for hazards that may cause a child to asphyxiate or choke.

a. _____

b. _____

c. _____

7. List three opportunities a nurse can use to teach students about safety.

a. _____

b. _____

c. _____

8. List five risks associated with the use of restraints.

a. _____

b. _____

c. _____

d. _____

e. _____

10. A patient with an indwelling catheter who gets up to go to the bathroom frequently has fallen and is placed in restraints for protection. Using the SBAR format, write an example of documenting the use of restraints on this patient.

S: _____

B: _____

A: _____

R: _____

11. Briefly discuss information that should be included on a safety event report, when it should be filled out, and who is responsible for recording the event.

_____

_____

_____

APPLYING YOUR KNOWLEDGE

CRITICAL THINKING QUESTIONS

1. Ask permission of friends or relatives with children living in the home to inspect their home for safety features appropriate to the children's ages. Check for poison control, fire prevention, fall protection, burn and shock protection, and so on. Share your results with the family, and explain to them what they need to do (if anything) to improve safety in their home. Reflect on the importance that different families attach to safety and its implication for your nursing practice.

2. Many people tend to take safety measures for granted. Draw on your experiences in conversations with nurses to identify safety risks for both nurses and patients in different practice settings. What can you do to minimize these risks?

3. A nurse has reminded an older adult multiple times to not bang on or pull at the IV in their nondominant arm. Discuss two strategies the nurse can use to maintain the IV.

REFLECTIVE PRACTICE: CULTIVATING QSEN COMPETENCIES

Use the following expanded scenario from Chapter 28 in your textbook to answer the questions below.

Scenario: Bessie, a 77-year-old woman, was recently discharged to her home after suffering a cerebrovascular accident (stroke). She lives alone in a small, one-bedroom apartment and uses a walker to ambulate. She says, "I have so much stuff crammed into this small apartment! I almost fell this morning going from my bedroom to the kitchen."

1. Patient-centered care/safety: What safety interventions might the nurse implement for this patient?

_____

_____

_____

2. Patient-centered care/safety: What would be a successful outcome for this patient?

_____

_____

_____

3. Patient-centered care/safety: What intellectual, interpersonal, and ethical/legal competencies are most likely to bring about the desired outcome?

_____

_____

_____

4. Teamwork and collaboration: What resources might be helpful for this patient?

_____

_____

_____

PRACTICING FOR NCLEX

MULTIPLE-CHOICE QUESTIONS

Circle the letter that corresponds to the best answer for each question.

1. A school nurse is preparing a teaching session on safety for parents of school-aged children. Which of these is an appropriate topic for the nurse to include for this age group?

   a. Selecting toys for the developmental level

   b. Providing drug, alcohol, and sexuality education

   c. Teaching stress reduction techniques

   d. Providing close supervision to prevent injuries

2. A nurse preceptor corrects the graduate nurse who is applying restraints to a patient. Which action by the new nurse requires correction by the preceptor?

   a. Padding the extremity prior to applying the restraint

   b. Explaining the procedure to the patient and family

   c. Tying the restraint in a secure double knot

   d. Maintaining the restrained extremity in an anatomical position

3. A nurse is filing a safety event report after an older adult patient tripped and fell while getting out of bed. Which action exemplifies an accurate step of this process?

   a. Adding the information in the safety event report to the patient medical record

   b. Calling the primary health care provider to fill out and sign the safety event report

   c. Providing an opinion of the patient's physical and mental condition contributing to the incident

   d. Documenting the patient's response, examination, and treatment of the patient after the incident

4. A nurse in the pediatric clinic is teaching parents when it is appropriate to move a child from a car seat to using a safety belt in the back seat of a vehicle with a lap and shoulder belt. Which finding will the nurse teach the parents indicates the child's readiness?

   a. The child's knees do not bend at the edge of the seat when back is against the vehicle's seat back.

   b. The seat belt stays low on the hips and is not resting on the soft part of the stomach.

   c. The shoulder belt does not lie on the collarbone or shoulder when fastened.

   d. The child's feet must touch the floor of the car when belted in with the lap and shoulder belt.

5. A nurse is assessing a patient who was exposed to botulism from contaminated food supplies. For which symptom will the nurse assess?

   a. Descending, symmetrical skeletal muscle paralysis

   b. Influenza-like symptoms

   c. Skin lesion with local edema that progresses, enlarges, ulcerates, and becomes necrotic

   d. Petechial hemorrhages

6. A nurse is caring for an older adult requiring wrist restraints after admission to the hospital for confusion and dehydration. The nurse notes reddened areas under the restraints where the patient tugs to free their arms. Which action will the nurse take next?

   a. Provide sedation and leave the restraints on.

   b. Remove the restraints, stay with the patient, and speak gently to them.

   c. Maintain the restraints, speak with her, explaining that she must calm down.

   d. Request the patient's family take her home because she is out of control.

7. A nurse working in a long-term care facility institutes interventions to prevent falls in older adults. Which intervention is an appropriate alternative to the use of restraints for ensuring patient safety and preventing falls?

   a. Involving family members in the patient's care

   b. Allowing the patient to use the bathroom independently

   c. Administering sedatives to prevent agitation

   d. Maintaining a high bed position to prevent the patient from getting out unassisted

8. A community health nurse is providing tips on child and home safety at a local health fair. What will the nurse include in the discussion?

   a. "Keep the phone number for the local poison control center next to the phone."

   b. "Install smoke detectors on every floor of the home."

   c. "Place medications on the highest shelf available."

   d. "Sleep with bedroom doors open to better hear children and older adults."

9. A nurse and nursing student are using the Get up and Go Test on an older adult. How does the nurse best explain the purpose of the tool to the student?

   a. "It determines readiness for discharge."

   b. "It assesses the risk for falling."

   c. "It provides information about readiness for physical therapy."

   d. "It evaluates for osteoporosis."

ALTERNATE-FORMAT QUESTIONS

Multiple-Response Questions

Circle the letters that correspond to the best answers for each question.

1. Nursing students are attending clinical in an acute care hospital during a fire drill. Which steps will the students follow to correctly use the RACE acronym? Select all that apply.

   a. R—Race to the front of the building to call for help.

   b. R—Rescue anyone in immediate danger.

   c. A—Activate the fire code system and notify the appropriate person.

   d. C—Check if the fire is contained or spreading to the hallways.

   e. C—Confine the fire by closing doors and windows.

   f. E—Extinguish the fire with an appropriate fire extinguisher.

2. A nurse is planning care for a patient with a history of frequent falls; the most recent was 30 minutes ago. When engaged in clinical reasoning related to fall prevention, which evidence will the nurse consider? Select all that apply

   a. A person with a history of falling is likely to fall again.

   b. Some people are more accident prone than others.

   c. Fires are responsible for most hospital incidents.

   d. Between 15% and 25% of falls result in fractures or soft tissue injury.

   e. A patient receiving diuretics or analgesics is at higher risk for falls.

   f. The reasonably prudent nurse is likely to be found liable if a patient is injured during a fall.

3. A nurse is teaching parents of toddlers how to prevent accidents and promote safety. Which age-appropriate interventions does the nurse include in the discussion? Select all that apply

   a. "Supervise the child closely to prevent injury."

   b. "Childproof the house to ensure that medications and poisonous products are locked."

   c. "Instruct the child to wear proper safety equipment when riding bicycles or scooters."

   d. "Do not leave the child alone in the bathtub or near water."

   e. "Provide drug, alcohol, and sexuality education."

   f. "Practice emergency evacuation measures with the child."

4. A nurse is applying restraints to a confused patient who has threatened the safety of their roommate. Which actions will the nurse use when applying restraints? Select all that apply.

   a. Checking facility policy for the application of restraints and securing a health care provider's order

   b. Choosing the most restrictive type of device that allows the least amount of mobility

   c. Padding bony prominences

d. For a restraint applied to an extremity, ensuring that the restraint is tight enough that a finger cannot be inserted between the restraint and the patient's wrist or ankle

e. Fastening the restraint to the side rail

f. Removing the restraint at least every 2 hours or according to facility policy and patient need

5. A community health nurse is providing education at the local community center on disaster preparedness. What will the nurse include in the teaching session? Select all that apply.

a. "Have emergency food supplies on hand."

b. "Assemble medications."

c. "Monitor sources that provide reliable information."

d. "Bring copies of insurance cards if leaving home."

e. "Develop a family disaster plan."

f. "Plan to carry antibiotics in case of a bioterrorist attack."

Sequencing Question

1. Place the following steps for applying restraints to a patient in the order in which they should occur.

a. Explain the reason for use of restraints to the patient and family.

b. Determine the need for restraints and assess patient's physical condition, behavior, and mental status.

c. Fasten restraint to the bed frame, not the bed rail.

d. Apply restraints according to manufacturer's directions.

e. Perform hand hygiene; document the reason for restraining the patient.

f. Perform hand hygiene.

g. Remove the restraint at least every 2 hours; reassure the patient at regular intervals and assess for signs of sensory deprivation.

h. Confirm facility policy for application of restraints and secure health care provider's order.

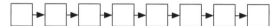

Prioritization Question

1. A nurse is working in a facility when they see smoke coming from the utility closet. Which action will the nurse take first? Circle the letter that corresponds to the best answer.

a. Pull the fire alarm

b. Call the security department

c. Remove patients from the vicinity

d. Obtain a fire extinguisher

CHAPTER 29

Complementary and Integrative Health

ASSESSING YOUR UNDERSTANDING

FILL IN THE BLANKS

1. A nurse planning care for a patient who believes in traditional Chinese medicine (TCM) helps the patient balance yin and _____, the belief that two opposing, yet complementary forces provide a natural order and interconnectedness with the universe.

2. A nurse's philosophy of patient care focuses on the body, mind, and emotions of the individual in order to heal the entire person. This nurse is practicing _____ nursing.

3. _____ consists of placing very thin, short, sterile needles at particular points believed to be centers of nerve and vascular tissue for purpose of pain management and restoring Qi.

4. A nurse guides a patient to use all five senses to focus on pleasant images to replace negative or stressful feelings promoting relaxation and healing. This nurse is engaging the patient in use guide _____.

5. A nurse recommends the use of _____ supplements, chemical compounds that contain ingredients believed to promote health, for a patient diagnosed with anorexia.

6. A nurse who provides a back massage using scented oils is using the complementary health approach (CHA) known as _____.

7. Nurses who use their hands on or near the body with the intent to heal are using a process of energy exchange known as therapeutic _____.

8. A nurse cautions a patient who wishes to use ginkgo biloba that this supplement should not be taken if the patient takes anticoagulants due to its effect on _____.

9. _____ medicine is a system in which medical doctors and health care professionals, such as nurses, pharmacists, and therapists, treat symptoms and diseases using drugs, radiation, or surgery.

10. The combination of complementary health and conventional health approaches in a coordinated manner refers to _____ health.

MATCHING EXERCISE

Match the term in Part A with its description in Part B.

PART A

a. Ayurveda

b. Yoga

c. Traditional Chinese medicine

d. Acupuncture

e. Qi gong

f. Homeopathy

PART B

_____ **1.** Uses thin, short, sterile needles, placed at meridians to restore balance and contribute to healing

_____ **2.** Supports and restores the body using techniques and medicines that are geared to strengthen the body's own healing ability

_____ **3.** Consists of a set of exercises that promote health through various physical postures

_____ **4.** System of postures, exercises (gentle and dynamic), breathing techniques, and visualization

_____ **5.** Balances body, mind, and spirit using key concepts of universal interconnectedness among people, their health, the universe, and the body's constitution and life forces

_____ **6.** Health and disease relate to a balance of yin and yang energy that shape the world and all life

SHORT ANSWER

1. Briefly describe the following CHAs and related nursing considerations.

    a. Ayurveda: _____

    _____

    Nursing considerations: _____

    b. Yoga: _____

    _____

    Nursing considerations: _____

    c. Qi gong: _____

    _____

    Nursing considerations: _____

    _____

2. Describe three mind–body therapies you might use for a patient experiencing unrelieved pain.

    a. _____

    _____

    b. _____

    _____

    c. _____

    _____

3. Describe the four scientific principles used in Therapeutic Touch.

    a. _____

    b. _____

    c. _____

    d. _____

4. Describe how the nursing care plan would differ for a patient diagnosed with leukemia when using Shamanism as a spiritual approach.

    _____

    _____

    _____

5. Explain how the following interventions can promote healing.

    a. Nutritional therapy: _____

    _____

    b. Aromatherapy: _____

    _____

    c. Music: _____

    _____

6. List and give an example of the four types or domains of CHA described by the National Center for Complementary and Alternative Medicine.

    a. _____

    _____

    b. _____

    _____

    c. _____

    _____

    d. _____

    _____

APPLYING YOUR KNOWLEDGE

CRITICAL THINKING QUESTION

1. Discuss how you might change your nursing plan to include CHA when caring for the following patients.

    a. Patient with end-stage AIDS receiving hospice care: _____

    _____

    _____

b. Resident living in a long-term care facility who has Alzheimer's disease: _____

_____

_____

REFLECTIVE PRACTICE: CULTIVATING QSEN COMPETENCIES

Use the following expanded scenario from Chapter 29 in your textbook to answer the questions below.

Scenario: Sylvia, a middle-aged woman, is scheduled for abdominal surgery next week. She comes to the outpatient clinic for preoperative evaluation and laboratory testing and says, "I'm really anxious about the surgery, but I don't want to take any medicines. Is there anything I can do to help me relax?"

1. Patient-centered care, safety, evidence-based practice: What type of CHA might the nurse suggest to promote relaxation for Sylvia?

_____

_____

_____

2. Evidence based practice, safety and informatics: What would be a successful outcome for Sylvia?

_____

_____

_____

3. Safety/evidence-based practice: What intellectual, technical, and interpersonal competencies are most likely to bring about the desired outcome?

_____

_____

_____

4. Teamwork and collaboration: What resources might be helpful for Sylvia?

_____

_____

_____

PRACTICING FOR NCLEX

MULTIPLE-CHOICE QUESTIONS

Circle the letter that corresponds to the best answer for each question.

1. A nurse works in an office with allopathic health care providers. For which patient would this type of medicine be most effective?
   a. Patient whose spinal cord was severed in a motor vehicle accident
   b. Patient diagnosed with eczema
   c. Patient who has chronic obstructive pulmonary disease
   d. Patient who has rheumatoid arthritis

2. A nurse is caring for a patient whose treatment has been based on the Ayurveda medical system. Which nursing intervention best incorporates the patient's beliefs into the nursing plan?
   a. Basing practice on the yin-yang theory
   b. Preparing the patient for exercises that help the patient regulate *qi*
   c. Helping the patient to balance their body, mind, and spirit
   d. Including the patient's shaman in the plan of care

3. A nurse is caring for a Native American male hospitalized following a myocardial infarction who asks to see their medicine man. Which of these reflects the nurse's best response?
   a. Informing the patient that he may visit with his medicine man upon discharge
   b. Supporting the patient's visit with the medicine man during their hospitalization
   c. Stating that while in the hospital, it is necessary to follow traditional medicine
   d. Asking the patient to concentrate on getting better and following their care plan

4. For which patient might the nurse need to alter the plan of care based on the principles of the patient's chosen medical system?
   a. Patient who visits a chiropractor
   b. Patient who believes in a strong mind–body connection
   c. Patient who is being treated by a naturopathic provider
   d. Patient who is being treated by an allopathic provider

5. A nurse is teaching a patient to use meditation techniques to promote mental calmness and physical relaxation. Which nursing intervention can the nurse use to facilitate this process?

a. Helping the patient to assume a specific, comfortable posture

b. Providing a stimulating environment in which to conduct the meditation

c. Teaching the patient to have multiple focal points

d. Promoting a closed attitude to avoid judgments and distractions

6. A nurse is caring for a patient who is experiencing moderate to severe pain postoperatively. To engage the patient's participation, which CHA will the nurse use to achieve effective pain control?

a. Acupuncture

b. Therapeutic touch

c. Botanical supplements

d. Guided imagery

ALTERNATE-FORMAT QUESTIONS

Multiple-Response Questions

Circle the letters that correspond to the best answers for each question.

1. A nurse who incorporates CHAs into their nursing practice is caring for a patient in a rehabilitation facility. Which CHA could the nurse discuss with this patient? Select all that apply.

a. Investigating herbs that may stimulate the patient's immune system

b. Encouraging the patient to join a yoga class when medically cleared

c. Administering pain medication prescribed by the primary care provider

d. Scheduling diagnostic tests for the patient

e. Teaching the patient how to meditate

f. Using guided imagery to relieve patient anxiety

2. A nurse uses healing touch when caring for hospitalized patients. For which patients would this practice be most appropriate? Select all that apply.

a. Patient with a surgical wound

b. Patient who has unrelenting pain

c. Patient whose energy field is unbalanced

d. Patient who is overweight

e. Patient who leaves the hospital against medical advice

f. Patient who is being prepared for a surgical procedure

3. Patients, families, health care providers, and health care institutions increasingly expect nurses to be knowledgeable about CHA and use them in their nursing practices. Which statements most accurately represent the role of CHA in nursing today? Select all that apply.

a. The knowledge base in nursing is expanding to include information on CHA.

b. Certification is available for nurses wishing to practice holistic nursing.

c. Graduate-level specialization in holistic nursing is available at some universities.

d. The development of CHA is market and patient driven.

e. CHA will eventually replace traditional nursing in many health care facilities.

f. Practitioners of CHA are strictly regulated by the government.

4. A nurse is teaching a patient about the use of herbs and supplements as part of an integrated treatment plan. What teaching points will the nurse include? Select all that apply.

a. "Go online to buy herbs and supplements."

b. "Whenever possible, buy products with more than one ingredient."

c. "Buy herbs and supplements that are standardized."

d. "Give the product adequate time to work."

e. "Be knowledgeable about the product and its therapeutic actions."

f. "Take a higher than usual dose of herbs to initiate the therapeutic effect."

5. A nurse is explaining the method of allopathic medicine to a patient. Which statements describe this approach to medicine? Select all that apply.

a. "Curing is accomplished by internal agents."

b. "Illness occurs in either the mind or the body, which are separate entities."

c. "Illness is a manifestation of imbalance or disharmony and is a process."

d. "Curing seeks to destroy the invading organism or repair the affected part."

e. "Healing is done by the patient."

f. "Health is the absence of disease."

6. A nurse is teaching an overweight patient a holistic approach to choosing foods. Which teaching points would the nurse include? Select all that apply.

   a. "Eat foods that are in season."

   b. "Avoid organically grown foods."

   c. "Reduce intake of refined and natural sugars."

   d. "Consider adopting a vegetarian diet."

   e. "Increase intake of dairy products."

   f. "Replace refined sugars with artificial sweeteners."

Prioritization Question

1. The nurse in the medical clinic is caring for a patient who takes echinacea, an herbal preparation, to prevent illness. Which of these situations requires the nurse to prioritize further education? Circle the letter corresponding to the best answer.

   a. Patient states that this may help ward off colds and illnesses

   b. Patient mentions they enjoy cooking with natural herbs and spices

   c. Patient states they will give this to their school-aged children this winter

   d. Patient states they take this supplement in the evening

CHAPTER 30

Medications

ASSESSING YOUR UNDERSTANDING

FILL IN THE BLANKS

1. A liquid medication called a(n) _____ should be shaken before use.

2. The _____ name is assigned by the manufacturer that first develops a drug and identifies the drug's active ingredient.

3. The _____ name is also called the brand name, which is selected by the pharmaceutical company (companies) that sell(s) the drug and is protected by trademark.

4. Clinical manifestations of a drug _____ can include rash, urticaria, fever, diarrhea, nausea, and vomiting; the most serious allergic effect is an anaphylactic reaction (anaphylaxis).

5. Drug _____ occurs when the body becomes accustomed to the effects of a particular drug over a period of time. Larger doses of the drug are needed to produce the desired effect.

6. _____ effects are specific groups of symptoms related to drug therapy that carry risk for permanent damage or death.

7. A(n) _____ effect (sometimes called *paradoxical effect*) is any unusual or peculiar response to a drug that may manifest itself by overresponse, under-response, or even the opposite of the expected response.

8. _____ drug effects have the potential to cause developmental defects in the embryo or fetus.

9. Body _____ area is expressed in square meters (m^2) and is used to calculate drug doses for infants, children, and others.

10. When administering otic medication to an adult, the nurse positions the pinna of the ear _____ and _____.

11. The nurse can expect a patient with liver disease to be at risk for _____ when taking a medication metabolized by the liver.

12. Because of the risk of small glass shards falling into the ampule, use a _____ needle to remove the medication from the vial and then discard it appropriately.

13. When considering mixing two medications in one syringe, first ensure that the two drugs are _____.

14. Insulin is typically available in multidose vials with a commonly used scale of U100. This designation means that _____ units of insulin are contained in 1 mL of solution.

15. The technique of adding a diluent to a powdered drug is called _____.

FILL IN THE BLANKS

Calculate the proper medication dose. Include a numeric answer and the units for administration (i.e., tablet(s), mL, etc.).

A health care provider has written prescriptions for the following medications. Based on the prescriptions, calculate how much you will administer on the line provided. Use both a numeric value and units (e.g., mL, tablet, etc.).

1. Prescription: gentamicin 60 mg IV. On hand: gentamicin 80 mg/2 mL. Administer:

   _____

   _____

2. Prescription: Mestinon 30 mg orally. On hand: Mestinon 60 mg/tab. Administer:

   _____

   _____

3. Prescription: amitriptyline 75 mg orally. On hand: amitriptyline 25 mg/tab. Administer:

   _____

   _____

4. Prescription: penicillin V 250 mg orally. On hand: penicillin V 500 mg/tab. Administer:

   _____

   _____

5. Prescription: naproxen 250 mg orally. On hand: naproxen 500 mg/tab. Administer:

   _____

   _____

6. Prescription: Pro-Banthine 15 mg orally. On hand: Pro-Banthine 5 mg/tab. Administer:

   _____

   _____

7. Prescription: Lanoxin 0.125 mg via NG tube. On hand: Lanoxin 0.250 mg/tab. Administer:

   _____

   _____

8. Prescription: furosemide 20 mg orally. On hand: furosemide 10 mg/tab. Administer:

   _____

   _____

9. Prescription: Dexamethasone 4 mg IV. On hand: Dexamethasone 8 mg/mL. Administer:

   _____

   _____

10. Prescription: levofloxacin 750 mg orally. On hand: capsules of 1 g, 500 mg, and 250 mg. Administer: _____

   _____

MATCHING EXERCISES

Matching Exercise 1

Match the term in Part A to the definition in Part B.

PART A

a. Trade
b. Drug classifications, or drug classes
c. Pharmacotherapeutics
d. Bioavailability
e. Loading dose

PART B

____ 1. Refers to groups of drugs that share similar characteristics, whether by their pharmaceutical or therapeutic properties

____ 2. These names are capitalized while generic names are presented in lowercase

____ 3. Larger than normal dose to quickly achieve the therapeutic effect

____ 4. Subtopic of pharmacology addressing "therapeutic uses and effects of drugs," also known as the clinical indication(s)

____ 5. Portion of a drug that reaches the systemic circulation and can act on the cells

Matching Exercise 2

Match the types of drug preparations in Part A with their descriptions listed in Part B.

PART A

a. Ointment
b. Capsule
c. Tablet
d. Elixir
e. Suppository
f. Syrup

PART B

___ **1.** Medication combined with water and sugar solution

___ **2.** Medication in a clear liquid containing water, alcohol, sweeteners, and flavoring

___ **3.** Semisolid preparation containing a drug to be applied externally; also called an *unction*

___ **4.** Small, solid dose of medication; compressed or molded; may be any size or shape, or enteric coated

___ **5.** Easily melted medication preparation in a firm base, such as gelatin, that is inserted into the body

___ **6.** Powder or gel form of an active drug enclosed in a gelatinous container; may also be called liquigel

Matching Exercise 3

Match the type of drug delivery in Part A to the body site in Part B.

PART A

a. Subcutaneous injection

b. Intramuscular injection

c. Intravenous injection

d. Intra-arterial injection

e. Inhalation

f. Intraosseous injection

PART B

___ **1.** Bone

___ **2.** Muscle

___ **3.** Artery

___ **4.** Vein

___ **5.** Below skin, fatty tissue

___ **6.** Pulmonary

SHORT ANSWER

1. List two categories for drug classification.

a. _____

b. _____

2. Explain the following processes by which drugs alter cell physiology.

a. Drug–receptor interactions: _____

_____

b. Drug–enzyme interactions: _____

_____

3. Give an example of how the following factors affect drug action.

a. Developmental stage of patient: _____

_____

b. Weight: _____

_____

c. Genetic factors: _____

_____

d. Cultural factors: _____

_____

e. Hepatic disease: _____

_____

f. Time of administration: _____

_____

4. Give three examples of situations in which you would question a medication prescription.

a. _____

b. _____

c. _____

5. Briefly describe the following four types of medication supply systems.

a. Stock supply system (computerized automated dispensing cabinets [ADCs]): _____

_____

b. Unit-dose dispensing system: _____

_____

c. Medication cart: _____

_____

d. Barcode-enabled medication administration (BCMA): _____

_____

6. Explain when and how the nurse carries out the three checks and eleven rights of administering medication.

a. Three checks: _____

_____

_____

b. Eleven rights: _____

_____

_____

7. Your patient tells you that they refuse to take the medication prescribed because it tastes "disgusting." List three techniques you could use to mask the taste.

   a. _____

   b. _____

   c. _____

8. Explain how the following factors would affect the type of equipment a nurse would choose for an injection.

   a. Route of administration: _____

   b. Viscosity of the solution: _____

   c. Volume to be administered: _____

   d. Body size: _____

   e. Type of medication: _____

9. List four steps that should be followed when a medication error occurs.

   a. _____

   b. _____

   c. _____

   d. _____

10. Describe the use of the following types of prepackaged medications.

   a. Ampules: _____

   b. Vials: _____

   c. Prefilled cartridges: _____

11. Fill in the missing information to explain how the following prescriptions would be administered. Use a pharmacology reference for medication information.

   a. Atenolol (Tenormin), 50 mg, PO BID, hold for BP less than 110 systolic

      Upon entering the room, the nurse introduces themselves and performs hand (1) _____. The nurse recognizes the medication name atenolol as the (2) _____ name, when the patient refers to it as Tenormin. Next, the nurse (3) _____ the patient using (4) _____ and (5) _____, comparing it to the eMAR. The nurse assesses the patient's (6) _____ signs prior to administration to avoid adverse reactions.

      The nurse teaches the patient that this medication is given by the (7) _____ route and will be given (8) _____ times daily. Prior to administering this antihypertensive medication, the nurse notes the blood pressure is 102/70. Based on this assessment, the nurse plans to (9) _____ the medication and (10) _____ the prescriber. Documentation in the MAR and electronic health record will include (11) _____, (12) _____, (13) _____, and (14) _____.

   b. Heparin 5,000 unit subcutaneously twice daily

      After hand hygiene and patient (1) _____, the nurse explains that the medication is being given to prevent blood clots and that the injection will be given in the (2) _____. The nurse then selects an appropriate syringe for the (3) _____ of medication (generally 1 or 3 mL). First, the nurse injects a volume of air equivalent to the volume of heparin needed, keeping the vial on a flat surface. The nurse then inverts the vial, withdrawing the medication, ensuring there are no air (4) _____ that could interfere with accurate dosing. The nurse performs the (5) _____ of the dose of medication and vial against the MAR (second check), and, prior to putting the vial away, checks the dose, syringe, and vial again (third check). The nurse gathers a fold of skin on the patient's abdomen and injects the medication at a 90-degree angle (45 degrees if the patient is extremely slender). When withdrawing the needle, the nurse applies (6) _____, without rubbing the injection site.

   c. NPH insulin 45 units daily SQ in the am

      After hand hygiene, active patient identification, and the first check of the vial of insulin against the eMAR, the nurse withdraws insulin from the vial using a(n) (1) _____ syringe.

Prior to administering the insulin injection, the nurse assesses the patient's (2) _____ blood glucose, whether they have (3) _____ or had beverages, and the (4) _____ routinely used at that time of day. The nurse continues (5) _____ glucose monitoring and observes for symptoms of (6) _____.

d. Nitroglycerin ointment (Nitro-Bid) 1/2 inch or 7.5 mg to anterior chest wall q8 hours

The nurse applies clean (1) _____; removes the old patch, folding it, medication side facing (2) _____; and wipes the area as needed. Using the supplied paper, the nurse measures out (3) _____ inch(es). The nurse writes the (4) _____, (5) _____, and their initials on a piece of tape long enough to cover the patch. The nurse places the patch on a new, non-(6) _____ area on the anterior chest wall and secures it with tape, then documents the removal

and new site of application. The nurse assesses the patient's blood (7) _____ before and after administration and for (8) _____ pain and dizziness.

e. Oxycodone 5 mg with acetaminophen 325 mg 1 tablet PO

q4 hours PRN for pain

When the patient reports pain, clarify the (1) _____ and (2) _____ of the patient's pain. Verify allergies and when the last doses were administered to ensure the (3) _____ interval has elapsed, and the maximum daily dose of acetaminophen is not (4) _____. Administer one tablet orally if indicated. Evaluate the medication's (5) _____ after administration. Assess for (6) _____ and presence of (7) _____.

12. You are preparing a patient for discharge who has prescriptions for ciprofloxacin at home. Identify the information you will need to provide medication education in the chart below. Use a pharmacology reference for medication information.

Method	Ciprofloxacin
Dosage range	
Possible route of administration	
Frequency/schedule	
Desired effects	
Possible adverse effects	
Signs and symptoms of toxic drug effects	
Special instructions	
Nursing/collaborative management of adverse effects	

13. Prior to administering medications, a nurse notes the therapeutic level of a medication is twice the therapeutic value. Explain what actions the nurse should take related to medication administration for the patient.

_____

_____

14. A nurse is preparing to carry out a prescription to draw a peak and trough level of the antibiotic vancomycin for a patient. Explain what actions the nurse will take to properly carry out this prescription.

_____

_____

15. A nurse retrieves a controlled substance from the automated dispensing cabinet. The system states that there are 25 tablets left and asks the nurse to confirm, but the nurse finds 24 tablets. What action must the nurse take to rectify the situation?

_____

_____

16. Per the 2020 National Patient Safety Goals, describe the steps the nurse takes to administer medications in a facility using barcode scanning with the electronic medication administration record.

_____

_____

APPLYING YOUR KNOWLEDGE

CRITICAL THINKING QUESTIONS

1. Think about your responsibilities when administering medication and then describe how you would respond in the following situations:

   a. A health care provider who is in a hurry prescribes a medication for your patient. After the provider leaves, you read the prescription and do not understand why your patient would need the medication prescribed. Because you are legally responsible for medications administered, what would you do?

   b. You bring a medication to a patient, who tells you, "That's not my pill." What should you do?

REFLECTIVE PRACTICE: CULTIVATING QSEN COMPETENCIES

Use the following expanded scenario from Chapter 30 in your textbook to answer the questions below.

Scenario: François is an older adult with a wound infection requiring intravenous antibiotic therapy. He is scheduled to receive his next dose at 1,000 hours. The medication delivered by the pharmacy is labeled with the correct drug and dose, but with a different patient's name.

1. Safety/teamwork and collaboration: How might the nurse use blended nursing skills to respond to this medication error? What resources might be helpful in preventing future errors?

_____

_____

2. Patient-centered care/safety: What would be a successful outcome for this patient?

_____

_____

3. Safety/evidence-based practice: What intellectual, technical, and ethical/legal competencies are most likely to bring about the desired outcome?

_____

_____

4. Informatics/safety: When the nurse scans the barcode, the system states that the medication and dose is correct. What action is safest, given the situation?

_____

_____

PRACTICING FOR NCLEX

MULTIPLE-CHOICE QUESTIONS

Circle the letter that corresponds to the best answer for each question.

1. A new graduate and preceptor are administering an intradermal tuberculin test. Which incorrect action by the graduate requires correction by the preceptor?

   a. Validating the patient's identity using name and date of birth

   b. Placing pressure on the site when a wheal or blister appears

c. Inserting the needle at a 10-degree angle with the bevel up during injection

d. Documenting the injection immediately after administration

2. A nurse is administering a subcutaneous injection of insulin to a patient. After agreeing on the injection site, which action would the nurse take next?

a. Identifying the appropriate landmarks for the site chosen

b. Cleansing the area around the injection site with alcohol

c. Using a firm, back-and-forth motion to cleanse the site

d. Removing the needle cap with their dominant hand, pulling it straight off

3. When a nurse is administering a subcutaneous injection to a patient, the needle pulls out of the skin when the skin fold is released. What action will the nurse take next?

a. Pull out and discard the needle in the appropriate sharps container.

b. Discard the equipment and start the procedure from the beginning, selecting a new site.

c. Engage the safety feature on the needle, discarding the syringe appropriately.

d. Document the incident and inform the primary care provider.

4. A nurse is administering an injection of insulin to a 5-year-old who has diabetes. Which statement by the nurse would take into consideration this child's developmental level?

a. "Don't worry, this won't hurt a bit."

b. "If you don't cry, I will give you a sticker."

c. "Try not to move, or this will hurt more."

d. "This will feel just like a little pinch."

5. A health care provider writes a prescription for an analgesic as: Morphine 2 mg IV PRN for a postoperative patient. What information does the nurse note is missing from the prescription?

a. The need to assess for pain every hour

b. How frequently the medication may be given

c. That this prescription is given one time only

d. To give the medication immediately

6. A home care nurse is teaching a patient with diabetes how to self-administer insulin. Which teaching point is most important to include in the teaching plan?

a. "Use the same area of the body at the same time every day."

b. "Rotate sites on the same part of the body for a week."

c. "Reuse syringes and needles up to three times."

d. "Store needles and syringes in a glass container."

7. During administration of an intramuscular injection, a nurse hits the patient's bone. What would be the appropriate initial response of the nurse to this situation?

a. Removing the needle and having another nurse stay with the patient while informing the primary care provider

b. Withdrawing the needle, applying a new needle to the syringe, and administering the injection in an alternate site

c. Documenting the incident according to facility policy and then removing the needle and syringe and discarding them

d. Removing the needle and discarding the needle and syringe, then calling the primary care provider

8. A nurse preparing medication for a patient is called away to an emergency. What action will the nurse take?

a. Have another nurse guard the preparations.

b. Put the medications back in the containers.

c. Have another nurse finish preparing and administering the medications.

d. Lock the medications in a room and finish them upon return.

9. A nurse is administering daily medications to a hospitalized patient. What action best describes active identification of the patient prior to administration?

a. Calling the patient by name and ensuring the patient states "yes"

b. Comparing the patient's ID bracelet to the MAR and patient's stated name

c. Checking the patient's health record, room number, and date of birth

d. Validating the patient's name with family or significant others

10. A camp nurse has a prescription to administer epinephrine to a child if stung by a bee. Which route of administration does the nurse anticipate using for this emergency?

a. Subcutaneous injection

b. Oral route

c. Transdermal patch

d. Nebulized inhalation

11. A nurse is administering a hepatitis B vaccination to an adult patient. What site will the nurse select for this injection?

a. Vastus lateralis

b. Deltoid muscle

c. Ventrogluteal

d. Dorsogluteal

12. A nurse is administering medications to an older adult patient. The nurse carefully monitors for drug toxicity due to which age-related factor?

a. Decreased adipose tissue and increased total body fluid in proportion to total body mass

b. Increased number of protein-binding sites

c. Increased kidney function, resulting in increased filtration and excretion

d. Decline in liver function and production of enzymes needed for drug metabolism

13. During administration of the antibiotic gentamicin, the patient develops hypotension, bronchospasms, and rapid, thready pulse. Which medications does the nurse plan to administer for this emergency?

a. Antibiotic, antihistamines, and isoproterenol

b. Bronchodilators, antihistamines, and vasodilators

c. Epinephrine, antihistamines, and bronchodilators

d. Antihistamines, vasodilators, and bronchoconstrictors

14. A patient has a prescription for azithromycin, 500 mg every 6 hours. The medication is available in 250-mg capsules. How many capsules will the nurse administer?

a. 1/2 capsule

b. 1 capsule

c. 2 capsules

d. 3 capsules

15. An oral preparation is prescribed for administration via nasogastric tube. Which nursing action is essential to promote safe medication administration?

a. Verifying the tube placement before administration

b. Having the patient swallow the pills around the tube

c. Flushing the tube with 30 mL saline before medication administration

d. Bringing the liquids to room temperature before administration

16. A nurse is preparing to administer an IM medication using the Z-track method? What action reflects proper injection technique?

a. Pulling the skin and tissue to the side before inserting the needle

b. Applying pressure to the injection site

c. Injecting the medication quickly, and steadily withdrawing the needle

d. Not massaging the site because it may cause irritation

17. Which of the following is essential when teaching the parents of a toddler to administer 5 mL or 1 teaspoon of an antibiotic suspension?

a. "Use the smallest teaspoon in the drawer."

b. "Use the child's favorite spoon."

d. "Use an infant dropper."

e. "Use a medication-measuring spoon."

18. A nurse and AP are caring for a group of surgical patients. Which activities can the nurse safely delegate to the AP?

a. Administering an oral antibiotic capsule

b. Documenting intake of liquids taken with medications

c. Administering oral acetaminophen for pain

d. Discussing injection site rotation with a patient with diabetes

19. A nurse is administering medications via nasogastric tube. Which medication must the nurse shake prior to measuring?

a. Medication dispensed in an ampule

b. IVPB medication

c. Insulin

d. Oral antibiotic in a suspension

20. How does a nurse convert 0.8 grams to milligrams?

a. Move the decimal point 2 places to the right.

b. Move the decimal point 3 places to the right.

c. Move the decimal point 2 places to the left.

d. Move the decimal point 3 places to the left.

21. A nurse is administering 7 AM medications to a patient. Using the eMAR below, what action is appropriate for the nurse to take?

Medication	Time	Administered	Withheld
Heparin 5,000 units subcutaneously every 12 hours	10 PM	AM	
Regular insulin 8 units subcutaneously	7 AM		
NPH 20 units subcutaneously	7 AM		

a. Obtaining a 3-mL syringe with 5/8-inch needle to administer heparin

b. Mixing the insulins in the same syringe, drawing up the regular insulin first

c. Injecting the insulin at a 45-degree angle

d. Placing the heparin injection 1 inch from the previous injection site

c. Checking that the dose selector is at 2 before dialing units of insulin for the dose

d. After administering the injection, pushing the button on the pen halfway in

e. Dialing the dose selector to 2 units to perform an "air shot" to get rid of bubbles

f. Administering the injection by holding the pen in the palm of their hand perpendicular to the forearm

ALTERNATE-FORMAT QUESTIONS

Multiple-Response Questions

Circle the letters that correspond to the best answers for each question.

1. A nurse is administering intramuscular injections to a group of patients on a surgical unit. Which actions are correct? Select all that apply.

a. Avoiding massaging the injection site after administering heparin

b. Selecting the deltoid for administration of 3 mL of IM antibiotic

c. Putting pressure on the injection site after using the Z-track technique

d. Administering a vaccine to an adult in the deltoid site

e. Raising a piggyback antibiotic higher than the main IV during infusion

f. Before administering insulin, ensuring the patient has eaten their meal

2. A nurse is teaching a patient how to use an insulin pen. Which steps reflect recommended procedure? Select all that apply.

a. After administering the injection, keeping the button depressed and counting to 3 before removal

b. Holding the pen upright and tap to force any air bubbles to the top

3. During medication administration through a drug-infusion lock using the saline flush, the patient complains of pain at the site. Which interventions will the nurse take at this time? Select all that apply.

a. Stopping the medication and assessing the site for signs of infiltration and phlebitis

b. Flushing the medication lock with normal saline again to recheck patency

c. If the site is within normal limits, resuming medication administration at a slower rate

d. Immediately stopping the medication, removing the medication lock, and restarting at a new site

e. Notifying the primary care provider that the site has been infiltrated

f. Finish administering the medication and then changing the medication lock

4. While administering an intermittent piggyback intravenous infusion of medication to a patient, a nurse observes a cloudy, white precipitate forming in the IV tubing. What actions will the nurse take? Select all that apply.

a. Assess the IV site for signs of infiltration or phlebitis.

b. Stop the IV and medication flow immediately.

c. Prime the secondary tubing by "backfilling" it.

d. Clamp the IV at the site nearest to the patient.

e. Replace the tubing on primary and secondary infusions.

f. Check for medication incompatibilities after administering.

5. A nurse is preparing to administer optic medications to a patient with glaucoma. What actions will the nurse take for correct administration? Select all that apply.

a. Perform hand hygiene and put on gloves.

b. Clean the patient's eyelids and lashes with a cotton ball soaked in water from the outer to inner canthus.

c. Tilt the patient's head back slightly if they are sitting, or place their head on a pillow if they are lying down.

d. Have the patient look up and focus on something on the ceiling.

e. Place their thumb near the margin of the patient's lower eyelid and exert pressure upward over the bony prominence of the cheek.

f. Squeeze the container and allow the prescribed number of drops to fall into the patient's cornea.

6. Which actions will the nurse perform when correctly instilling otic medications? Select all that apply.

a. Inserting the tip of the medication container or dropper into the auditory canal

b. Cleansing the external ear with cotton balls moistened with water or normal saline solution

c. After administration, positioning the patient in bed on their affected side for 5 minutes

d. Withdrawing the medication into the dropper, returning the excess to the stock bottle

e. Pulling the cartilaginous portion of the pinna down and back in a child younger than age 3 years

f. Gently pressing the tragus a few times

7. Which actions will the nurse perform when administering a subcutaneous injection correctly? Select all that apply.

a. Cleansing the injection site with an antimicrobial swab using soft up-and-down motions

b. Removing the needle cap by pulling it straight off

c. Pinching the area surrounding the injection site or spreading the skin taut at the site

d. Injecting the needle quickly at a 45- to 90-degree angle

e. Withdrawing the needle gently, at the same angle when a wheal appears

f. Withdrawing the needle quickly at the same angle at which it was inserted

8. A nurse is reviewing medication prescriptions for a patient. Which are the expected components of a medication prescription? Select all that apply.

a. Patient's name and a secondary identifier (date of birth, medical record number)

b. Date and the time when the prescription is written

c. Brand name of the drug to be administered

d. Dosage of the drug, stated in either the apothecary or metric system

e. Route by which the drug is to be administered, only if there is more than one route possible

f. Signature of the nurse carrying out the prescription

9. A nurse is working on a unit with a patient in room 2 named John Smith and a patient in room 8 named John Smith. Which actions will the nurse take when administering medications to these patients?

a. Ask each patient, "Is your name John Smith"?

b. Check each patient's armband for the patient's name.

c. Ask each patient if these are their correct medications.

d. Ask each patient the year of their birth.

e. Ensure the medications are appropriate to the patient's conditions.

f. Ask each patient their medical record number.

Theory to Practice

1. A nurse is planning to administer a subcutaneous injection of a medication to a patient who is 5 ft tall and weighs 82 lb. Which needle angle and depth would be most appropriate for this patient? Circle the letter of the correct needle.

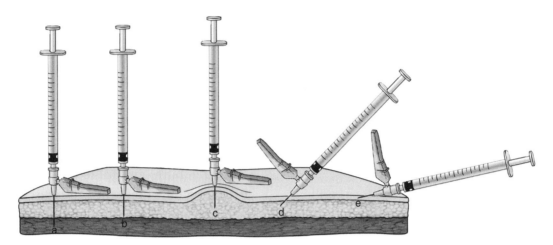

Prioritization Question

1. The nurse is evaluating the outcome of an analgesic medication administered 30 minutes ago. Which question will the nurse ask first? Circle the letter corresponding to the best answer.

   a. "Do you have any medication allergies?"

   b. "Do you have any questions about the medication?"

   c. "What time of day do you take this medication at home?"

   d. "Can you rate the severity of your pain for me?"

31

Perioperative Nursing

ASSESSING YOUR UNDERSTANDING

FILL IN THE BLANKS

1. Caring for patients prior to, during, and after _____ is known as perioperative nursing.

2. A patient who is brought to the emergency department with internal bleeding is scheduled for surgery. This type of surgery is classified as surgery based on its _____.

3. A patient who schedules knee replacement surgery is having a planned surgery, also known as _____ surgery.

4. Surgery is classified as minor or major based on the degree of _____.

5. As the surgeon makes an incision in a patient undergoing gallbladder surgery, it is expected that the patient is in the _____ phase of general anesthesia.

6. A nurse teaches a patient scheduled for a colonoscopy that they will most likely receive _____ sedation.

7. _____ consent is a patient's voluntary agreement to undergo a particular procedure or treatment after receiving the appropriate information in everyday language from the health care provider.

8. _____ directives allow patients to specify instructions for health care treatment should they be unable to communicate these wishes postoperatively.

9. During The Joint Commission protocol known as the _____ protocol, the surgical team members agree on the identity of the patient, the correct surgical site, and the procedure that will be performed.

10. After completion of surgery and emergence from anesthesia, the patient is transferred to the _____.

11. The _____ is the body's first line of defense against infection.

12. The nurse directs the patient without an indwelling urinary catheter to _____ prior to receiving preoperative medications.

13. Urinary retention is suspected when a patient voids in small, _____ amounts.

14. During a surgical procedure with general anesthesia, an _____ tube may be inserted to administer the anesthetic gases and maintain patent air passages.

MATCHING EXERCISES

Matching Exercise 1

Match the title in Part A with the role of the nurse listed in Part B. Answers may be used more than once.

PART A

a. Scrub nurse

b. Circulating nurse

c. RNFA

d. APRN

PART B

___ **1.** Member of the sterile team who maintains surgical asepsis while draping and handling instruments and supplies

___ **2.** Actively assists the surgeon by providing exposure, hemostasis, and wound closure

___ **3.** Coordinates care activities and collaborates with health care providers and nurses in all phases of perioperative and postanesthesia care

___ **4.** Assesses the patient on admission to the operating room and collaborates in safely positioning the patient on the operating bed

___ **5.** Integrates case management, critical paths, and research into care of the surgical patient

___ **6.** Assists with monitoring the patient during surgery, provides additional supplies, and maintains environmental safety

Matching Exercise 2

Match the appropriate monitoring in Part A with the complication listed in Part B. Answers may be used more than once, and some items have multiple answers.

PART A

a. Measuring inspiration via incentive spirometer

b. Monitoring white blood cells

c. Measuring output of drainage devices

d. Observing for calf swelling

e. Assessing for tachycardia and hypotension

f. Auscultating for crackles in the lung fields

PART B

___ **1.** Pneumonia

___ **2.** Thrombophlebitis

___ **3.** Shock

___ **4.** Wound infection

___ **5.** Atelectasis

SHORT ANSWER

1. Briefly describe the time period for the following stages of the perioperative period.

a. Preoperative phase: _____

_____

b. Intraoperative phase: _____

_____

c. Postoperative phase: _____

_____

2. Give a brief description of the following types of surgery.

a. Based on urgency: _____

_____

_____

b. Based on degree of risk: _____

_____

_____

c. Based on purpose: _____

_____

_____

3. Describe the following three phases of anesthesia.

a. Induction: _____

_____

b. Maintenance: _____

_____

c. Emergence: _____

_____

4. Your patient is undergoing surgery to remove a lump from their breast. List six areas of information the nurse ensures are given to the patient when securing informed consent.

a. _____

b. _____

c. _____

d. _____

e. _____

f. _____

5. Indicate how each of the health problems places the patient at greater risk for postoperative complications.

a. Cardiovascular problems: _____

_____

_____

b. Pulmonary disorders: _____

_____

_____

c. Kidney and liver dysfunction: _____

_____

_____

d. Endocrine disorders: _____

_____

_____

6. Explain how you would help your patient overcome the following fears experienced in the preoperative phase.

a. Fear of the unknown: _____

_____

_____

b. Fear of pain and death: _____

_____

_____

c. Fear of changes in body image and self-concept: _____

_____

7. Describe the nurse's role related to screening tests in the preoperative period.

_____

_____

_____

_____

8. Describe how you would prepare a preoperative patient for the following conditions.

a. Surgical events and sensations: _____

_____

b. Pain management: _____

_____

9. Describe how you would prepare a patient on the day of surgery in the following areas.

a. Hygiene and skin preparation: _____

_____

_____

b. Elimination: _____

_____

_____

c. Nutrition and fluids: _____

_____

_____

d. Rest and sleep: _____

_____

_____

10. Give three examples of expected outcomes for a patient during the intraoperative phase.

a. _____

b. _____

c. _____

11. Briefly outline the assessments and interventions performed by the nurse in the PACU.

_____

_____

_____

_____

12. Prepare a teaching plan for a postoperative patient who is returning to their home. Include the family in your planning.

_____

_____

_____

_____

13. Give an example of how the following factors may present a greater surgical risk for some patients.

a. Developmental considerations: _____

_____

b. Medical history: _____

_____

c. Medications: _____

_____

d. Previous surgery: _____

_____

e. Lifestyle: _____

_____

f. Nutrition: _____

_____

_____

g. Activities of daily living: _____

_____

h. Sociocultural needs: _____

_____

14. Explain what assessment information a nurse in the PACU would document for a patient in the postoperative phase using the following guidelines.

   a. Vital signs: _____

   _____

   b. Color and temperature of skin: _____

   _____

   c. Level of consciousness: _____

   _____

   d. Intravenous fluids: _____

   _____

   e. Surgical site: _____

   _____

   f. Tubes and drains: _____

   _____

   g. Pain management: _____

   _____

   h. Position and safety: _____

   _____

   i. Comfort: _____

   _____

15. Give an example of two nursing interventions you could institute for a patient to alleviate the following postoperative problems.

   a. Nausea and vomiting: _____

   _____

   b. Thirst: _____

   _____

   c. Hiccups: _____

   _____

   d. Surgical pain: _____

   _____

APPLYING YOUR KNOWLEDGE

CRITICAL THINKING QUESTION

1. Mentally walk through a preoperative assessment for the patients described below. Develop a brief nursing care plan for each patient based on the data collected. Be sure to include preoperative care, intraoperative care, and postoperative care in your planning. Individualize the care and priorities based on differences in each patient's presentation.

   a. A 52-year-old patient who smokes a pack of cigarettes a day is scheduled to undergo coronary artery bypass surgery. The patient is overweight and says they rarely find time to exercise.

   b. A 35-year-old patient is scheduled to undergo surgery to remove a colon tumor. They underwent radiation therapy 6 weeks before the surgery date. They have a family history of colon cancer.

REFLECTIVE PRACTICE: CULTIVATING QSEN COMPETENCIES

Use the following expanded scenario from Chapter 31 in your textbook to answer the questions below.

  Scenario: Molly, a 38-year-old woman who is scheduled for a vaginal hysterectomy later in the day, arrives at the hospital at 0630. With tears in her eyes and wringing her hands, she states, "I really didn't sleep very much last night. I kept thinking about the surgery."

1. Patient-centered care: How might the nurse use blended nursing skills to implement the perioperative plan of care in a manner that respects the patient's human dignity and addresses her fears and concerns about the surgical experience?

   _____

   _____

   _____

2. Patient-centered care/evidence-based practice: What would be a successful outcome for this patient?

   _____

   _____

   _____

3. Evidence-based practice/safety: What intellectual, interpersonal, and/or ethical/legal competencies are most likely to bring about the desired outcome?

   _____

   _____

   _____

4. Teamwork and collaboration/evidence-based practice: What resources might be helpful for Molly?

_____

_____

_____

PRACTICING FOR NCLEX

MULTIPLE-CHOICE QUESTIONS

Circle the letter that corresponds to the best choice for each question.

1. A nurse expects a patient to receive what type of regional anesthesia for a cesarean delivery?
   a. Inhalation
   b. Epidural
   c. Topical
   d. Local infiltration with lidocaine

2. A nurse plans to accompany a surgeon to the patient's bedside to witness informed consent. Which situation requires further collaboration with the health care provider?
   a. The patient is confused or has received sedation.
   b. The nurse recognizes their signature is a part of a legal document which is subject to review in court.
   c. Due to the emergent nature of surgery, the health care provider documented consent obtained via telephone.
   d. The surgeon takes responsibility for securing informed consent.

3. An infant is scheduled for heart surgery. When developing the postoperative care plan, which surgical risk associated with infants does the nurse prioritize?
   a. Delayed wound healing
   b. Hypothermia or hyperthermia
   c. Congestive heart failure
   d. Gastrointestinal upset

4. A patient scheduled for surgery tells the nurse they are taking an aminoglycoside antibiotic for a kidney infection. Knowing this medication can promote neuromuscular weakness when combined with anesthesia,

the nurse plans to monitor for what postoperative complication?
   a. Hemorrhage
   b. Electrolyte imbalances
   c. Cardiovascular collapse
   d. Respiratory depression

5. A nurse is caring for a surgical patient who has diabetes mellitus. Which assessment does the nurse prioritize?
   a. Monitoring fluid and electrolyte balance
   b. Assessing wound healing
   c. Observing for respiratory depression
   d. Evaluating for altered metabolism and drug excretion

6. When preparing an obese patient for cardiac surgery, what teaching will the nurse prioritize?
   a. How to prevent delayed wound healing and wound infection
   b. Need for IV fluid and electrolytes to restore their balance
   c. Use of the incentive spirometer and frequent repositioning
   d. Reporting redness of the chest incision

7. A nurse is providing preoperative teaching for a patient regarding pain management. Which teaching point is most appropriate to include?
   a. "Be sure to ask for your 'as needed' PRN medication when the pain becomes severe."
   b. "If your pain is not relieved, ask your nurse to order a different medication."
   c. "You will receive pain medication by injection as long as you are not permitted to eat."
   d. "Most hospitals no longer use injectable pain control methods."

8. A nurse and preceptor are caring for patients in the PACU. Which action by the new nurse requires intervention by the preceptor?
   a. Instructing the patient to cough
   b. Encouraging the patient to breathe shallowly
   c. Assisting the patient with leg exercises
   d. Turning the patient in bed

9. A nursing student and primary nurse are performing assessments in the PACU. What observation does the preceptor teach the student would take priority during postanesthesia recovery?

   a. Stridor

   b. Pain

   c. Wound infection

   d. Edema

10. A nurse is providing care to a patient post cardiac surgery. What intervention will best prevent cardiovascular complications?

    a. Positioning the patient in bed with pillows placed under his knees

    b. Keeping the patient from ambulating until the day after surgery

    c. Implementing leg exercises and turning the patient in bed every 2 hours

    d. Keeping the patient cool and uncovered to prevent pyrexia

11. A nurse notes a PACU is displaying signs and symptoms of blood loss, including tachycardia and hypotension. What action will the nurse take first?

    a. Removing extra covers on the patient to keep temperature down

    b. Placing the patient in a flat position with legs elevated 45 degrees

    c. Discontinuing the IV fluids and medications

    d. Placing the patient in the prone position

12. The surgeon entered a prescription for a patient to remain NPO until surgery. What does the nurse teach the patient is the purpose of this prescription?

    a. Prevents infection

    b. Promotes effective circulation

    c. Promotes wound healing

    d. Prevents aspiration

13. In which position does the surgical nurse plan to place a patient undergoing minimally invasive surgery of the lower abdomen or pelvis?

    a. Trendelenburg position

    b. Sims position

    c. Lithotomy position

    d. Prone position

14. A nurse on a medical-surgical unit is caring for a patient who is displaying signs and symptoms of a pulmonary embolus. What is the priority intervention for this patient?

    a. Obtaining a prescription for rapid intravenous hydration

    b. Instructing the patient to perform Valsalva maneuver

    c. Assisting the patient to the Fowler position

    d. Encouraging the patient to ambulate every 2 to 3 hours

15. A postsurgical patient is experiencing decreased lung sounds, dyspnea, cyanosis, crackles, restlessness, and apprehension. Which action will the nurse take first?

    a. Request a prescription for a chest x-ray.

    b. Discuss antibiotic therapy with the health care provider.

    c. Assess the pulse oximetry reading.

    d. Apply sequential compression devices and antiembolism stockings.

ALTERNATE-FORMAT QUESTIONS

Multiple-Response Questions

Circle the letters that correspond to the best answers for each question.

1. A staff nurse is orienting to the PACU. Which actions would the nurse expect to perform in this area? Select all that apply.

   a. Preparing the patient for home care

   b. Informing the patient that surgical intervention is necessary

   c. Transferring the patient to the recovery room

   d. Admitting the patient to the recovery area

   e. Assessing for complications as the patient emerges from anesthesia

   f. Arranging for a rehabilitative program for the patient

2. A nurse is caring for a patient whose anesthesia plan is for regional anesthesia. Which methods could the nurse expect the patient to receive? Select all that apply.

   a. Inhalation

   b. Spinal block

   c. Intravenous

   d. Oral route

   e. Nerve block

   f. Epidural block

3. A nurse accompanies the surgeon to the bedside to witness them obtaining informed consent from the patient. What information must be provided to a patient to obtain informed consent? Select all that apply.

   a. Description of the procedure or treatment, along with potential alternative therapies

   b. Name and qualifications of the nurse providing perioperative care

   c. Underlying disease process and its natural course

   d. Explanation of the risks involved and how often they occur

   e. Explanation that a signed consent form is binding and cannot be withdrawn

   f. Customary insurance coverage for the procedure

4. What factors would the nurse consider when assessing postoperative patients? Select all that apply.

   a. Infants are at a greater risk from surgery than are middle-aged adults.

   b. Infants experience a slower metabolism of drugs that require renal biotransformation.

   c. Muscle relaxants and narcotics have a shorter duration of action in infants.

   d. Older adults have decreased renal blood flow, necessitating careful monitoring of fluid and electrolyte status and input and output.

   e. Older adults have an increased gastric pH and require monitoring of nutritional status during the perioperative period.

   f. Older adults have an increased hepatic blood flow, liver mass, and enzyme function that prolongs the duration of medication effects.

5. A nurse is making postoperative rounds with the surgeon. What factors should the nurse consider when assessing patients for postsurgical risks? Select all that apply.

   a. Cardiovascular diseases increase the risk for dehydration after surgery.

   b. Patients with respiratory disease may experience acid–base imbalance after surgery.

   c. Kidney and liver diseases influence the patient's response to anesthesia.

   d. Diabetes increases the risk for hypoglycemia after surgery.

   e. Endocrine diseases increase the risk for slow surgical wound healing.

   f. Pulmonary disorders increase the risk for hemorrhage and hypovolemic shock after surgery.

6. A nurse is assessing preoperative patients. Which patients will require follow-up with the surgeon preoperatively? Select all that apply.

   a. Patient taking a daily diuretic

   b. Patient receiving an oral anticoagulant the evening before surgery

   c. Adolescent patient with asthma and using a mini-nebulizer treatment with a bronchodilator

   d. Patient who received a sedative the night before surgery

   e. Patient taking oral adrenal steroids who is NPO

7. A charge nurse is reviewing presurgical screening tests for patients on the unit. Which findings require follow-up by the nurse? Select all that apply.

   a. Elevated white blood cell count, indicating an infection

   b. Decreased hematocrit and hemoglobin level, indicating bleeding or anemia

   c. Hyperkalemia, indicating possible renal failure

   d. Low creatinine levels, indicating an increased risk for cardiac problems

   e. Abnormal urine constituents, indicating infection or fluid imbalances

   f. Increased hemoglobin level, indicating infection

8. A nurse on a surgical unit is caring for a patient who had abdominal surgery yesterday. Which nursing interventions will the nurse include in the postoperative care plan? Select all that apply.

   a. Teaching the patient to suppress urges to cough in order to protect the incision

   b. Encouraging the patient to take frequent shallow breaths to improve lung expansion and volume

   c. Placing the patient in a semi-Fowler position to perform deep-breathing exercises every 1 to 2 hours

   d. Encouraging the patient to lie in bed with the incision facing upward to prevent pressure on sutures

e. Teaching the patient appropriate leg exercises to increase venous blood return from the legs

f. Encouraging the patient to use incentive spirometry 10 times each waking hour

Sequencing Questions

1. Place the following guidelines for teaching a patient deep breathing in the order in which they would be performed.

   a. Ask the patient to inhale through the nose gently and completely.

   b. Place the patient in semi-Fowler position with the neck and shoulders supported.

   c. Ask the patient to exhale gently and completely.

   d. Repeat this exercise three times every 1 to 2 hours.

   e. Ask the patient to place their hands over the rib cage so that they can feel their chest rise as their lungs expand.

   f. Ask the patient to exhale as completely as possible through the mouth with lips pursed (as if whistling).

   g. Ask the patient to hold their breath for 3 to 5 seconds and mentally count "one, one thousand, two, one thousand, etc."

   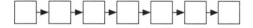

2. Place the following guidelines for teaching a patient effective coughing in the order in which they would be performed.

   a. Ask the patient to "hack out" for three short breaths.

   b. Repeat the exercise every 2 hours while awake.

   c. Place the patient in a semi-Fowler position, leaning forward, and provide a pillow or bath blanket to splint the incision.

   d. Ask the patient to cough deeply once or twice and take another deep breath.

   e. Ask the patient to take a quick breath with their mouth open.

   f. Ask the patient to inhale and exhale deeply and slowly through the nose three times.

   g. Ask the patient to take a deep breath and hold it for 3 seconds.

   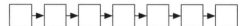

Prioritization Question

1. A nurse is caring for a group of postoperative patients. Which patient will the nurse assess first? Circle the letter corresponding to the best answer.

   a. Patient reporting pain when coughing

   b. Patient with blood pressure 108/62, pulse 78

   c. Patient expectorating clear mucus

   d. Patient reporting unilateral calf pain

Hygiene

ASSESSING YOUR UNDERSTANDING

FILL IN THE BLANKS

1. The _____ is the largest organ in the body.

2. Inflammation of the tissue that surrounds the teeth is referred to as _____.

3. Nurses should carefully inspect the feet of patients who have _____.

4. Infestation with lice is called _____.

5. Individuals with extreme obesity have _____ care needs.

6. _____ refers to a strong mouth odor.

7. Nurses are able to use self-contained bathing systems consisting of a plastic bag containing 8 to 10 premoistened washcloths that do not require _____.

8. Ticks embedded in the patient's skin may transmit Rocky Mountain spotted fever or _____ disease and should be removed with a tweezer.

9. During perineal care, avoid applying _____, which may become a medium for bacterial growth.

10. Acne results from pores clogged by dead skin cells and _____, another name for oil.

MATCHING EXERCISES

Match the oral diseases/conditions in Part A, with their description in Part B.

PART A

a. Stomatitis

b. Halitosis

c. Plaque

d. Glossitis

e. Cheilosis

f. Caries

PART B

____ 1. Ulceration of the lips, often caused by vitamin B complex deficiencies

____ 2. Inflammation of the tongue

____ 3. Formation of cavities

____ 4. Strong mouth odor

____ 5. Invisible, destructive bacterial film that builds up on teeth; leads to the destruction of tooth enamel

____ 6. Inflammation of the oral mucosa; may be caused by pathogens, trauma, irritants, nutritional deficiencies

CORRECT THE FALSE STATEMENTS

Mark the item "T" for true or "F" for false. If false, correct the underlined word or words to make the statement true in the space provided.

____ 1. The <u>sebaceous glands</u> secrete cerumen, which consists of heavy oil and brown pigment, into the external ear canals. _____

____ 2. Patients with dehydration or NPO status should receive oral care every <u>1 to 2 hours</u> and as needed. _____

____ 3. When performing hygiene on a <u>circumcised</u> male, the nurse must retract the <u>foreskin</u> before cleansing, and pull it back into place when finished. _____

____ 4. A nurse ensures the patient's comfort after lunch and offers assistance to nonambulatory patients with toileting, handwashing, and oral care during <u>afternoon</u> care (PM care). _____

____ 5. Before leaving the patient's bedside, the nurse should ensure that the bed is in its <u>highest</u> position. _____

____ 6. The odor of perspiration occurs when <u>bacteria</u> act on the skin's normal secretions. _____

____ 7. <u>Dry</u> skin is especially bothersome during adolescence. _____

____ 8. When providing perineal care for a female patient, the nurse separates the <u>labia</u> and moves the washcloth from the pubic area toward the anal area. _____

____ 9. A health care provider who treats foot disorders is known as a <u>pediatrician</u>. _____

____ 10. Depending on the patient's self-care abilities, the nurse offers assistance with toileting, oral care, bathing, back massage, special skin care measures, cosmetics, dressing, and positioning for comfort during the <u>afternoon care</u> schedule. _____

SHORT ANSWER

1. Briefly describe how the following factors may influence personal hygiene behaviors.
   a. Culture: _____
   _____
   b. Socioeconomic class: _____
   _____
   c. Spiritual practices: _____
   _____
   d. Developmental level: _____
   _____
   e. Health state: _____
   _____
   f. Personal preference: _____
   _____

2. List four specific nursing activities that assist patients with self care deficits to meet their daily needs.
   a. _____
   b. _____
   c. _____
   d. _____

3. A parent brings their 6-month-old infant to a well-baby clinic for immunizations. When assessing the infant, you notice dirty skin folds and a scaly scalp. What nursing actions are appropriate for the nurse to take?
   _____
   _____
   _____

4. Describe the activities the nurse would perform in the following scheduled care time periods.
   a. Early morning care: _____
   _____
   _____
   b. Morning care (AM care): _____
   _____
   _____
   c. Afternoon care (PM care):_____
   _____
   _____

d. Hour-of-sleep care (HS care): _____

_____

_____

e. As-needed care (PRN care): _____

_____

_____

5. List the benefits of bathing.

_____

_____

_____

6. Describe how you would assist a patient on bed rest with bathing when they state that they are able to wash themselves.

_____

_____

_____

7. Discuss advantages of a towel bath and the types of patients who might benefit.

_____

_____

_____

8. Describe the conditions for which you would assess when providing hygiene/care for the following areas.

a. Lips: _____

_____

b. Buccal mucosa: _____

_____

c. Gums: _____

_____

d. Tongue: _____

_____

e. Hard and soft palates: _____

_____

f. Eyes: _____

_____

g. Ears: _____

_____

h. Nose: _____

_____

9. Briefly describe the care necessary for a patient with:

a. Hearing aids: _____

_____

b. Dentures: _____

_____

10. List variables known to cause nail and foot problems.

_____

_____

_____

_____

_____

APPLYING YOUR KNOWLEDGE

CRITICAL THINKING QUESTIONS

1. Think about nurses' responsibility to assist patients with daily hygiene. Then reflect on how you would respond in the following situations. See if your classmates would respond as you do.

a. Same-age, opposite-sex patient requires total assistance with hygiene:

_____

b. Patient confined to bed but able to assist with hygiene refuses to do so:

_____

c. Older adult incontinent patient refuses your offer to assist with perineal care:

_____

2. While nurse may provide a backrub to patients for pain or other reasons, for what type(s) of patient problem is a backrub contraindicated?

3. Interview patients of different backgrounds or cultures to find out how they perform their daily hygiene routine. Note how their routine is similar to or different from your personal routine. What would you do to assist these people if they were placed in your care?

REFLECTIVE PRACTICE: CULTIVATING QSEN COMPETENCIES

Use the following expanded scenario from Chapter 32 in your textbook to answer the questions below.

Scenario: Sonya is an older Hispanic woman who has had a stroke (brain attack) resulting in right-sided paralysis. She is being discharged from the hospital and will now live with her daughter, who will be her primary caregiver. Her daughter is eager to learn everything she can about caring for her mother and asks numerous questions, including the best way to help her mother with personal hygiene.

1. Patient-centered care/safety: With what assessments and teaching will Sonya and her daughter need help to meet Sonya's hygiene needs?

2. Patient-centered care: What would be a successful outcome for this patient?

3. Patient-centered care/evidence-based practice: What intellectual, technical, and interpersonal competencies are most likely to bring about the desired outcome?

4. Patient-centered care/teamwork and collaboration: What resources might be helpful for Sonya and her daughter?

PATIENT CARE STUDY

Use this care study to apply your knowledge by completing the nursing Process Worksheet found in Appendix A.

Scenario: Dominic, a 78-year-old retiree with a history of Parkinson's disease, lives alone in a small home. He was recently hospitalized for cardiac dysrhythmia and pacemaker placement. The home health care nurse visits 1 week post discharge to monitor the surgical site and medication monitoring. The nurse observes that the patient is disheveled, and there are multiple stains on his clothing. Several food items are in various stages of preparation on the kitchen counter, and some appear to have spoiled. The patient has several days' growth of beard, and a body odor is apparent. He is pleasant and oriented to place and person but cannot identify the time or day of the week: "I lose track of what day it is. Time is not important when you are my age. The most important

thing to me right now is to be able to take care of myself and stay in this house near my friends." There is a walker visible in a corner of the living room, but the patient ambulates slowly around the house with a minimum of difficulty and does not use the walker. He comments that he keeps busy "reading, watching old movies, and going to senior center activities with friends who stop by for me." His daughter, who lives several hours away, visits him every weekend and prepares his medications for the week in a plastic container that is easy for him to open. The nurse observes that all the medications appeared to have been taken to date. "I don't mess around with my medicines. One helps my heart, and the others keep me from shaking."

PRACTICING FOR NCLEX

MULTIPLE-CHOICE QUESTIONS

Circle the letter that corresponds to the best answer for each question.

1. A nurse is teaching an adolescent with negative body image how to manage acne. What does the nurse include in the teaching plan?
   a. Gently squeeze the infected areas to release the infection.
   b. Wash your face less frequently to avoid removing beneficial oils.
   c. Keep your hair off your face and wash your hair daily.
   d. Use cosmetics and emollients to cover the condition.

2. A nurse in a long-term care facility is discussing oral care with a forgetful patient who wears dentures. What reminder should the nurse provide?
   a. Keeping dentures out for long periods permits the gum line to change, affecting denture fit.
   b. It is best to wrap your dentures in a tissue or a disposable wipe when not in use.
   c. Do not store your dentures in water because the plastic material may warp.
   d. Brush the dentures with powder and rinse thoroughly with hot water.

3. A nurse is providing perineal care for patients in a hospital setting. Which action is most appropriate?
   a. Cleansing from most-contaminated to least-contaminated area
   b. Avoiding retracting the foreskin in an uncircumcised male
   c. Drying the cleaned areas and applying an emollient as indicated
   d. Applying powder liberally to the area to prevent the growth of bacteria

4. A nurse is supervising a new AP who is providing hygiene to a patient with diabetes. Which action does the nurse explain is appropriate when providing foot care?
   a. Soaking the feet in a solution of mild soap and tepid water
   b. Drying the feet thoroughly; applying moisturizer on the tops and bottoms
   c. Using a nail clipper or scissors to trim the nails
   d. Shaving off any corns or calluses

5. A nurse on a telemetry unit is caring for a patient receiving the anticoagulant warfarin. Which instruction about hygiene is appropriate to give this patient?
   a. Brush your teeth after every meal.
   b. You will need to wait to go home to wash your hair.
   c. Electric razors are recommended for patients receiving anticoagulants.
   d. You may remove the heart monitor to bathe or shower.

6. A nurse caring for the skin of patients of different age groups should consider which accurately described condition?
   a. An infant's skin and mucous membranes are protected from infection through natural immunity.
   b. Secretions from skin glands are at their maximum from age 3 years onward.
   c. The skin becomes thicker and more leathery with aging and is prone to wrinkles and dryness.
   d. An adolescent's skin ordinarily has enlarged sebaceous glands and increased glandular secretions.

7. A nurse in a university's student health clinic provides teaching about sexual and genitourinary health. Which teaching by the nurse is correct?
   a. "Douching is not necessary as it can change the pH of the normally acidic vagina."
   b. "Wipe the perineal area back to front after using the toilet."
   c. "Avoid using a condom during sexual intercourse."
   d. "It is inappropriate to ask sexual partners about previous STIs."

8. A nurse is assisting the AP with hygiene and perineal care for a patient experiencing urinary and fecal incontinence. Which of these actions takes priority?
   a. Cleansing the skin with an antibacterial soap
   b. Rinsing the skin with hot water to kill pathogens
   c. Applying a skin barrier
   d. Applying an adult brief or diaper

9. A nurse is attempting to bathe a patient with dementia who is uncooperative and screams during bathing. Which nursing actions can the nurse use to relieve distress?
   a. Beginning by washing the hair as it is often the most distressing
   b. Placing the patient in the shower
   c. Playing the patient's favorite music
   d. Firmly telling the patient they must bathe today

10. Nursing students in a critical care experience perform oral hygiene for patients receiving mechanical ventilation and sedation. In postconference, the professor asks the students to state the rationale for meticulous oral hygiene in this population. Which answer demonstrates the student understands this concept?
    a. "Patients who receive sedation will be unable to brush their teeth."
    b. "Diligent mouth care decreases the incidence of ventilator-associated pneumonia."
    c. "Meticulous oral hygiene prepares the patients for visiting hours."
    d. "Meticulous oral hygiene prevents dental caries."

ALTERNATE-FORMAT QUESTIONS

Multiple-Response Questions

Circle the letters that correspond to the best answers for each question.

1. A school nurse is preparing educational materials for parents after an outbreak of pediculosis. Which information is essential to include? Select all that apply
   a. Household members should not share hairbrushes, combs, or barrettes.
   b. Use an OTC pediculicide per package instructions.
   c. Adults living with children who have pediculosis should avoid shaking hands.
   d. Dry clean all bedding, clothing, and towels.
   e. Stuffed animals may be sealed in a plastic bag for 2 weeks.

2. A nurse working in a dermatology practice discusses protective measures to prevent sun damage. Which points will the nurse emphasize? Select all that apply
   a. Apply a sunscreen with a protection factor (SPF) of 15 or lower.
   b. Avoid spending time in direct sun, especially between 10 AM and 2 PM.
   c. Cover the skin with long sleeves and a broad-brimmed hat.
   d. Use sunscreen on infants under 6 months old to prevent burning.
   e. Wear sunglasses with a UVA/UVB rating of at least 50% each.
   f. If sunscreen is labeled water resistant, it will not need to be reapplied.

3. Which nursing interventions are correct when teaching APs in a residential facility about oral care? Select all that apply.
   a. Use a hard toothbrush to remove plaque from the teeth.
   b. Brush teeth every 2 hours.
   c. Avoid cleaning the tongue with a toothbrush.
   d. An automatic toothbrush may be used to remove debris and plaque from teeth.
   e. Never use water-spray units to assist with oral hygiene.
   f. If desired, the patient may use sodium bicarbonate as cleaning agents for short-term use.

4. For which of these patients would the nurse anticipate using chlorhexidine gluconate (CHG) for bathing?
   a. Patient with a central venous catheter
   b. Preoperative patient for cardiac surgery later that day
   c. Patient being discharged after a kidney infection
   d. Patient receiving mechanical ventilation
   e. Pregnant patient in early labor
   f. Patient in the neonatal intensive care unit

5. A graduate nurse and preceptor are providing care for a patient's eyes and ears. Which actions by the graduate require correction by the preceptor? Select all that apply.
   a. Cleansing the eye from the inner canthus to the outer canthus using a wet, warm cotton ball
   b. Applying artificial tears solution twice a day when the blink reflex is decreased or absent
   c. Using a protective shield to protect the eyes when the blink reflex is absent
   d. Using boric acid to remove excess secretions from the eyes
   e. Cleansing the patient's external ear with a washcloth-covered finger
   f. Cleansing the inner ear of cerumen with a cotton-tipped swab

Prioritization Question

1. A nurse delegates bathing to the AP on an intermediate care unit. Which patient will the nurse ask the AP to bathe first?
   a. Patient who just arrived on the unit after 32 hours in the ED
   b. Patient reporting chest pain
   c. Patient who had urinary incontinence
   d. Patient demanding a bath

CHAPTER 33

Skin Integrity and Wound Care

ASSESSING YOUR UNDERSTANDING

FILL IN THE BLANKS

1. The nurse is changing the dressing covering a patient's surgical incision. This type of wound will heal by _____ intention.

2. The nurse notes swelling and pain at an incision site. These symptoms are most likely caused by an accumulation of blood and plasma called a(n) _____.

3. A patient's wound is in the inflammatory cellular phase, meaning that _____ and _____, or phagocytic cells, arrive first to ingest bacteria and cellular debris.

4. The new tissue found in the proliferative phase of wound healing, that is red, highly vascular, and bleeds easily is documented as _____ tissue.

5. The nurse reviews a radiologic imaging report stating that the patient has an abnormal passage extending from one internal organ into another. The nurse gives the oncoming nurse reports on this condition, referring to the abnormality as a(n) _____.

6. When cleaning a wound, the nurse typically chooses sterile 0.9% sodium _____ as the cleansing solution.

7. The nurse anchors a bandage by wrapping it around the patient's body part overlapping the previous bandage turn. This procedure is the _____ turn method of bandage wrapping.

8. A nurse assessing a patient's wound notes blackened area of tissue necrosis in the wound base. The nurse documents that the wound has _____ present.

9. A covering placed over or into a wound to protect and/or promote healing is known as a(n) _____.

10. The nurse explains to the patient that a cloth or elasticized device that fastens together with Velcro, called a _____, will be given to them to support the wound after surgery.

MATCHING EXERCISES

Matching Exercise 1

Match the term in Part A with its definition in Part B.

PART A

a. Dehiscence

b. Scar

c. Evisceration

d. Granulation tissue

e. Wound

f. Epithelialization

PART B

_____ **1.** New tissue, pink-red in color, composed of fibroblasts and small blood vessels that fill an open wound when it starts to heal

_____ **2.** Natural act of healing of dermal and epidermal tissue in which a protective membrane forms over a wound

_____ **3.** Disruption in the normal integrity of the skin

_____ **4.** Avascular collagen tissue that does not sweat, grow hair, or tan in sunlight

_____ **5.** Partial or total disruption of wound layers

_____ **6.** Protrusion of viscera through the incisional area

Matching Exercise 2

Match the term in Part A with its definition in Part B.

PART A

a. Sanguineous wound drainage

b. Exudate

c. Purulent wound drainage

d. Serous wound drainage

e. Black wounds

f. Hemorrhage

PART B

_____ **1.** Wound drainage made up of white blood cells, liquefied dead tissue debris, and both dead and live bacteria

_____ **2.** Wounds characterized by oozing from the tissue covering the wound, often accompanied by purulent drainage

_____ **3.** Composed of fluid and cells that escape from the blood vessels and are deposited in or on tissue surfaces

_____ **4.** May occur from a slipped suture, a dislodged clot from stress at the suture line, infection, or the erosion of a blood vessel by a foreign body (such as a drain)

_____ **5.** Wound drainage that is composed of the clear, serous portion of the blood and drainage from serous membranes

_____ **6.** Wound drainage that consists of large numbers of red blood cells and looks like blood

Matching Exercise 3

Match the wound care dressings and wraps in Part A with their description/indication listed in Part B. Answers may be used more than once.

PART A

a. Telfa

b. Transparent films

c. ABDs, Surgipads

d. Drain sponge or Sof-Wick

e. Gauze dressings

PART B

_____ **1.** Type of dressing often used over intravenous sites, subclavian catheter insertion sites, and noninfected healing wounds

_____ **2.** Special gauze that covers the incision line and allows drainage to pass through and be absorbed by the center absorbent layer

_____ **3.** Used to prevent outer dressings from adhering to the wound and causing further injury when removed

_____ **4.** Precut halfway to fit around drains or tubes

_____ **5.** Commonly used to cover wounds; they come in various sizes and are commercially packaged as single units or in packs

_____ **6.** Placed over the smaller gauze to absorb drainage and protect the wound from contamination or injury

SHORT ANSWER

1. List six major functions of the skin.

   a. _____

   b. _____

   c. _____

   d. _____

   e. _____

   f. _____

2. Describe how the following mechanisms contribute to pressure injury development.

   a. External pressure: _____

   _____

   b. Friction and shearing forces: _____

   _____

3. Give an example of how the following factors could promote development of a pressure injury.

   a. Nutrition: _____

   _____

   b. Hydration: _____

   _____

   c. Moist skin _____

   _____

   d. Mental status: _____

   _____

   e. Age: _____

   _____

   f. Immobility: _____

   _____

4. The visiting nurse notes a stage 2 pressure injury developing on a patient's coccyx. Develop a nursing care plan for this patient that involves the family in the treatment of the injury.

   _____

   _____

   _____

   _____

5. Briefly describe the phases of wound healing.

   a. Hemostasis: _____

   _____

   b. Inflammatory phase: _____

   _____

   c. Proliferative phase: _____

   _____

   d. Maturation phase: _____

   _____

   _____

6. List three goals that the nurse could enter on a care plan for patients who are at risk for pressure injury or impaired skin integrity.

   a. _____

   b. _____

   c. _____

7. Give two examples of interview questions that could be asked to assess a patient's skin integrity in the following areas.

   a. Overall appearance of the skin: _____

   _____

   _____

   b. Recent changes in skin condition: _____

   _____

   c. Activity/mobility: _____

   _____

   _____

   d. Nutrition: _____

   _____

   e. Pain: _____

   _____

   f. Elimination: _____

   _____

8. Describe how you would assess the following aspects of wound healing.

   a. Appearance: _____

   _____

   b. Wound drainage: _____

   _____

   c. Pain: _____

   _____

   d. Sutures and staples: _____

   _____

9. Discuss the purposes for wound dressings.

   _____

   _____

10. Describe the RYB color classification and interventions for these open wounds.

a. R = red = protect: _____

_____

_____

b. Y = yellow = cleanse: _____

_____

_____

c. B = black = debride: _____

_____

_____

11. Briefly describe the use of the following methods of applying heat and any advantages or disadvantages.

a. Hot water bags or bottles: _____

_____

b. Electric heating pad: _____

_____

c. Aquathermia pad: _____

_____

d. Chemical heat packs: _____

_____

e. Warm moist compresses: _____

_____

f. Sitz baths: _____

_____

g. Warm soaks: _____

_____

12. State the purpose of a drain inserted during a surgical procedure.

_____

_____

APPLYING YOUR KNOWLEDGE

CRITICAL THINKING QUESTIONS

1. Explain nursing care to prevent pressure injuries in the following patients.

a. Comatose 35-year-old male

b. Frail older adult who is confined to bed

c. Premature infant on life support

2. Follow the wound care nurse or nurse on a surgical unit, assisting with wound care and dressing changes. Ask the patients how the wound has affected their mobility, sensory perception, activity, nutrition, and exposure to friction and shear.

REFLECTIVE PRACTICE: CULTIVATING QSEN COMPETENCIES

Use the following expanded scenario from Chapter 33 in your textbook to answer the questions below.

Scenario: Sam, a 56-year-old, has been admitted to the hospital for aggressive treatment of a bone infection that has not responded to usual treatment methods. Sam is 5 ft 4 inches tall and weighs more than 300 lb. They tell you, "Last time I was here, my skin got really irritated, and I developed several skin wounds."

1. Patient-centered care/evidence-based practice: What nursing intervention would be appropriate to prevent skin irritation and the development of pressure injuries for Sam?

_____

_____

_____

2. Patient-centered care: What would be a successful outcome for this patient?

_____

_____

_____

3. Evidence-based practice: What intellectual, technical, and interpersonal competencies are most likely to bring about the desired outcome?

_____

_____

_____

4. Teamwork and collaboration: What resources might be helpful for Sam?

_____

_____

_____

PATIENT CARE STUDY

Use this care study to apply your knowledge by completing the Nursing Process Worksheet found in Appendix A.

Scenario: Mrs. Chijioke, an 88-year-old woman who lives alone, was brought to the hospital after being found by neighbors at the bottom of her cellar steps. A hip fracture was surgically repaired 3 days ago. The nurse notes redness of coccyx, heels, and elbows which blanches with pressure and returns to normal color quickly when pressure is released. Although Mrs. Chijioke can be lifted out of bed into a chair, she spends most of the day in bed, lying on her back. At 5 ft tall and 89 lb, Mrs. Chijioke looks lost in the hospital bed. Her eyes are bright, and she usually attempts a warm smile, but she is weak and lies motionless for hours. Her skin is wrinkled and paper-thin, and her arms are bruised from unsuccessful attempts at intravenous therapy. She was dehydrated on admission after 48 hours on the floor and is receiving nutritional, fluid, and electrolyte support. With a long history of diabetes, the patient is now spiking a fever of 102.2°F (39°C), which concerns the nurse.

PRACTICING FOR NCLEX

MULTIPLE-CHOICE QUESTIONS

Circle the letter that corresponds to the best answer for each question.

1. A nurse receives in report that a patient who is being treated for self-inflicted wounds has anorexia. What finding poses the greatest risk for poor wound healing?
   a. Albumin level of 3.1 mg/dL
   b. Total lymphocyte count of 1,160/mm³
   c. Body weight decrease of 5%
   d. Arm muscle circumference 90% of standard

2. A nurse on a neurology unit notes a stage 1 pressure injury on their patient's back. What nursing intervention is most appropriate?
   a. Place an ABD pad over the area to protect the skin on the patient's back.
   b. Use a ring cushion to protect reddened areas from additional pressure.
   c. Increases the amount of time the head of the bed is elevated.
   d. Encourage the patient to get out of bed to a chair several times a day.

3. When providing wound care and cleansing for a postoperative incision, which nursing action reflects the proper procedure?
   a. Using a moistened gauze, wiping outward from the wound in lines parallel to it
   b. Providing friction when cleaning the wound to loosen dead cells
   c. Swabbing the wound with povidone–iodine to prevent infection
   d. Irrigating the wound from the bottom to the top

4. A nurse is changing the dressing of a patient with a gunshot wound. What nursing intervention is appropriate?
   a. Applying continuous wet-to-dry dressings
   b. Keeping skin surrounding the injury moist to prevent breakdown
   c. Selecting a dressing that absorbs exudate and maintains a moist environment
   d. Packing the wound cavity tightly with dressing material

5. While giving a back rub to an older adult, a nurse notices a midthoracic stage 2 pressure injury. What action will the nurse take next?
   a. Place a sterile dressing over the pressure injury.
   b. Use a wet-to-dry dressing on the pressure injury.
   c. Apply a nonadherent dressing and change every 3 hours.
   d. Cleanse the site with normal saline.

6. A nurse is caring for a patient who has a Penrose drain placed during abdominal surgery. What daily drain management will the nurse plan for?
   a. Careful cleansing around the sutures with a swab and povidone solution prior to shortening the drain
   b. Emptying and suctioning the device, following the manufacturer's directions prior to shortening the drain
   c. Using sterile forceps and a twisting motion, pulling the drain out a short distance and cutting off the end of the drain with sterile scissors
   d. Compressing the container with the port open, then sealing the port before shortening the drain

7. When caring for a patient with a pressure injury that is superficial such as an abrasion, blister, or shallow crater, which documentation is most appropriate to enter in the health record?

a. Stage 1

b. Stage 2

c. Stage 3

d. Stage 4

8. A nurse carries out a prescription to apply a heating pad to a patient experiencing neck pain. Which nursing action is performed correctly?

a. Using a safety pin to attach the pad to the bedding

b. Covering the heating pad with a heavy blanket

c. Placing the heating pad under the patient's neck

d. Applying the pad for 20 to 30 minutes, assessing regularly

9. A wound nurse regularly assesses for patients at risk for pressure injuries in a hospital setting. Which patient would the nurse identify is at highest risk for developing a pressure injury?

a. Newborn

b. Patient with cardiovascular disease

c. Older adult with arthritis

d. Critical care patient

10. A nurse discusses shearing forces in the development of pressure injury with a group of nursing students. Which patient would the students identify is most likely to develop a pressure injury from shearing forces?

a. Patient sitting in a chair who slides down

b. Patient lifting themselves up on their elbows

c. Patient lying on wrinkled sheets

d. Patient remaining on their back all day

11. A nurse in the burn unit is assessing the patient's wounds. Which of these wounds does the nurse anticipate will heal by primary intention?

a. Surgical incision with sutures and edges well approximated

b. Large wound with considerable tissue loss allowed to heal naturally

c. Wound left open for several days to allow edema to subside

d. New wound with eschar that becomes infected

12. A nurse is performing this step of I&O and drainage assessment for a postoperative patient. What step will the nurse take next?

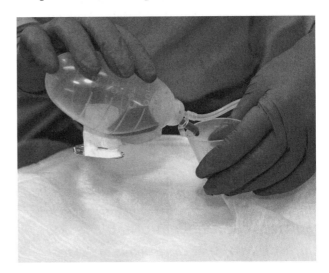

a. Compress the drain.

b. Irrigate the drain with saline.

c. Discard the drainage.

d. Document serous drainage in the health record.

13. A nurse is caring for a patient with a stage 4 pressure ulcer that has recently become malodorous with increased purulent drainage. Which statement by the AP requires the nurse to follow up?

a. "I'm concerned about the patient; they didn't eat much today."

b. "I will wait to change the sheets until you perform wound care."

c. "I helped the patient order television service; they couldn't read the instructions."

d. "The patient's blood glucose is 104 mg/dL."

ALTERNATE-FORMAT QUESTIONS

Multiple-Response Questions

Circle the letters that correspond to the best answers for each question.

1. A nursing student and wound care nurse are performing assessments on a group of patients at risk for delayed wound healing. Which patients do they identify as at risk? Select all that apply.
   a. Older adult who is bedridden
   b. Patient with a peripheral vascular disorder
   c. Patient with obesity
   d. Patient who consumes a diet high in vitamins A and C
   e. Patient taking corticosteroids
   f. School-aged child with a surgical incision

2. A nurse on a medical-surgical unit is assessing a patient's surgical wound. Which assessments of wound complications are accurately described? Select all that apply.
   a. Symptoms of wound infection appear within 1 to 2 weeks after surgery.
   b. Dehiscence is present when there is a partial or total disruption of wound layers.
   c. Evisceration occurs when the viscera protrudes through the incisional area.
   d. Delayed wound healing develops in thin patients due to a thinner layer of tissue cells.
   e. An increased serosanguineous drainage between postoperative days 4 and 5 is a sign of an impending evisceration.
   f. Postoperative fistula formation most often results from an infection or abscess.

3. A nurse appropriately documents which of these wounds are healing normally without complications? Select all that apply.
   a. The edges of the incision appear clean and well approximated with a crust.
   b. After 2 weeks, the wound edges appear normal and heal together.
   c. Increased swelling and drainage have developed.
   d. The wound is without redness or warmth upon palpation.
   e. Exudate develops early due to the inflammatory response.
   f. The incision is painful with purulent drainage.

4. In which situations has the nurse used a dressing properly? Select all that apply.
   a. Placed a Surgipad directly over an incision
   b. Placed transparent dressings over an ABD to help keep the wound dry
   c. Placed a transparent dressing over a central venous access device insertion site
   d. Used appropriate aseptic techniques when changing a dressing
   e. Placed Sof-Wick around a drain insertion site
   f. Applied Telfa to a wound to keep drainage from passing through to a secondary dressing

5. Which interventions reflect appropriate care when providing care for a patient with a draining wound? Select all that apply.
   a. Administering a prescribed analgesic 30 to 45 minutes before changing the dressing
   b. Changing the dressing midway between meals
   c. Placing protective ointment or paste to clean skin surrounding the draining wound
   d. Applying a layer of protective ointment or paste on top of the previous layer during dressing changes
   e. Placing an absorbent dressing material as the first layer of the dressing
   f. Using a nonabsorbent material over the first layer of absorbent material

6. A nurse is using the RYB wound classification system to document patient wounds. Which wounds would the nurse document as a Y (yellow) wound? Select all that apply.
   a. Reflects the color of normal granulation tissue
   b. Characterized by oozing from the tissue covering the wound
   c. Has beige drainage
   d. Requires wound cleaning and irrigation
   e. Covered with thick eschar
   f. Treated by using sharp, mechanical, or chemical debridement

7. The nurse is teaching a patient at risk for pressure injuries and their family about preventing pressure injuries. What information is correct to include in the discussion? Select all that apply.

   a. "Pressure injuries usually occur over bony areas where body weight is distributed over a small area without much fatty tissue."

   b. "Most pressure injuries occur over the trochanter and calcaneus."

   c. "A pressure injury doesn't typically appear within the first 2 days of immobility."

   d. "The skin can tolerate considerable pressure without cell death, but for short periods only."

   e. "The duration of pressure rather than the amount of pressure plays a larger role in pressure injury formation."

8. Which would be appropriate actions for the nurse to take when cleaning and dressing a pressure injury? Select all that apply.

   a. Cleaning the wound with each dressing change, pressing firmly to remove necrotic tissue

   b. Using povidone–iodine or hydrogen peroxide to irrigate and clean the injury

   c. Using whirlpool treatments, if ordered, until the injury is considered clean

   d. Keeping the injury tissue moist and the surrounding skin dry

   e. Using a dressing that absorbs exudate but maintains a moist healing environment

   f. Packing wound cavities densely with dressing material to promote tissue healing

9. Which nursing interventions reflect appropriate use of heat or cold therapy? Select all that apply.

   a. Making more frequent checks of the skin of an older adult using a heating pad

   b. Applying a heating pad on a sprained wrist in the acute stage

   c. Instructing the patient to lean or lie directly on the thermal device

   d. Filling an ice bag with small pieces of ice to about two thirds full

   e. Covering a cold pack with a cotton sleeve to keep it in place on an arm

   f. Applying moist cold to a patient's eye for 40 minutes every 2 hours

10. Which actions would a nurse be expected to perform when applying a saline-moistened dressing to a patient's pressure wound? Select all that apply.

    a. Putting on clean gloves and squeezing excess fluid from the gauze dressing before packing it tightly in the wound

    b. Positioning the patient to promote cleanser or irrigation solution to flow from the clean end of the wound toward the dirtier end

    c. Carefully and gently removing tape; using a silicone-based adhesive remover to help remove if resistance is met

    d. Applying a dry, sterile gauze pad over the wet gauze, then placing an ABD pad over the gauze pad

    e. Using clean technique, opening the supplies and dressings and placing the fine mesh gauze into the basin, saturating the gauze with the prescribed solution

    f. Loosely packing the moistened gauze into the wound using forceps or cotton-tipped applicators to press the gauze into all wound surfaces

11. A wound care nurse is providing staff education on negative pressure wound therapy. Which wounds does the nurse teach are candidates for the device?

    a. Dry wounds with minimal drainage

    b. Slow-healing chronic wounds

    c. New postoperative incisions

    d. Wounds colonized with bacteria

    e. Wounds with heavy drainage

Sequencing Question

1. Place the following steps for collecting a wound culture in the order in which they should be performed.

   a. Using aseptic technique, don sterile gloves and clean wound. Remove sterile gloves.

   b. Explain the procedure to patient; gather equipment; perform hand hygiene.

   c. Apply clean dressing to wound.

   d. Perform hand hygiene. Remove all equipment and make patient comfortable.

   e. Remove gloves from inside out, and discard them in plastic waste bag. Perform hand hygiene.

f. Twist cap to loosen swab in Culturette tube, or open separate swab and remove cap from culture tube, keeping inside uncontaminated. Put on clean glove or new sterile glove, if necessary.

g. Label specimen container appropriately, attach laboratory requisition to tube with a rubber band or place tube in a plastic bag with requisition attached; send to lab within 20 minutes.

h. Carefully insert swab into wound and rotate the swab several times. Use another swab if collecting specimen from another site.

i. Place swab in Culturette tube, being careful not to touch outside of container. Twist cap to secure; if using Culturette tube, crush ampule of medium at bottom of tube.

j. Don clean disposable gloves. Remove dressing and assess wound and drainage.

k. Record collection of specimen, appearance of wound, and description of drainage in chart.

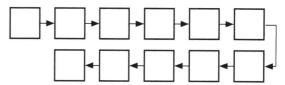

Activity

ASSESSING YOUR UNDERSTANDING

FILL IN THE BLANKS

1. The framework of bones, joints, and cartilage is called the _____ system.

2. The attachment of a muscle to the more stationary bone is called the site of _____; the attachment to the more movable bone is the site of _____.

3. When a person is standing, their center of gravity is located in the center of their pelvis, midway between the _____ and the _____ pubis.

4. Orthopedics refers to the correction or prevention of disorder of body structures used in _____.

5. _____ are permanent contractions of a muscle, unless exercise, joint motion, and good posture are maintained.

6. _____ is an age-related problem in which bone destruction exceeds bone formation and results in thin bones that fracture easily.

7. Exercise using muscle contraction with resistance is referred to as _____ exercise.

8. Immobility causing venous stasis may lead to _____ formation.

9. A patient who has been immobile may develop a decrease in muscle size referred to as _____.

10. A patient displaying hypotonicity or decreased muscle tone can be documented as having _____.

11. Impaired muscle strength or weakness is termed _____; absence of strength secondary to nervous impairment is called _____.

12. When teaching the patient with a right knee injury to walk with a cane, in which hand will the nurse instruct the _____ patient to hold the cane?

IDENTIFICATION

1. Identify the bed-lying positions illustrated below by placing the names of the positions on the lines provided.

a. _____

b. _____

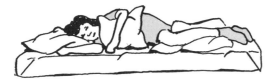

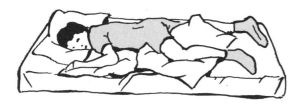

c. _____

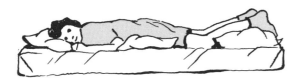

d. _____

e. _____

MATCHING EXERCISES

Matching Exercise 1

Match the type of joint listed in Part A with the examples listed in Part B. Not all answers will be used.

PART A

a. Ball-and-socket joint
b. Condyloid joint
c. Gliding joint
d. Hinge joint
e. Pivot joint
f. Saddle joint

PART B

____ 1. Joints between the axis and atlas and the proximal ends of the radius and ulna

____ 2. Carpal bones of the wrist; tarsal bones of the feet

____ 3. Wrist joint

____ 4. Joint between the trapezium and metacarpal of the thumb

____ 5. Shoulder and hip joints

Matching Exercise 2

Match the term used to describe body positions and movements in Part A with its definition listed in Part B. Not all answers will be used.

PART A

a. Flexion
b. Extension
c. Adduction
d. Dorsiflexion
e. Pronation
f. Abduction
g. Supination

PART B

____ 1. Assumption of a prone position

____ 2. Lateral movement of a body part away from the midline of the body

____ 3. Bending the hand or foot backward

____ 4. State of being bent

____ 5. State of being in a straight line

____ 6. Lateral movement of a body part toward the midline of the body

Matching Exercise 3

Match the condition related to muscle mass listed in Part A with its definition listed in Part B.

PART A

a. Hypertrophy
b. Muscle tone
c. Hypotonicity
d. Spasticity
e. Hemiparesis
f. Quadriplegia

PART B

____ 1. Increased muscle mass resulting from exercise or training

____ 2. Increased tone that interferes with movement

____ 3. Slight residual tension that remains in a normal resting muscle with an intact nerve supply

___ **4.** Weakness of half of the body

___ **5.** Decreased tone that results from disuse or neurologic impairment

___ **6.** Paralysis of the arms and legs

CORRECT THE FALSE STATEMENTS

Mark the item "T" for true or "F" for false. If false, correct the underlined word or words to make the statement true in the space provided.

___ **1.** The bones of the jaw and spinal column are classified as <u>short bones</u>. _____

___ **2.** In a <u>gliding joint</u>, articular surfaces are flat; flexion–extension and abduction-adduction are permitted. _____

___ **3.** <u>Ligaments</u> are tough, fibrous bands that bind joints together and connect bones and cartilage. _____

___ **4.** It is a <u>nerve impulse</u> that stimulates muscles to contract. _____

___ **5.** <u>Body dynamics</u> are the efficient use of the body as a machine and as a means of locomotion. _____

___ **6.** <u>Tonus</u> is the term used to describe the state of slight contraction or the usual state of skeletal muscles. _____

___ **7.** The <u>narrower</u> a base of support and the lower the center of gravity, the greater the stability of the object. _____

___ **8.** The <u>labyrinthine</u> sense informs the brain of the location of a limb or body part as a result of joint movements stimulating special nerve endings in muscles, tendons, and fascia. _____

___ **9.** The <u>cerebral motor cortex</u> integrates semivoluntary movements such as walking, swimming, and laughing. _____

___ **10.** Rehabilitative exercises for knee or elbow injuries are examples of <u>isokinetic</u> exercises. _____

___ **11.** <u>Atelectasis</u> is an incomplete expansion or collapse of lung tissue. _____

___ **12.** <u>Footdrop</u> is a complication of immobility in which the foot cannot maintain itself in the perpendicular position, heel–toe gait is impossible, and the patient experiences extreme difficulty in walking. _____

___ **13.** Should a patient faint or begin to fall while walking, the nurse should stand with their feet apart to create a wide base of support and rock the pelvis out on the <u>opposite</u> side the patient. _____

___ **14.** When a patient stands between the back legs of a walker, the walker should extend from the floor to the patient's hip joint; the patient's elbows should be flexed about <u>30 degrees</u>. _____

___ **15.** A nurse should <u>lift</u> an object to be moved to reduce the energy needed to overcome the pull of gravity. _____

___ **16.** Circling the arm at the shoulder, such as during a serve in tennis is called <u>hyperflexion</u>. _____

___ **17.** When a seated person looks at the ceiling, their cervical spine is <u>pronated</u>. _____

___ **18.** When caring for a patient with foot drop, the patient's foot is in <u>dorsiflexion</u>. _____

___ **19.** A nurse documents that the patient with a left hip fracture is is lying with the leg rotated outward and the toes pointing away from midline as "the left leg is in <u>external rotation</u>." _____

___ **20.** The Katz Index of Independence in Activities of Daily Living is used to measure the <u>child's</u> capacity to care for oneself and assist nurses to detect subtle changes in health and prevent functional decline. _____

SHORT ANSWER

1. Briefly explain the effects of exercise and immobility on the body systems listed in the table below. Write your answers in the spaces provided in the table.

Body System	Effects of Exercise	Effects of Immobility
Cardiovascular		
Respiratory		
Gastrointestinal		
Urinary		
Musculoskeletal		
Metabolic		
Integumentary		
Psychological Well-Being		

2. List three functions performed by the muscles through contraction.

a. _____

b. _____

c. _____

3. Describe the four steps the nervous system completes to stimulate muscles to contract.

a. _____

_____

b. _____

_____

c. _____

_____

d. _____

_____

4. Briefly describe the following concepts of ergonomics.

a. Body alignment or posture: _____

_____

b. Balance: _____

_____

c. Coordinated body movement: _____

_____

5. List four guidelines for the use of ergonomics when a person is at work.

a. _____

_____

b. _____

_____

c. _____

_____

d. _____

_____

6. Briefly describe how the following types of exercise provide health benefits to patients and give an example of each.

a. Aerobic exercises: _____

_____

b. Stretching exercises: _____

_____

c. Strength and endurance exercises:

_____

_____

d. Activities of daily living: _____

_____

7. List four psychological benefits of regular exercise.

a. _____

b. _____

c. _____

d. _____

8. Briefly describe how the following devices are used to promote correct alignment or alleviate discomfort on body parts.

a. Pillows: _____

_____

b. Mattresses: _____

_____

c. Adjustable bed: _____

_____

d. Bed side rails: _____

_____

e. Trapeze bar: _____

_____

f. Cradle: _____

_____

g. Sandbags: _____

_____

h. Trochanter rolls: _____

_____

I. Hand/wrist splints or rolls: _____

_____

9. Describe how you would teach a patient the following exercises or positions.

a. Quadriceps setting exercise and drills: ____

_____

_____

b. Pushups: _____

_____

c. Dangling: _____

_____

10. A patient visits the health care provider's office for pain and stiffness related to degenerative joint disease (osteoarthritis). Describe how you would assess, diagnose, and plan an exercise program for this patient.

a. Physical assessment: _____

_____

_____

_____

b. Diagnosis: _____

_____

_____

_____

c. Exercise program: _____

_____

_____

_____

11. Give two examples of normal and abnormal findings when assessing the mobility status of a patient in the following areas.

a. General ease of movement:

Normal: _____

_____

Abnormal: _____

_____

b. Gait and posture:

Normal: _____

_____

Abnormal: _____

_____

c. Alignment:

Normal: _____

_____

Abnormal: _____

_____

d. Joint structure and function:

Normal: _____

_____

Abnormal: _____

_____

   e. Muscle mass, tone, and strength:
Normal: _____

_____

Abnormal: _____

_____

   f. Endurance:
Normal: _____

_____

Abnormal: _____

_____

APPLYING YOUR KNOWLEDGE

CRITICAL THINKING QUESTIONS

1. Visit a physical therapy department and observe how the physical therapists assist patients with mobility. Interview several patients to find out how mobility issues have affected their lives. If possible, assist with some of the exercise routines, and try some of the exercises yourself. Reflect on what you learned about mobility and exercise, especially that which you can use for patients you care for.

2. Using a partner, practice placing each other into the following positions: Fowler's, supine, prone, lateral side-lying, and Sims'. What did this teach you about the experience of being positioned that will be helpful in your practice? Discuss each position for health risks that may arise from the following factors: comfort level, body alignment, and pressure points.

3. Try maneuvering on a busy street while on crutches or in a wheelchair. How does impaired mobility affect your ability to perform everyday chores? How did the public react to your impaired mobility? What effects might a permanent disability have on patients, and how can you promote their coping?

REFLECTIVE PRACTICE: CULTIVATING QSEN COMPETENCIES

Use the following expanded scenario from Chapter 34 in your textbook to answer the questions below.

Scenario: Kelsi is a 10-year-old girl in the pediatric unit as a result of a skiing accident. Unconscious at the present time, she may or may not regain consciousness. Kelsi is on bed rest. She requires frequent positioning to maintain correct body alignment as well as passive range-of-motion exercises to maintain her range of motion.

1. Patient-centered care/safety: What patient teaching might the nurse incorporate into the plan of care to help Kelsi's parents minimize the complications of immobility for their daughter?

_____

_____

_____

2. Patient-centered care/evidence-based practice: What would be a successful outcome for this patient?

_____

_____

_____

3. Patient-centered care/evidence-based practice: What intellectual, technical, interpersonal, and ethical/legal competencies are most likely to bring about the desired outcome?

_____

_____

_____

4. Teamwork and collaboration: What resources might be helpful for this family?

_____

_____

_____

PATIENT CARE STUDY

Use this care study to apply your knowledge by completing the nursing Process Worksheet found in Appendix A.

Scenario: Robert Witherspoon, a 42-year-old university professor, presents for a checkup shortly after his father's death. His father died of complications of coronary artery disease. Mr. Witherspoon is 5 ft 9 inches tall, weighs 235 lb, has a decided "paunch," and reports that until now he has made no time for exercise because he preferred to use his free time reading or listening to classical music. He enjoys French cuisine, rich desserts, and has a total cholesterol level of 310 mg/dL (optimal is under 200 mg/dL). He admits being frightened by his father's death and is appropriately concerned about his elevated cholesterol level. "I guess I've never given much thought to my health before, but my dad's death changed all that," he tells you. "I know that coronary artery disease runs in families, and I can tell you that I'm not ready to pack it all in yet. Tell me what I have to do to fight this thing. Now, I'm recognizing the wisdom of his health behaviors and wondering if diet and exercise won't do the trick for me. Can you help me design an exercise program that will work?"

PRACTICING FOR NCLEX

MULTIPLE-CHOICE QUESTIONS

Circle the letter that corresponds to the best answer for each question.

1. A nurse is performing range-of-motion exercises on a patient who is on bed rest. What action will the nurse take when the patient states: "I'm just a little short of breath with these exercises today."
   a. Encourage the patient to finish the exercises and then reevaluate the nursing plan.
   b. Stop the exercises and reevaluate the nursing care plan.
   c. Finish the exercises and report the incident to the primary care provider.
   d. Modify the number of repetitions for each exercise and then modify the plan.

2. While performing ROM, the nurse moves a patient's arm from an extended position to a position at the side of the patient's body. What term does the nurse use to describe this movement?
   a. Adduction
   b. Abduction
   c. Circumduction
   d. Flexion

3. To protect their backs, which motions are appropriate for nurses to use when moving an object?
   a. Balancing their head over their shoulders, leaning forward, and relaxing the stomach muscles when moving an object
   b. Using the muscles of the back to help provide the power needed in strenuous activities
   c. Using the internal girdle and a long midriff to stabilize the pelvis and to protect the abdominal viscera when stooping, reaching, lifting, or pulling
   d. Lifting rather than sliding, rolling, pushing, or pulling objects, reducing the energy required to lift against the pull of gravity

4. A nurse is assisting a patient from a bed to a wheelchair. Which nursing action is most appropriate?
   a. Discouraging the patient from helping with the transfer
   b. Administering pain medication following the transfer
   c. Grabbing and holding the patient by their arms
   d. Using assistive devices to lift over 35 lb of patient weight

5. The nurse uses gait belts when assisting patients to ambulate. Which patient would be a likely candidate for this assistive device?
   a. Cooperative patient who has leg strength
   b. Patient who has an abdominal incision
   c. Postoperative thoracotomy patient
   d. Patient on extended bed rest

6. The home care nurse is providing education to a patient who is bedridden and their family. The nurse teaches them to increase fluids and turn in bed to lessen risk for which complication of immobility?

   a. Pulmonary fibrosis

   b. Increasing circulating fibrinolysin

   c. Predisposition to renal calculi

   d. Increased metabolic rate

7. A community health nurse is promoting exercise and activities for older adults. Which teaching point is most appropriate?

   a. "Quickly increase the repetitions for arm and leg exercises."

   b. "Warm up before beginning exercises and to cool down after exercising."

   c. "Continue to exercise especially if feeling weakness, to build up stamina."

   d. "Force joints to meet or exceed their natural limit before modifying exercises."

8. A nurse is assessing an ambulatory patient's gait. Which nursing documentation best describes their mobility status?

   a. Straight line can be drawn from the ear through the shoulder and hip.

   b. Patient displays full range of motion in arms and legs.

   c. Arms swing freely in alternation with legs.

   d. Adequate muscle mass, tone, and strength are present.

9. A patient will be ambulating for the first time since undergoing cardiac surgery. What safety consideration is most important?

   a. Tell the patient if they are fearful of walking, to look at their feet to ensure correct positioning.

   b. If the patient can lift their legs a few inches off the bed, they do not have sufficient muscle power to permit walking.

   c. Avoid assisting a patient with initial postoperative ambulation without a physical therapist present.

   d. If the patient begins to fall, slide them down your body to the floor, and protect their head.

10. A nurse is caring for a patient with paresis of the lower extremities after a spinal injury. Which intervention will the nurse use to prevent thromboembolism?

    a. Getting the patient out of bed to the chair at least once daily

    b. Observing for swelling and edema of the lower extremities

    c. Applying a thromboembolism stocking and providing ROM

    d. Encouraging intake of 2 to 3 L of water and fluids each day

11. A nurse receives in report that their postoperative patient had an episode of lightheadedness and was unable to get out of bed to the chair as ordered. What action will the oncoming nurse take before transferring the patient to the chair?

    a. Provide an abdominal binder.

    b. Assess orthostatic vital signs.

    c. Ask for the AP to assist with the transfer.

    d. Encourage the patient to eat lunch.

12. A nurse recommends aerobic exercise for a patient who is overweight. Which exercise would the nurse suggest?

    a. Swimming

    b. Lifting weights

    c. Yoga

    d. Stretching exercises

13. A nurse is performing range-of-motion exercises on a patient's arm. The nurse starts by lifting the patient's arm forward to above their head. What action would the nurse perform next?

    a. Move their opposite arm forward to above their head.

    b. Return their arm to the starting position at the side of their body.

    c. Rotate their lower arm and hand so that their palm is up.

    d. Move their arm across the body as far as possible.

14. During range-of-motion exercises, the nurse presses the sole of a patient's foot toward the mattress and then pushes the foot upward. Which type of movement is this nurse promoting by these actions?
   a. Internal and external rotation of the ankle
   b. Dorsiflexion and plantar flexion of the ankle
   c. Flexion and extension of the ankle
   d. Inversion and eversion of the ankle

15. A nurse is caring for an older adult with kyphosis. Which position will the nurse recommend to best prevent skin breakdown in that area?
   a. Supine
   b. Prone
   c. Side lying
   d. Low Fowler's

16. A nurse in the emergency department is teaching a patient how to walk with crutches. Which teaching point is a recommended guideline for this activity?
   a. "Ensure you are not putting pressure on your axilla (armpit) when walking."
   b. "Prevent crutches from getting closer than 3 inches to your feet."
   c. "Do not climb stairs while using crutches."
   d. "The handgrip for the crutches should be even with your waist."

ALTERNATE-FORMAT QUESTIONS

Multiple-Response Questions

Circle the letters that correspond to the best answers for each question.

1. Which exercises would the nurse recommend when planning isometric exercise for a patient recovering from prolonged bed rest? Select all that apply.
   a. Jogging
   b. Range-of-motion exercises
   c. Contracting the quadriceps
   d. Bicycling
   e. Contracting and releasing the gluteal muscles

2. A nurse is promoting body movements for a patient during range-of-motion exercises. Which of these actions represent flexion? Select all that apply.
   a. Bending the hand or foot backward and forward
   b. Turning the sole of the foot toward the midline, then turning the sole of the foot outward
   c. Bending the leg and bringing the heel toward the back of the leg and then returning the leg to the straight position
   d. Curling the toes downward and then straightening them out
   e. Moving the head from side to side, then bringing the chin toward each shoulder
   f. Extending the leg and lifting it upward, then returning the leg to the original position

3. A community health nurse is providing a wellness program that includes teaching the benefits of exercise. Which teaching points would the nurse include? Select all that apply.
   a. "Exercise increases resting heart rate and blood pressure."
   b. "Exercise increases intestinal tone."
   c. "Exercise increases the efficiency of the metabolic system."
   d. "Exercise increases blood flow to the kidneys."
   e. "Exercise decreases appetite."
   f. "Exercise decreases the rate of carbon dioxide excretion."

4. A nurse is assisting a patient recovering from a motor vehicle accident to ambulate with a cane. What patient outcomes indicate proper use of the cane? Select all that apply.
   a. Holding the cane with the same hand as the leg needing support
   b. Holding the cane with the dominant hand; switching hands when fatigued
   c. Beginning with weight evenly distributed between the feet and cane
   d. Bending over the cane for support
   e. Ensuring the patient's arm using the cane is extended when walking
   f. Stating that they will request a rubber tip to prevent slipping

5. A nurse on the neurology unit assesses patients' mobility. What abnormal findings will the nurse enter in the electronic health record? Select all that apply.

   a. Increased joint mobility

   b. Flaccidity

   c. Circumducted gait

   d. Contracture

   e. Full range of motion

   f. Paresis

6. A nurse is caring for patients on an orthopedic unit with alterations in mobility. Which nursing interventions are recommended for these patients? Select all that apply.

   a. Instructing the patient to lie in the prone position for increased cardiac workload

   b. Instructing those with ineffective respiratory expansion to lie in the supine position

   c. Suggesting patients with orthostatic hypotension to sleep sitting up or in an elevated position

   d. Performing ROM exercises every 2 hours for impaired physical mobility

   e. Increasing fluid intake and fiber for patients experiencing constipation

   f. Repositioning those with impaired skin integrity at least every 1 to 2 hours

7. Which nursing actions would the nurse perform when assisting patients with passive ROM exercises? Select all that apply.

   a. Raising the bed to the highest position

   b. Adjusting the bed to the flat position or as low as the patient can tolerate

   c. Hyperextending each joint, then returning them to the resting position

   d. Performing each exercise 10 to 15 times

   e. Moving each joint in a smooth, rhythmic manner

   f. Using a flat palm to support joints during ROM exercises

Rest and Sleep

ASSESSING YOUR UNDERSTANDING

FILL IN THE BLANKS

1. _____ refers to a condition in which the body is in a decreased state of activity with the outcome of feeling refreshed.

2. A state of rest accompanied by altered consciousness and relative inactivity is referred to as _____.

3. The nurse explains to a patient that two systems in the brainstem known as the _____ activating system and the _____ synchronizing region are believed to work together to control the cyclic nature of sleep.

4. Predictable fluctuations in sleep, vital signs, hormone secretion cycle every 24 hours is known as _____ rhythm.

5. Nurses who are exposed to light working the night shift may develop _____ work disorder, in which peak physiologic activity may occur between 2200 and 0600 when they try to rest.

6. Shortened sleep duration in childhood is related to an increased risk of _____ during childhood or later.

7. A patient who reports difficulty falling asleep, intermittent sleep, or early awakening from sleep is experiencing a sleep disorder known as _____.

8. During apnea, the blood _____ level drops, typically causing irregular pulse and increased blood pressure.

9. When patients are in stages III and IV of sleep, representing about 10% of total sleep time, they are experiencing deep-sleep states termed _____ or slow-wave sleep.

10. A parent tells the pediatric nurse that their child experiences patterns of waking from sleep at night and they are unaware of their environment. This type of sleep disorder is a(an) _____.

11. Sleeping more than normal during the day, a condition characterized by excessive sleep, is termed _____.

12. Falling asleep standing up and having an uncontrollable desire to sleep is known as _____.

MATCHING EXERCISES

Matching Exercise 1

Match the term in Part A with its definition of the sleep disorder listed in Part B.

PART A

a. Insomnia

b. Narcolepsy

c. Sleep apnea

d. Somnambulism

e. Enuresis

f. Sleep deprivation

PART B

____ 1. Bedwetting during sleep

____ 2. Difficulty falling asleep, intermittent sleep, or early awakening from sleep

____ 3. Periods of no breathing between snoring intervals

_____ **4.** Decrease in the amount, consistency, and quality of sleep

_____ **5.** Sleepwalking

_____ **6.** Condition characterized by excessive sleep, particularly during the day

Matching Exercise 2

Match the stage of NREM sleep listed in Part A with the characteristics of that stage listed in Part B. Some answers may be used more than once.

PART A

a. Stage I

b. Stage II

c. Stage III

d. Stage IV

PART B

_____ **1.** Deep sleep from which an individual cannot be aroused with ease

_____ **2.** Transitional stage between wakefulness and sleep

_____ **3.** Metabolism slows and the body temperature is low

_____ **4.** Involuntary muscle jerking may occur and awaken the sleeper

_____ **5.** Depth of sleep increases, and arousal becomes increasingly difficult

_____ **6.** Constitutes 50% to 55% of sleep

CORRECT THE FALSE STATEMENTS

Mark the item "T" for true or "F" for false. If false, correct the underlined word or words to make the statement true in the space provided.

_____ **1.** During sleep, stimuli from the cortex are <u>minimal</u>. _____

_____ **2.** Sleep stages III and IV are deep-sleep states termed <u>delta sleep or slow-wave sleep</u>. _____

_____ **3.** Any time a person is awakened from sleep, they will return <u>to point in the sleep cycle where they were disturbed</u>. _____

_____ **4.** Most people go through <u>8 to 10</u> cycles of sleep each night. _____

_____ **5.** On average, infants require <u>10 to 12</u> total hours of sleep each day. _____

_____ **6.** During times of stress, REM sleep <u>decreases</u> in amount, which tends to add to anxiety and stress. _____

_____ **7.** A small <u>protein</u> snack before bedtime is recommended for patients with insomnia. _____

_____ **8.** Exercise that occurs within a 2-hour interval before normal bedtime <u>promotes</u> sleep. _____

_____ **9.** The administration of a <u>larger midafternoon dose</u> of asthma medication may prevent attacks that commonly occur at night during sleep. _____

_____ **10.** People with RLS should avoid alcohol, caffeine, and any OTC <u>analgesics</u> that may aggravate the symptoms of RLS. _____

_____ **11.** <u>Narcolepsy</u> refers to periods of no breathing between snoring intervals. _____

SHORT ANSWER

1. List three benefits of sleep.

   a. _____

   b. _____

   c. _____

2. List the average amount of sleep required for the following age groups and two interventions to minimize sleep disturbance.

   a. Infants

      Amount of sleep: _____

      Interventions: _____

   b. Children

      Amount of sleep: _____

      Interventions: _____

   c. Adults

      Amount of sleep: _____

      Interventions: _____

   d. Older adults

      Amount of sleep: _____

      Interventions: _____

3. Briefly describe how the following factors influence sleep.

   a. Physical activity: _____

   _____

   b. Psychological stress: _____

   _____

c. Motivation: _____

_____

d. Culture: _____

_____

e. Diet: _____

_____

f. Alcohol and caffeine: _____

_____

g. Smoking: _____

_____

h. Environmental factors: _____

_____

i. Lifestyle: _____

_____

j. Exercise: _____

_____

k. Illness: _____

_____

l. Medications: _____

_____

4. List the assessment data needed when obtaining a sleep history from a patient when a sleep disturbance is reported.

_____

_____

_____

_____

5. Describe four findings that indicate a patient is getting sufficient rest to provide energy for the day's activities or can validate the existence of a sleep disturbance that is decreasing the quantity or quality of sleep.

a. _____

b. _____

c. _____

d. _____

6. Describe how you would prepare a restful environment for a home health care patient who is experiencing a sleep disorder.

_____

_____

_____

7. Write a sample nursing diagnosis for the following sleep problems.

a. An older adult patient in a long-term care facility is bored during the day and takes a nap in the afternoon and early evening. They have difficulty sleeping at night.

_____

_____

b. A nurse working rotating shifts in the emergency room complains of being sleepy all the time but cannot sleep when they lie down after work.

_____

_____

8. Describe how each of the following is affected by REM sleep.

a. Eyes: _____

b. Muscles: _____

c. Respirations: _____

d. Pulse: _____

e. Blood pressure: _____

f. Gastric secretions: _____

g. Metabolism: _____

h. Sleep cycle: _____

9. Give an example of a question you would ask a patient to assess for the following sleep factors.

a. Usual sleeping and waking times: _____

_____

b. Number of hours of undisturbed sleep:

_____

_____

c. Quality of sleep: _____

_____

d. Number and duration of naps: _____

_____

e. Energy level: _____

_____

f. Means of relaxing before bedtime: _____

_____

_____

g. Bedtime rituals: _____

_____

CHAPTER 35 REST AND SLEEP   **227**

h. Sleep environment: _____
_____

i. Pharmacologic aids: _____
_____

j. Nature of a sleep disturbance: _____
_____

k. Onset of a disturbance: _____
_____

l. Causes of a disturbance: _____
_____

m. Severity of a disturbance: _____
_____

n. Symptoms of a disturbance: _____
_____

o. Interventions attempted and results:
_____
_____

10. Explain the different presentations of sleep apnea in children versus adults.
_____
_____
_____

APPLYING YOUR KNOWLEDGE

CRITICAL THINKING QUESTION

1. What interprofessional interventions could be developed to promote healthy sleep–rest patterns in the hospital environment?

REFLECTIVE PRACTICE: CULTIVATING QSEN COMPETENCIES

Use the following expanded scenario from Chapter 35 in your textbook to answer the questions below.

Scenario: Charlie is an 86-year-old man who has recently been admitted to a long-term care facility. He tells his daughter that "even though I go to bed around 9 pm, I don't fall asleep until after midnight and then I'm up twice to go to the bathroom and have a lot of trouble falling back to sleep." His daughter has mentioned to the nurse that her father spends a lot of time napping during the day.

1. Patient-centered care/evidence-based practice: What nursing interventions might the nurse employ to help alleviate Charlie's sleep disturbances?
_____
_____
_____

2. Patient-centered care/evidence-based practice: What would be a successful outcome for this patient?
_____
_____
_____

3. Patient-centered care/evidence-based practice: What intellectual, interpersonal, and ethical/legal competencies are most likely to bring about the desired outcome?
_____
_____
_____

4. Teamwork and collaboration: What resources might be helpful for Charlie?
_____
_____
_____

PATIENT CARE STUDY

Use this care study to apply your knowledge by completing the Nursing Process Worksheet found in Appendix A.

You are a nurse in a family practice clinic. Scenario: Gina Cioffi, a 23-year-old graduate nurse, has been in her position as a critical care staff nurse at a large tertiary medical center for 3 months. "I was so excited about working three 12-hour shifts a week when I started this job, thinking I'd have lots of time for other things I want to do, but I'm not sure anymore," she says. "I've been doing extra shifts when we're short-staffed because the money is so good. Now, I'm always tired and all I think about is how soon I can get back to bed. Worst of all, when I do finally get into bed, I often can't fall asleep, especially if things have been busy at work and someone 'went bad'." Looking at Gina, you notice dark circles under her eyes and are suddenly struck

Copyright © 2023 by Wolters Kluwer. *Study Guide for Fundamentals of Nursing: The Art and Science of Person-Centered Nursing Care*, 10th edition.

by the change in her appearance from when she first started working. At that time, she "bounced into work" looking fresh each morning, and her features were always animated. Now, her skin is pale, her hair and clothes look rumpled, and the "brightness" that was so characteristic of her earlier is strikingly absent. With some gentle questioning, you discover that she frequently goes out with new friends she has made at the hospital when her shift is over, and she sometimes goes for 48 hours without sleep. "I know I've gotten myself into a rut. How do I get out of it? I used to think my sleep habits were bad at school, but this is a hundred times worse because there never seems to be time to crash. I just have to keep on going."

PRACTICING FOR NCLEX

MULTIPLE-CHOICE QUESTIONS

Circle the letter that corresponds to the best answer for each question.

1. A nurse in a long-term care facility notes that a patient sleeps for abnormally long times. After researching sleep disorders, the nurse learns that which area of this patient's brain may have suffered damage?
   a. Cerebral cortex
   b. Hypothalamus
   c. Medulla
   d. Midbrain

2. A pediatric nurse teaches parents about normal sleep patterns in children. Which of the following teaching points should the nurse include?
   a. "Daytime napping decreases during the preschool period; most children no longer nap by the age of 5."
   b. "Report any eye movements, groaning, or grimacing by their infant during sleep periods."
   c. "Waking from nightmares or night terrors is common during the adolescent stage."
   d. "Parents can help alleviate the child's fears and awareness of possible death while sleeping."

3. What interview question would be the best choice for a nurse to use to assess for recent changes in a patient's sleep–wakefulness pattern?
   a. "In what way does the sleep you get each day affect your everyday living?"
   b. "How much sleep do you think you need to feel rested?"
   c. "What do you usually do to help yourself fall asleep?"
   d. "Do you usually go to bed and wake up about the same time each day?"

4. A nurse is able to arouse a patient who needs to go for a test relatively easily. Which stage of sleep is this patient most likely experiencing?
   a. Stage I
   b. Stage II
   c. Stage III
   d. Stage IV

5. A nurse on the night shift delays vital sign assessment suspecting the patient is in REM sleep. On which patient cue did the nurse likely base this decision?
   a. Eyes darting back and forth quickly
   b. Slow, regular breathing
   c. Awakening to soft footsteps
   d. Lower blood pressure

6. A nurse on a surgical unit is planning interventions to promote sleep. Which intervention is the best choice for these patients?
   a. Encouraging the patients to take a shower or bath before bedtime
   b. Having the patients set an alarm clock so that they are not worried about getting up
   c. Creating a warm, dark environment in the patients' rooms
   d. Offering a small bedtime snack with a carbohydrate and protein

7. A patient with restless leg syndrome reports a creeping, crawling, or tingling sensation in their legs and the need to constantly move their legs during sleep. What teaching is appropriate for this patient?
   a. "Sleeping pills such as sedatives can be useful."
   b. "Try stretching the legs at bedtime."

c. "Discuss a narcotic analgesic with the health care provider."

d. "Ask your health care provider if you can take an OTC antihistamine."

8. A nurse in a long-term care facility is assessing a group of patients' risks for altered sleep and rest. Which of these patients does the nurse identify for follow up?

a. Patient who walks 20 minutes each day

b. Patient taking medication for hypothyroidism

c. Patient who frequently reports nocturia

d. Patient who requests acetaminophen for arthritis prior to sleep

9. A nurse in a pediatric practice is assessing an adolescent brought by their parent for fatigue and daytime sleepiness problems. Which of these questions related to the teen's lifestyle would the nurse ask?

a. "What kind of grades do you typically earn?"

b. "What time do you go to bed and wake up?"

c. "What do you dislike about school"

d. "Are you having crawling sensations in your legs?"

10. A patient with frequent insomnia asks the nurse about the natural sleep aid melatonin. Which education by the nurse is appropriate?

a. "Melatonin should be taken by 6 pm to be effective."

b. "This medication facilitates sleep, but not sleep maintenance."

c. "You shouldn't take this medication if you are overweight."

d. "Melatonin is an OTC herb that promotes sleep."

11. When educating a patient with insomnia, the nurse would suggest which intervention?

a. "Nap frequently during the day to make up for the lost sleep at night."

b. "Exercise vigorously before bedtime to promote drowsiness."

c. "Eliminate caffeine and alcohol in the evening."

d. "Avoid foods high in carbohydrates before bedtime."

12. A new patient in the medical-surgical unit scheduled for an exploratory laparotomy in the morning reports difficulty sleeping. Which nursing action would the nurse use first?

a. Help the patient maintain a normal bedtime routine and time for sleep.

b. Provide an opportunity for the patient to talk about concerns.

c. Offer prescribed sleep medication.

d. Bring the patient a warm glass of milk at bedtime.

ALTERNATE-FORMAT QUESTIONS
Multiple-Response Questions
Circle the letters that correspond to the best answers for each question.

1. Nurses on a particularly busy hospital unit are carrying out an evidence-based practice project to promote a restful environment. Which interventions will the nurses include? Select all that apply.

a. Maintaining a brighter room during daylight hours and dimming lights in the evening

b. Keeping the room warm and providing earplugs and eye masks if requested

c. Decreasing the volume on alarms, pages, telephones, and staff conversations

d. Scheduling nursing procedures separately to avoid tiring out the patients

e. Medicating for pain if needed

f. Keeping the doors to the patients' rooms open

2. A nurse is teaching a patient about nonpharmacologic measures to alleviate restless leg syndrome. Which teaching points would the nurse include in the plan? (Select all that apply.)

a. "Drinking a cup of coffee before bed can help relieve the tingling sensations."

b. "Applying heat or cold to the extremity can help relieve the symptoms."

c. "An alcoholic beverage is recommended before bed to help you relax."

d. "Biofeedback and transcutaneous electrical nerve stimulation can help relieve symptoms."

e. "Massaging the legs may relieve symptoms."

3. A nurse is providing patient teaching for the parents of an overweight child diagnosed with obstructive sleep apnea. What treatment measures would the nurse explain during the teaching session? Select all that apply.

   a. Plan to increase activity and promote weight loss

   b. Treatment with intranasal antibiotics

   c. Trial of sedative-hypnotic medications

   d. Continuous passive airway pressure machine

   e. Counseling for depression

4. A nurse is teaching the practice of stimulus control to a patient who has insomnia. The nurse would include which teaching points in the teaching plan? Select all that apply.

   a. Recommending that the patient use the bedroom for sex and sleep only

   b. Leaving the bedroom if they cannot fall asleep within 20 minutes and returning when sleepy

   c. Getting up the same time every day, no matter what time they fell asleep

   d. Napping during the day if unable to sleep during the night

   e. Exercising moderately 1 hour before going to bed

   f. Encouraging one or two alcoholic drinks to promote relaxation before bedtime

5. A nurse explains cognitive behavioral therapy (CBT) to a patient who is experiencing chronic insomnia. Which statements by the nurse best describe this therapy? Select all that apply.

   a. "Sedatives and hypnotics are used in conjunction with CBT."

   b. "You will meet with a therapist to work through any maladaptive sleep beliefs."

   c. "Used with other complementary therapies, CBT is very successful."

   d. "Pharmacologic approaches should be attempted prior to CBT to resolve the insomnia."

   e. "CBT may include progressive muscle relaxation measures and stimulus control."

   f. "Sleep restrictions at night will help eliminate prolonged night awakenings."

6. A nurse caring for a patient with hypersomnia assesses for underlying causes of the sleep disorder. What are the possible causes to consider? Select all that apply.

   a. Another sleep disorder, such as sleep apnea

   b. Depression

   c. Malnourishment

   d. Alcohol abuse

   e. Some medications

   f. Eating disorders

CHAPTER 36

Comfort and Pain Management

ASSESSING YOUR UNDERSTANDING

FILL IN THE BLANKS

1. _____ is a defense mechanism that indicates the patient is experiencing a problem.

2. Because pain is a(n) _____ experience, it is present when the individual reporting states that it is present.

3. Peripheral receptors that respond to mechanical, thermal, and chemical noxious stimuli are referred to as _____.

4. Endogenous opioid neuromodulators called _____ and _____ can produce analgesic effects.

5. Pain sensations from the site of injury or inflammation are conducted to the spinal cord and then the brain in a process known as _____.

6. _____ pain is generally rapid in onset and is protective, disappearing when the situation is resolved.

7. A patient with inflammation and infection in the gallbladder reports right shoulder pain. This is an example of _____ pain.

8. Phantom limb pain is an example of _____ pain.

9. Patients may have difficulty localizing and describing _____ pain.

10. Terms such as dull, sharp, or diffuse are used to describe the _____ of pain.

MATCHING EXERCISES

Matching Exercise 1

Match the term in Part A with its description in Part B.

PART A

a. Psychogenic

b. Allodynia

c. Diabetic neuropathy

d. Visceral

e. Chronic

f. Intractable

PART B

____ 1. Pain that occurs following a normally weak or nonpainful stimulus, such as a light touch or a cold drink

____ 2. Pain that is resistant to therapy and persists despite a variety of interventions

____ 3. Pain that is poorly localized and originates in body organs, the thorax, cranium, and abdomen

____ 4. Pain that may be limited, intermittent, or persistent but lasts for 6 months or longer and interferes with normal functioning

____ **5.** Pain for which no physical cause can be identified, but can be as intense as that from a physical event

____ **6.** Metabolic and vascular changes damage peripheral and autonomic nerves causing numbness, prickling, or paresthesias

Matching Exercise 2

Match the type of pain in Part A with the appropriate example in Part B. Answers may be used more than once.

PART A

a. Cutaneous

b. Deep somatic

c. Visceral

d. Referred

PART B

____ **1.** Pain associated with cancer of the uterus

____ **2.** Pain associated with a knee injury

____ **3.** Pain associated with stomach ulcers

____ **4.** Neck or jaw pain associated with a myocardial infarction (heart attack)

____ **5.** Pain associated with a burn injury

____ **6.** Pain associated with a fractured humerus

Matching Exercise 3

Match the term in Part A with the appropriate nonpharmacologic pain relief method listed in Part B.

PART A

a. Distraction

b. Biofeedback

c. Acupressure

d. TENS

e. Cutaneous stimulation

f. Placebo

PART B

____ **1.** Requires the patient to focus attention on something other than the pain

____ **2.** Machine with a signal helps the patient learn by trial and error to control the supposed involuntary body mechanisms that may cause pain

____ **3.** Use of the fingertips to create gentle but firm pressure to usual acupuncture sites

____ **4.** Electrical stimulation of large-diameter fibers to inhibit the transmission of painful impulses carried over small-diameter fibers

____ **5.** Application of cold, ice or heat

____ **6.** Administration or use is ethically questionable

SHORT ANSWER

1. Read the situation below, write a three-part health problem statement, then describe behavioral, physiologic, and affective responses to pain that you might observe.

Situation: A patient underwent a cesarean birth yesterday and uses their call light to request something for their incisional pain. You assess them holding their lower abdomen and wincing when they move.

Health Problem:

Etiology:

Signs and Symptoms:

2. Briefly describe the chemical process proposed to occur when tissue is injured.

_____

_____

_____

3. Explain why referred pain can be transmitted to a cutaneous (skin) site different from its origin.

_____

_____

_____

4. Explain the mechanism of the gate control theory and how it is believed to control pain.

_____

_____

_____

5. Give an example of how the following factors may influence a patient's pain experience.

a. Culture/ethnicity: _____

_____

b. Family, biologic sex, or age: _____

_____

c. Religious beliefs: _____
_____

d. Environment and support people: _____
_____

e. Anxiety and other stressors: _____
_____

f. Past pain experience: _____
_____

6. Describe how you would respond to a patient who tells you the following about their surgical pain experience.

a. "I count on you to know when I'm in pain and will do something to relieve it." _____
_____

b. "I'll wait as long as possible to ask for something for pain, I'm afraid I may become addicted." _____
_____

c. "It's natural to have pain when you get older. It's just something I've learned to live with." _____
_____

7. Give an example of a question you could ask when assessing for the following characteristics of pain.

a. Duration of pain: _____
_____

b. Quantity and intensity of pain: _____
_____

c. Quality of pain: _____
_____

d. Physiologic indicators of pain: _____
_____

8. What is your perception of the use of placebos for a patient demanding a drug. Is lying to the patient ever justifiable? What impact could this action have on the nurse–patient relationship? What nursing judgment will you make when receiving a prescription for a placebo for your patient?
_____
_____
_____
_____

9. How would you modify your means of assessing for pain in the following patients?

a. Patient with a cognitive impairment:
_____
_____

b. 5-year-old patient: _____
_____

c. Older adult: _____
_____

APPLYING YOUR KNOWLEDGE

CRITICAL THINKING QUESTIONS

1. When caring for a patient with chronic pain, discuss what care decisions you will make when a patient requesting pain medication rates their pain 9/10? The patient is talking with family and ate 50% of their lunch an hour ago.
Medication Administration Record
Oxycodone/acetaminophen 2 tabs every 4 hours prn moderate pain
Morphine 2 mg IV prn every 4 hours prn severe pain

2. During your clinical rotation, you care for a patient with end-stage cancer experiencing severe pain. The nurse tells you the patient has received all the pain medication that has been prescribed; they cannot administer more medication without a doctor's order. How could you provide additional comfort measures? How would you advocate for effective pain management for this patient? Reflect on how your competence in pain management could affect this patient's quality of life in their last days?

3. Compare and contrast two pain assessment tools available (e.g., in your textbook) in the areas of physical assessment, pain scales, location and duration of the pain, coping measures, pain management, and the effect of pain on daily living.

REFLECTIVE PRACTICE: CULTIVATING QSEN COMPETENCIES

Use the following expanded scenario from Chapter 36 in your textbook to answer the questions below.

Scenario: Carla is a 72-year-old woman who has a history of type 2 diabetes and associated diabetic neuropathy. She reports pain in her lower extremities that is at times sharp but is generally dull. She also reports that she has relatively new periods of numbness and tingling. Carla is becoming increasingly worried that this constant pain is going to take over her life. She reports that an increase in stress and anxiety seems to be making the pain even worse.

1. Patient-centered care/safety: What nursing interventions might the nurse use to help manage this patient's pain associated with diabetic neuropathy?

   _____

   _____

   _____

2. Patient-centered care/evidence-based practice: What would be a successful outcome for this patient?

   _____

   _____

   _____

3. Patient-centered care/evidence-based practice: What intellectual competencies are most likely to bring about the desired outcome?

   _____

   _____

   _____

4. Teamwork and collaboration: What resources might be helpful for Carla?

   _____

   _____

   _____

PATIENT CARE STUDY

Use this care study to apply your knowledge by completing the Nursing Process Worksheet found in Appendix A.

Scenario: Tabitha Wilson, a 24-month-old infant with AIDS, is hospitalized with infectious diarrhea. She is well known to the pediatric staff, and there is concern that she might not pull through this admission. She has suffered many of the complications of AIDS and is no stranger to pain. Currently, the skin on her buttocks is raw and excoriated, and tears stream down her face whenever she is moved. Her blood pressure also shoots up when she is touched. The severity of her illness has left her extremely weak and listless, and her foster mother reports that she no longer recognizes her child. When alone in her crib, she seldom moves, and she moans softly. Several nurses have expressed great frustration caring for Tabitha because they find it hard to perform even simple nursing measures like turning, diapering, and weighing her when they see how much pain these procedures cause.

PRACTICING FOR NCLEX

MULTIPLE-CHOICE QUESTIONS

Circle the letter that corresponds to the best answer for each question.

1. A nurse implements cutaneous stimulation for a patient as part of a strategy for pain relief. Which nursing action exemplifies the use of this technique?

   a. Playing soft music in the patient's room

   b. Assisting the patient to focus on something pleasant

   c. Providing a back massage before bed

   d. Teaching the patient deep-breathing techniques

2. A nurse is visiting a patient at home who is recovering from a bowel resection. The patient complains of constant pain and discomfort and displays signs of depression. When assessing this patient for pain, what should be the nurse's focal point?

   a. Judging whether the patient is experiencing pain or depression

   b. Beginning pain medications before the pain is too severe

c. Administering a placebo and performing a reassessment of the pain

d. Reviewing and revising the pain management plan

3. During interprofessional rounds, the team discusses a patient recovering from an above-the-knee amputation with continued severe pain in spite of receiving opioid analgesics. The nurse suggests adding an adjuvant medication. What is the best example of an adjuvant?

a. Medication used for breakthrough pain, when around-the-clock dosing is used

b. Substance without therapeutic effect, believed to provide comfort

c. Anticonvulsant medication for neuropathic pain that can enhance the action of the opioid

d. Device the patient can activate when pain occurs to deliver a preset dose of analgesic

4. A nurse on a surgical unit is evaluating prescriptions for patients who will receive postoperative PCA. The nurse contacts the provider to discuss alternate pain management for which patient whose condition is inappropriate for PCA?

a. Child in grade school

b. Patient with dementia

c. Adolescent undergoing an appendectomy

d. Patient in labor who may need a cesarean section

5. A nurse is teaching a novice nurse about the therapeutic effects of laughter. Which example correctly identifies one of these effects?

a. It activates the immune system.

b. It increases the level of epinephrine.

c. It decreases heart rate.

d. It causes shallow breathing.

6. A patient who recently underwent amputation of a leg complains of pain in the amputated extremity. What would be the nurse's best response?

a. "Your leg can't hurt because the leg has been amputated."

b. "Your pain is a phenomenon known as 'ghost pain'."

c. "Your pain is a real experience."

d. "You are experiencing central pain syndrome."

7. Prior to administering an opioid medication, the nurse assesses that the patient is occasionally drowsy, drifting off to sleep during conversation, but easy to arouse. What action will the nurse take?

a. Administer naloxone.

b. No action is needed; this is an expected effect.

c. Increase fluid intake.

d. Suggest a lower dose of medication.

8. Which means of pain control is based on the gate control theory?

a. Biofeedback

b. Distraction

c. Hypnosis

d. Acupuncture

9. A nurse is assessing a patient for the chronology of the pain she is experiencing. What is an appropriate interview question to obtain this data?

a. "How does the pain develop and progress?"

b. "How would you describe your pain?"

c. "How would you rate the pain on a scale of 1 to 10?"

d. "What do you do to alleviate your pain and how well does it work?"

10. A patient complains of severe pain following a mastectomy. The nurse would expect to administer what type of pain medication to this patient?

a. NSAIDs

b. Corticosteroids

c. Opioid analgesics

d. Nonopioid analgesics

11. A nurse on a medical-surgical unit administers pain medication to patients. Which patient would benefit from a PRN drug regimen as an effective method of pain control?

a. Patient experiencing acute pain

b. Patient in the early postoperative period

c. Patient experiencing chronic pain

d. Patient in the postoperative stage with occasional pain

12. A nurse is providing preoperative patient education regarding the use of analgesics. Which principle is important to emphasize?

    a. "Try not to develop an addiction or dependence."

    b. "Use nonpharmacologic therapies as adjuncts to the medical regimen."

    c. "It is easier to prevent severe pain with prescribed medication than treat it."

    d. "Remaining still and quiet to prevent pain is desirable."

13. Three days after surgery, a patient continues to have moderate to severe incisional pain. Based on the gate control theory, what action should the nurse take?

    a. Administer pain medications in smaller doses but more frequently.

    b. Decrease external stimuli in the room during painful episodes.

    c. Reposition the patient and gently massage the patient's back.

    d. Advise the patient to try to sleep following administration of pain medication.

14. A nurse is treating a young school-aged child who is in pain but cannot verbalize characteristics of the pain. What would be the nurse's best intervention in this situation?

    a. Take no action if the child offers no complaints.

    b. Have the child use a doll to act out their pain experience.

    c. Administer antianxiety medication to treat fear of pain.

    d. Use distraction to prevent the child from noticing their pain.

15. When caring for a patient receiving an opioid medication via PCA, which instruction is essential to provide the patient and family?

    a. "This medication is very strong, we will be checking your vital signs frequently."

    b. "The medication may make you sleepy."

    c. "Only the patient may press the button for pain medication."

    d. "If your mouth becomes dry, we can swab your mouth with water."

ALTERNATE-FORMAT QUESTIONS

Multiple-Response Questions

Circle the letters that correspond to the best answers for each question.

1. A nurse in the emergency department cares for multiple patients experiencing pain. Which patients would the nurse document as having acute pain? Select all that apply.

    a. Patient experiencing a heart attack

    b. Patient with diabetic neuropathy

    c. Patient reporting signs and symptoms of appendicitis

    d. Fall victim with a broken ankle

    e. Patient with rheumatoid arthritis

    f. Patient who has bladder cancer

2. A nurse is providing a back massage to a patient who is having trouble sleeping. Which nursing actions are performed appropriately? Select all that apply.

    a. Massaging the patient's shoulder, entire back, areas over iliac crests, and sacrum with light vertical stroking motions

    b. Kneading the patient's skin using continuous grasping and pinching motions

    c. Assisting the patient to a prone position and draping the patient with the bath blanket

    d. Completing the massage with short, stroking movements that eventually become heavier in pressure

    e. Applying warmed lotion to patient's shoulders, back, and sacral area

    f. Placing hands at the base of the spine, stroking upward to the shoulder and back down to the buttocks

3. A nurse recognizes common pain syndromes that cause neuropathic pain. Which patient conditions would the nurse place at risk for this type of pain? Select all that apply.

    a. Tooth abscess

    b. Postherpetic neuralgia

    c. Phantom limb pain

    d. Diabetic neuropathy

    e. Lung cancer

    f. Complex regional pain syndrome

4. Nurses assess patients' responses to pain. Which represent physiologic responses? Select all that apply.

   a. Exaggerated weeping and restlessness

   b. Protecting the painful area

   c. Increased blood pressure

   d. Muscle tension and rigidity

   e. Nausea and vomiting

   f. Grimacing and moaning

5. A nurse is initiating PCA for a postoperative patient whose family is visiting. What information should the nurse give the patient and family? Select all that apply.

   a. Tell the family members to push the button to treat pain when the patient appears uncomfortable.

   b. Inform the patient that pushing the button delivers a specified dose of medication.

   c. Tell the patient that this method results in inconsistent blood levels of analgesic.

   d. Teach that the pump will not deliver medication during the "lock-out" interval, for safety.

   e. Explain that the carbon dioxide monitor is to detect early signs of respiratory depression.

Prioritization Question

1. A nurse working on a surgical unit is reviewing vital signs taken by the AP. Which patient will the nurse prioritize for assessment? Circle the letter that corresponds to the best answer.

   a. Patient reporting postoperative pain 7/10 with a blood pressure of 156/88

   b. Patient with cancer reporting pain scaled as 6/10

   c. Postcolostomy patient reporting pain 3/10 whose respiratory rate is 8

   d. Patient moaning in pain, requesting pain medication for abdominal pain

37

Nutrition

ASSESSING YOUR UNDERSTANDING

FILL IN THE BLANKS

1. The study of nutrients and how they are handled by the body is called
   _____.

2. What is the body mass index (BMI) for a 220-lb man who is 6 ft 3 inches tall?
   _____

3. According to the BMI guidelines published by the NHLBI, a person with a BMI >30 indicates _____.

4. A patient with a negative nitrogen balance is in a _____ state.

5. The nurse teaches patients to avoid manufactured, partially hydrogenated liquid oils, referred to as _____ fats, which raise serum cholesterol.

6. Vitamins do not provide _____ but are needed for the metabolism of carbohydrates, proteins, and fats.

7. The fat-soluble vitamins are
   _____, _____, E, and _____.

8. The nurse in the community discusses healthy eating using MyPlate food guidelines. This schematic includes what food groups:
   _____, _____, complex _____, and dairy.

9. The nurse teaches a patient that it is recommended that carbohydrates provide _____% to _____% of calories for adults, focusing on complex carbohydrates, such as whole grains.

10. Most health care experts recommend that protein intake should contribute _____% to _____% of total caloric intake.

11. An adult's total body weight is _____% to _____% water.

12. Dysphagia is associated with an increased risk for _____, the misdirection of oropharyngeal secretions or gastric contents into the larynx and lower respiratory tract.

13. _____ metabolism is the energy required to carry on the involuntary activities of the body at rest—the energy needed to sustain the metabolic activities of cells and tissues.

14. _____ are specific biochemical substances used by the body for growth, development, activity, reproduction, lactation, health maintenance, and recovery from injury or illness.

15. A patient who has anorexia has a _____ of _____.

16. _____ minerals that have recommended dietary intake established include iron, zinc, manganese, chromium, copper, molybdenum, selenium, fluoride, and iodine.

Matching Exercises

Matching Exercise 1

Match the nutrient in Part A to the type of function it performs in Part B. Answers may be used more than once.

PART A

a. Carbohydrates

b. Protein

c. Fat

PART B

____ **1.** Spares protein so it can be used for other functions

____ **2.** Promotes tissue growth and repair

____ **3.** Prevents ketosis from inefficient fat metabolism

____ **4.** When metabolized, it burdens the kidneys

____ **5.** Delays glucose absorption

____ **6.** Forms antibodies

Matching Exercise 2

Match the function on the left side of the chart with the mineral listed in Part A. List one food source for each mineral.

PART A

a. Calcium

b. Phosphorus

c. Iron

d. Sodium

e. Iodine

f. Chloride

Mineral Function	Mineral	Food Source
1. Bone and tooth formation, blood clotting, nerve transmission, muscle contraction		
2. Major ion of extracellular fluid; fluid balance; acid–base balance		
3. Bone and tooth formation; acid–base balance; energy metabolism		
4. Component of HCl in stomach; fluid balance; acid–base balance		
5. Component of thyroid hormones		
6. Oxygen transported by way of hemoglobin; constituent of enzyme systems		

MATCHING EXERCISE 3

Match the terms listed in Part A with their definition listed in Part B.

PART A

a. Macronutrients

b. Micronutrients

c. Calories

d. Basal metabolism

e. RDA

f. MyPlate Food Guide

PART B

_____ **1.** Measurement of energy in the diet

_____ **2.** Recommendation for average daily amounts that healthy population groups should consume over time

_____ **3.** Graphic device designed to represent a total diet and provide a firm foundation for health

_____ **4.** Essential nutrients that supply energy and build tissue

_____ **5.** Amount of energy required to carry on the involuntary activities of the body at rest

_____ **6.** Vitamins and minerals that are required in much smaller amounts to regulate and control body processes

SHORT ANSWER

1. Briefly explain the body's state of nitrogen balance.

_____

_____

_____

2. Explain the difference between the following fatty acids and give an example of each. Note effects on serum cholesterol levels and health.

    a. Saturated fats: _____

_____

_____

    b. Unsaturated fats: _____

_____

    c. Trans fats: _____

_____

_____

3. Briefly describe the nutritional needs of the following age groups:

    a. Infancy: _____

_____

_____

    b. Toddlers and preschoolers: _____

_____

_____

    c. School-aged children: _____

_____

_____

    d. Adolescents: _____

_____

_____

    e. Adults: _____

_____

_____

    f. Pregnant persons: _____

_____

_____

    g. Older adults: _____

_____

_____

4. Complete the table below that depicts the function and recommended percentage of the diet for the energy nutrients.

Nutrient	Function	Recommended %
a. Carbohydrates		
b. Proteins		
c. Fats		
d. Vitamins		
e. Minerals		
f. Water		

5. List four dietary interventions to increase peristalsis which prevents or treats constipation.
a. _____
b. _____
c. _____
d. _____

6. Briefly describe the following eating disorders and the typical manifestations.
a. Anorexia nervosa: _____

b. Bulimia: _____

7. Give an example of how the following variables may affect a patient's nutritional needs.
a. Biologic sex: _____

b. State of health: _____

c. Alcohol abuse: _____

d. Medications: _____

e. Religion: _____

f. Economics: _____

8. Describe the following methods of collecting dietary data.
a. Food diaries: _____

b. 24-hour diet recall: _____

c. Food frequency record: _____

_____

9. Describe how a nurse would assess a patient who is using home health care services for adequate nourishment.

_____

_____

_____

10. List three teaching strategies a nurse may use to assist with adherence to prescribed dietary practices.

a. _____

b. _____

c. _____

11. Describe the following types of diets, noting their nutritional value, and give an example of the types of food provided in each.

a. Clear-liquid diet: _____

_____

b. Full-liquid diet: _____

_____

c. Low-fiber diet: _____

_____

12. Briefly describe why a nasointestinal or jejunal feeding tube may be used.

_____

_____

_____

APPLYING YOUR KNOWLEDGE

CRITICAL THINKING QUESTIONS

1. You are caring for a patient who is NPO for an extended period related to pancreatitis and now received TPN. Using the nursing process, summarize your nursing care focusing on managing the patient's parenteral nutrition.

2. During your clinical experience or with a friend, conduct a 24-hour dietary recall. Is the patient or person following a prescribed or therapeutic diet? Does the person's diet include the recommended number of servings of foods from MyPlate? Is the diet high or low in fat? What education might this person need?

REFLECTIVE PRACTICE: DEVELOPING QSEN COMPETENCIES

Use the following expanded scenario from Chapter 37 in your textbook to answer the questions below.

Scenario: William Johnston, a 42-year-old executive, is newly diagnosed with high blood pressure and high cholesterol. He confides that his health has been the last thing on his mind and that his health habits are less than admirable. "I usually eat on the run, often fast food, or big dinners with lots of alcohol. I can't remember the last time I worked out or did any exercise, unless running from my car to the train counts! I guess it's no wonder I've gained a few pounds over the years!"

1. Patient-centered care/safety: What patient teaching might the nurse provide to help William meet his nutritional and exercise needs?

_____

_____

2. Patient-centered care: What would be a successful outcome for this patient?

_____

_____

3. Evidence-based practice: What intellectual, interpersonal, and ethical/legal competencies are most likely to bring about the desired outcome?

_____

_____

_____

4. Teamwork and collaboration: What resources might be helpful for this patient?

_____

_____

_____

PATIENT CARE STUDY

Use this care study to apply your knowledge by completing the Nursing Process Worksheet found in Appendix A.

Scenario: Mr. Church, a 74-year-old White man, is being admitted to the geriatric unit of the hospital for pneumonia. He was diagnosed with Alzheimer's disease 4 years ago, and 1 year ago, he was admitted to a long-term care facility. His wife of 49 years informs the admitting nurse that she instigated his admission to the hospital because she was alarmed by his shortness of breath and weight loss. Assessment reveals a 6-ft 1-inch tall, emaciated man who weighs 149 lb. His wife reports that he has lost 20 lb in the past 2 months. The staff at the long-term care facility report that he was eating his meals, and his wife validated that this was the case, but there is no clear calorie count. Mrs. Church nods her head vigorously when asked if her husband had seemed more agitated and hyperactive recently. Mr. Church has dull, sparse hair; pale, dry skin; and dry mucous membranes.

PRACTICING FOR NCLEX

MULTIPLE-CHOICE QUESTIONS

Circle the letter that corresponds to the best answer for each question.

1. A nurse and patient are planning the diet for the patient needing a quick source of energy due to frequent episodes of hypoglycemia (low blood sugar). What nutrient that provides quick energy will the nurse recommend?
   a. Carbohydrates
   b. Vitamins
   c. Minerals
   d. Water

2. A nurse is assessing a group of patients' BMR. Which patient would the nurse suspect would have an increased BMR?
   a. Older adult
   b. Patient with a fever
   c. Patient NPO before surgery
   d. Patient sleeping

3. A nurse is performing a nutritional assessment of an obese patient who visits a weight control clinic. What information should the nurse take into consideration when planning a weight reduction plan for this patient?
   a. To lose 1 lb/wk, the daily intake should be decreased by 200 calories.
   b. One pound of body fat equals approximately 5,000 calories.
   c. Psychological reasons for overeating should be explored, such as eating for boredom.
   d. Obesity is treatable, and 50% of obese people who lose weight keep it off for 7 years.

4. What consideration based on biologic sex would a nurse make when planning a menu for a male patient with well-defined muscle mass?
   a. Men have a lower need for carbohydrates.
   b. Men have a higher need for minerals.
   c. Men have a higher need for proteins.
   d. Men have a lower need for vitamins.

5. When caring for a patient with a small-bore feeding tube, the nurse plans to verify tube placement by aspirating gastric contents for pH testing. What nursing action will the nurse use to aspirate the gastric secretions?
   a. Using a small syringe and inserting 10 mL of sterile water
   b. Injecting air boluses into the tube with a large syringe and slowly applying negative pressure to withdraw fluid
   c. Continuing to instill air until fluid is aspirated
   d. Placing the patient in the Trendelenburg position to facilitate the fluid aspiration process

6. A nurse is working on an acute care unit where many patients have nasogastric, gastrostomy or jejunostomy tubes for feedings. To prevent complications, the nurse should regularly assess and trend what measurement?
   a. Tube length
   b. Color of gastric fluid
   c. Gastric fluid pH
   d. Daily weight

7. When caring for a patient with poor dentition and difficulty chewing, which dietary recommendation will the nurse make to help the patient maintain optimal nutrition?

a. Gastrostomy feeding

b. Full-liquid diet

c. Mechanically altered, soft diet

d. Higher fat diet

8. Which nursing action is essential for the nurse to perform when safely administering enteral feeding?

a. Adding food dye to the feeding as a means of detecting aspirated fluid during suction

b. Assessing gastric residual before each feeding or every 4 to 8 hours during continuous feeding

c. Monitoring bowel sounds at least four times per shift to ensure the presence of peristalsis

d. Preventing contamination during enteral feedings by using an open system

9. A nurse on a surgical unit is assessing the nutritional needs of patients. The nurse suggests TPN for which of these patients?

a. Patient with serum albumin level of 2.5 g/dL or less

b. Patient with residual of more than 100 mL

c. Patient with intestinal surgery with no bowel sounds

d. Patient with presence of dumping syndrome

10. A visiting nurse is at the home of a patient receiving home TPN for malabsorption after bowel surgery and their spouse. What finding is essential for the nurse to report to the health care provider?

a. Anorexia

b. Low-grade fever

c. Inability to state the purpose of TPN

d. Hypoactive bowel sounds

11. A nurse has aspirated 100 mL of gastric residual for a patient receiving continuous tube feeding at 75 mL/hr. Which action will the nurse take next?

a. Discard the gastric residual using standard precautions.

b. Place the tube feeding on hold for 2 hours.

c. Recommend initiating total parenteral nutrition.

d. Return the residual and flush the tube.

12. A nurse and an AP are caring for a patient post stroke. Which instruction will the nurse give the AP as they prepare to feed the patient?

a. Provide mouth care after the meal.

b. Do not exceed 15 minutes for feeding.

c. Stop if the patient begins coughing forcefully.

d. The patient can recline during feeding.

13. A nurse at a health fair is providing education on cardiovascular risks and body fat distribution. What can best assess abdominal adiposity?

a. Weight

b. Waist circumference

c. Caloric intake

d. Presence of diabetes

ALTERNATE-FORMAT QUESTIONS

Multiple-Response Questions

Circle the letters that correspond to the best answers for each question.

1. A nurse working on a medical-surgical unit is performing nutritional screening. Which patients will the nurse identify as having risk for anorexia? Select all that apply.

a. Patient with depression

b. Patient with preference for fried food

c. Patient receiving chemotherapy

d. Patient requesting an evening snack

e. Patient with loss of smell and taste

f. Patient with poorly controlled pain

2. Students attending clinical in a family medical practice are learning about nutritional requirements and BMR. Which patients will the students identify as having an increased BMR? Select all that apply.

a. Toddler having a growth spurt

b. Older adult in a long-term care facility

c. Adolescent fasting to lose weight

d. School-aged child with a fever

e. Adult going through a divorce

f. Adult with hypersomnia

3. When a nurse attempts to aspirate gastric residual from a PEG tube prior to intermittent tube feeding, they find that the tube is clogged. What are appropriate nursing interventions in this situation? Select all that apply.

a. Using warm water and gentle pressure to remove the clog

b. Flushing with a carbonated beverage

c. Using the tube's stylet to unclog the tube

d. When necessary, replacing the tube

e. Reminding all staff to adequately flush the tube after each feeding

f. Changing the dressing on the feeding tube using clean technique

4. A nurse in a long-term care facility collaborates with the dietician to assess residents for adequate nutrition. Which strategies will the nurse recommend to address age-related changes affecting nutrition? Select all that apply.

a. Avoid cold liquids with decreased peristalsis in the esophagus.

b. Serve a variety of foods and textures for loss of sense of taste and smell.

c. Avoid eating right before bedtime for gastroesophageal reflux.

d. Eat a high-fiber diet for slowed intestinal peristalsis.

e. Encourage patients with lower glucose tolerance to eat more simple carbohydrates.

f. Offer large, frequent meals for reduction in appetite and thirst sensation.

5. A home health care nurse is teaching a patient and caregivers how to administer an enteral feeding. Which teaching points are appropriate? Select all that apply.

a. Discard gastric residuals to prevent an acid–base imbalance.

b. Be careful not to rotate the guard at the gastric tube insertion after cleaning around it.

c. Check for leaking of gastric contents around the insertion site.

d. Clean around the gastric tube with soap and water, making sure it is adequately rinsed.

e. Maintain elevation of head of the bed during gastric feeding and for an hour after.

f. Mark the tube at the level of the abdominal wall in indelible ink and validate frequently.

6. A nurse is caring for a patient receiving total parenteral nutrition. Which actions will the nurse include in the care plan? Select all that apply.

a. Administer the TPN using an inline filter via an infusion pump.

b. Plan to use the same catheter lumen with each tubing change.

c. Maintain a gauze dressing firmly over the site, changing weekly.

d. Expect a weight gain of 1 lb per day.

e. Monitor blood glucose levels as prescribed.

f. Assess vital signs, platelet levels, and serum protein.

7. When caring for the patient receiving nasogastric enteral feedings, which nursing actions will best prevent complications? Select all that apply.

a. Elevating the head 30 to 45 degrees during the feeding and 1 hour afterward

b. Giving larger, less frequent feedings

c. Flushing the tube before and after feeding

d. Cleaning and moistening the nares and applying a lubricant

e. Changing the delivery set every other day according to facility policy

f. Holding the feeding for gastric residual of more than 250 mL

Prioritization Question

1. The nurse on a surgical unit is caring for a group of patients receiving parenteral feedings. What patient will the nurse plan to assess first? Circle the letter corresponding to the best answer.

a. Patient with a temperature of 100°F

b. Patient with a dressing soiled with 2-cm dried blood

c. Patient unresponsive since admission

d. Patient needing teaching for surgery later today

Urinary Elimination

ASSESSING YOUR UNDERSTANDING

FILL IN THE BLANKS

1. Continued incontinence of urine past the age of toilet training is documented in the medical record as _____.

2. The process of _____ is the act of emptying the bladder, urination, or voiding.

3. When assessing the urinary system of a newborn, the newborn should have _____ to _____ wet diapers daily.

4. The nurse records the patient who has involuntary, uncontrolled loss of urine from the bladder as experiencing urinary _____.

5. A urinary _____ is a surgical procedure that creates an alternate route for urine excretion.

6. The nurse documents the patient's report of getting up multiple times a night to void as _____.

7. A patient having a delay or difficulty in initiating voiding is said to experience _____.

8. Generally, a clean-catch urine specimen should be collected _____.

9. A patient with an obstruction in the urinary tract may require insertion of a _____, or thin catheter or tube that provides a pathway for the flow of urine.

ASSESSING YOUR UNDERSTANDING

MATCHING EXERCISES

Matching Exercise 1

Match the terms associated with micturition in Part A with their definitions listed in Part B.

PART A

a. Urinary retention

b. Stress incontinence

c. Urge incontinence

d. Overflow incontinence

e. Autonomic bladder

PART B

_____ 1. Involuntary loss of urine associated with an abrupt and strong desire to void

_____ 2. Involuntary loss of urine related to an increase in intra-abdominal pressure during coughing, sneezing, laughing, or other physical activities

_____ 3. Involuntary loss of urine associated with overdistention and overflow of the bladder

_____ 4. Occurs when urine is produced normally but not appropriately excreted from the bladder

_____ 5. Voiding by reflex only

Matching Exercise 2

Match the color of urine listed in Part A with the medication that produces that color listed in Part B. Answers may be used more than once.

PART A

a. Pale yellow

b. Orange, orange-red, or pink

c. Green or green-blue

d. Brown or black

e. Red

PART B

____ **1.** Diuretics

____ **2.** Injectable iron compounds

____ **3.** Amitriptyline

____ **4.** Phenazopyridine

____ **5.** Anticoagulants

____ **6.** Vitamin B complex

SHORT ANSWER

1. Describe how the following factors affect micturition.

    a. Developmental considerations: _____

    _____

    b. Food and fluid: _____

    _____

    c. Psychological variables: _____

    _____

    d. Activity and muscle tone: _____

    _____

    e. Pathologic conditions: _____

    _____

    f. Medications: _____

    _____

2. List four factors that indicate a child is ready for toilet training.

    a. _____

    b. _____

    c. _____

    d. _____

3. Describe special urinary considerations that should be included in the nursing history for the following patients.

    a. Infants and young children: _____

    _____

    b. Older adults: _____

    _____

    c. Patients with limited or no bladder control or urinary diversions: _____

    _____

    d. Patient receiving dialysis: _____

    _____

4. Describe how you would examine the following areas of the urinary system when performing a physical assessment.

    a. Kidneys: _____

    _____

    b. Bladder: _____

    _____

    c. Urethral orifice: _____

    _____

    d. Skin integrity and hydration: _____

    _____

    e. Urine: _____

    _____

5. List four expected outcomes that denote normal voiding in a patient.

    a. _____

    b. _____

    c. _____

    d. _____

6. Explain how the following factors influence a patient's voiding patterns.

    a. Schedule: _____

    _____

    b. Privacy: _____

    _____

    c. Position: _____

    _____

    d. Hygiene: _____

    _____

7. List three reasons for catheterization.

a. _____

b. _____

c. _____

8. List two expected outcomes for a patient with a urinary diversion or stoma appliance.

a. _____

b. _____

APPLYING YOUR KNOWLEDGE

CRITICAL THINKING QUESTIONS

1. Develop a teaching plan to teach a postsurgical patient with male genitalia and their partner how to perform self-catheterization in a home setting. What factors are likely to influence the success of your teaching plan?

REFLECTIVE PRACTICE: CULTIVATING QSEN COMPETENCIES

Use the following expanded scenario from Chapter 38 in your textbook to answer the questions below.

Scenario: Midori Morita, age 69, is taking care of her 70-year-old husband at home. Mrs. Morita asks, "Should I talk with my husband's doctor about getting a urinary catheter? Ever since he came home from the hospital this last time, he seems unable to use the urinal. He dribbles urine constantly, and I can't keep up with the laundry. He had a catheter in the hospital."

1. Patient-centered care/evidence-based practice/safety: How might the nurse respond to Mrs. Morita's remarks regarding her husband's home care?

_____

_____

_____

2. Patient-centered care/evidence-based practice/safety: What would be a successful outcome for this patient?

_____

_____

_____

3. Evidence-based practice: What intellectual, technical, interpersonal, and/or ethical/legal competencies are most likely to bring about the desired outcome?

_____

_____

_____

4. Teamwork and collaboration: What resources might be helpful for the Morita family?

_____

_____

_____

PATIENT CARE STUDY

Use this care study to apply your knowledge by completing the nursing Process Worksheet found in Appendix A.

Scenario: Mr. Eisenberg, age 84, was admitted to a long-term care facility when his wife of 62 years died. He has two adult children, neither of whom feels prepared to care for him the way his wife did. "We don't know how Mom did it year after year," his son says. "After he retired from his law practice, he was terribly demanding, and it just seemed nothing she did for him pleased him. His Parkinson's disease does make it a bit difficult for him to get around, but he's able to do a whole lot more than he is letting on. He's always been this way." The aides have reported to you that Mr. Eisenberg is frequently incontinent of both urine and stool during the day, as well as during the night. He is alert and appears capable of recognizing the need to void or defecate and signaling for any assistance. His son and daughter report that this was never a problem at home and that he was able to go into the bathroom with assistance. He has been depressed about his admission to the home and seldom speaks, even when directly approached. He has refused to participate in any of the floor social events since his arrival.

PRACTICING FOR NCLEX

MULTIPLE-CHOICE QUESTIONS

Circle the letter that corresponds to the best answer for each question.

1. A nurse is assessing a middle-adult female who states that they notice an involuntary loss of urine following a coughing episode. What is the most appropriate response by the nurse?
   a. "This can happen after childbirth or menopause. I can teach you pelvic floor exercises called Kegel exercises to help."
   b. "This is typical of reflex incontinence. Have you had damage to your spinal cord in the past?"
   c. "It's unusual to experience total incontinence unless you had any surgeries or trauma to that area."
   d. "Transient incontinence often results from your medications; have you received diuretics or IV fluids lately?"

2. A nurse explains the purpose of performing a bladder scan after the patient voids. What explanation is most appropriate?
   a. It tests for a urinary tract infection.
   b. It determines if urinary retention is present.
   c. It treats urinary incontinence.
   d. It assesses kidney function.

3. A nurse is caring for a patient who had surgery to remove a bladder tumor. How does the nurse explain the purpose of continuous bladder irrigation to the patient?
   a. It collects a sterile, postoperative urine specimen.
   b. It reduces postoperative pain.
   c. It prevents clots from blocking the catheter.
   d. It prevents postoperative infection.

4. A nurse in the operating room is preparing to insert an indwelling catheter prior to a patient undergoing surgery. What is the most important principle the nurse adheres to when performing this procedure?
   a. Asepsis is essential, as the bladder is normally a sterile cavity.
   b. The external opening to the urethra should always be sterilized.

   c. Pathogens introduced into the bladder will remain in the bladder.
   d. Underfilling the balloon can promote infection.

5. A nurse is teaching a patient with female genitalia how to collect a clean-catch urine specimen. What education is most appropriate for the nurse to provide?
   a. "First, cleanse the urinary opening with the antiseptic wipe from front to back."
   b. "Collect the first 10 mL of urine voided in the sterile specimen container."
   c. "Place the container near the meatus and collect at least 3 oz of urine."
   d. "Collect all the urine in the container until the bladder is empty."

6. A nurse is choosing a collection device to collect urine for a urinalysis from a bedridden male patient? What device will the nurse ask the patient to use?
   a. Specimen hat
   b. Large urine collection bag
   c. Bedpan
   d. Urinal

7. A patient is being treated for a bladder infection and dehydration. The patient has developed urge incontinence and skin excoriation. What nursing intervention is the priority for this patient?
   a. Telling the patient the incontinence is typically temporary due to the infection
   b. Asking the patient to be mindful of the need to urinate and you will promptly assist them
   c. Keeping the perineal and groin areas clean and dry and applying skin barrier or protectant
   d. Encouraging the patient to restrict fluids to reduce incontinence

8. A nurse preceptor and new graduate nurse are inserting an indwelling catheter into the urinary bladder. Which action by the new graduate is performed correctly?
   a. Cleaning the urinary meatus with a cotton ball and alcohol, using a different cotton ball with each stroke
   b. Assisting the patient to a prone position with their knees flexed, their feet about 2 ft apart, and their legs abducted

c. Using the dominant hand, holding the catheter 12 inches from the tip and inserting it slowly into the urethra.

d. Inflating the catheter balloon by slowly injecting the entire volume of sterile water supplied in prefilled syringe

9. A nurse assessing an older adult finds that the patient has had four urinary tract infections in the past year. What physiologic change of aging would the nurse suspect is the cause?

a. Decreased bladder contractility

b. Diminished ability to concentrate urine

c. Decreased bladder muscle tone

d. Neurologic weakness

10. A physician has ordered the collection of a fresh urine sample for a 24-hour urine collection for analysis. To properly perform this procedure, which action will the nurse take?

a. Keeping each voided specimen in a separate container

b. Discarding the last voided specimen of the 24-hour period

c. Planning to use a straight catheterization each time the patient reports the urge to void

d. Discarding the first voided urine of the day

11. A nurse is caring for a patient who has a kidney stone obstructing their ureter and causing a kidney infection. A ureteral stent insertion is planned until infection resolves. How will the nurse explain the purpose of the stent to the patient?

a. "A catheter, a small flexible tube, will be placed through your urinary opening into your bladder for several days to weeks until healing occurs."

b. "The surgeon will make a small opening above your pubic area to insert a catheter to drain your urine."

c. "This surgery will divert urine from the ureter to an opening onto the skin of your abdomen."

d. "The stent is a soft hollow tube, temporarily inserted into the ureter to allow drainage of urine from the ureter until you can have the stone removed."

12. A nurse notes a patient's urine is turbid in appearance, with a sharp odor, and the patient has a temperature of 99.8°F. What action will the nurse recommend?

a. Sending a specimen for culture and sensitivity

b. Obtaining a urine specific gravity

c. Initiating antibiotic therapy

d. Initiating straight catheterization

13. Which instruction to a patient collecting a clean-catch, midstream urine specimen is essential to give the patient?

a. "Wear sterile gloves."

b. "Wipe the perineal area back to front."

c. "Do not touch the inside of the container or lid."

d. "Void first in the cup, then the rest in the toilet."

14. The nurse is teaching a patient about an intravenous pyelogram. Which statement by the patient requires follow up with the health care provider?

a. "I'm concerned what they might find."

b. "During my heart catheterization, I started wheezing."

c. "I will drink plenty of fluids when I return."

d. "I didn't have anything to eat today."

ALTERNATE-FORMAT QUESTIONS
Multiple-Response Questions
Circle the letters that correspond to the best answers for each question.

1. A nurse is preparing a patient for an intravenous pyelogram (IVP). Which nursing actions will the nurse use to prepare the patient for this procedure? Select all that apply.

a. Telling the patient not to void before the test

b. Withholding or limiting foods before testing

c. Giving an enema the day of the examination

d. Restricting fluids after the examination

e. Obtaining the patient's allergy history

f. Monitoring I & O after the examination

2. A nurse is collecting a urine specimen for urinalysis. What actions will the nurse take when collecting the specimen? Select all that apply.

   a. Explaining the need to insert a temporary catheter to obtain the urine

   b. Teaching the patient to collect a sterile, midstream urine specimen

   c. Noting that a female patient is menstruating on the laboratory slip

   d. Using strict aseptic technique when collecting and handling urine specimens

   e. Leaving the specimen at room temperature for a 24-hour period

   f. Allowing the patient to void into a bedpan, urinal, or specimen hat

3. A nurse is assessing the freshly voided urine of a patient. What characteristics of the urine indicate a urinary problem? Select all that apply.

   a. Amber color

   b. Ammonia-like odor

   c. pH of 6.0

   d. Clear

   e. Purulent

   f. Cloudy

4. A nurse is performing a physical assessment of a patient's urinary system. Which nursing actions are appropriate during this assessment? Select all that apply.

   a. Placing the patient in a supine position when using a bedside bladder scanner

   b. Measuring the height of the edge of the bladder below the symphysis pubis

   c. Inspecting the urethral orifice for any signs of inflammation, discharge, or foul odor

   d. Placing all male patients in the dorsal recumbent position to clearly visualize the meatus

   e. Retracting the foreskin of an uncircumcised male patient to visualize the meatus

   f. Assessing the patient's urine for color, odor, clarity, and the presence of any sediment

5. A nurse is assessing a patient's bladder volume using an ultrasound bladder scanner. Which actions will the nurse take? Select all that apply.

   a. Gently palpating the patient's symphysis pubis

   b. Placing a generous amount of ultrasound gel midline on the patient's abdomen, about 1 to 1.5 inches above the symphysis pubis

   c. Ensuring the scanner head directional icon is pointed away from the patient's head

   d. Aiming the scanner head slightly downward toward the coccyx

   e. Adjusting the scanner head to center the bladder image on the crossbars

   f. Pressing and holding the END button until it beeps three times showing the bladder volume on the screen

6. A nurse is catheterizing a male urinary bladder, and urine leaks out of the meatus around the catheter. What actions would the nurse perform next? Select all that apply.

   a. Increase the size of the indwelling catheter.

   b. Ensure the smallest-sized catheter with a 10-mL balloon is used.

   c. Consider an evaluation for urinary tract infection if problem does not resolve.

   d. Ensure that the correct amount of solution was used to inflate the balloon.

   e. If underfill is suspected, attempt to push the catheter further into the bladder.

   f. Assess the patient for diarrhea.

7. A nurse is changing a stoma appliance on an ileal conduit. Which nursing actions are appropriate? Select all that apply.

   a. Gently removing the appliance, starting at the top and keeping the abdominal skin taut

   b. Removing the appliance faceplate by pulling it from the skin rather than pushing

   c. Applying a silicone-based adhesive remover by spraying or wiping as needed

   d. Cleansing the skin around stoma with alcohol on a gauze pad

   e. Ensuring the skin around stoma is thoroughly dry by patting it dry

   f. Applying the faceplate by using firm, even pressure for approximately 1 minute

Hot Spot Questions

1. Place an X on figures A and B below to identify the female and male urethras.

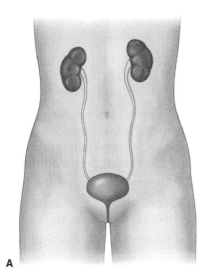

A

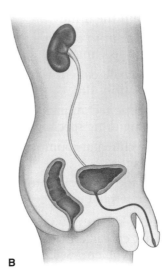

B

2. Place an X on the figure below to identify the location of the external sphincter.

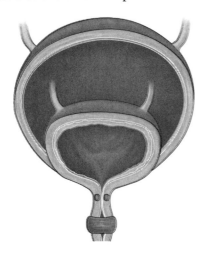

3. Place an X on the figure below to identify the urinary bladder.

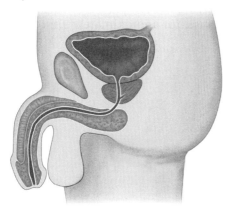

4. Place an X on the figure below to mark the spot where a suprapubic catheter would be inserted into the bladder.

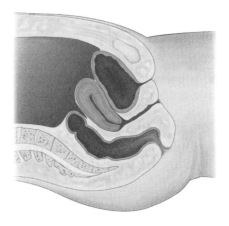

Bowel Elimination

ASSESSING YOUR UNDERSTANDING

FILL IN THE BLANKS

1. The gastrointestinal tract extends from mouth to _____.

2. The stomach churns food and pushes the partially digested food called _____ into the small intestine.

3. The components of the small intestine include the duodenum, _____, and _____.

4. The _____ valve marks the beginning of the large intestine (colon).

5. The autonomic nervous system controls contraction of the intestine, creating waves of _____ to move waste along the length of the bowel for excretion.

6. When a person passes gas, the nurse documents this using the professional term, _____.

7. The _____ maneuver refers to bearing down to defecate, the increased pressures in the abdominal and thoracic cavities result in decreased blood flow to the atria and ventricles, thus temporarily lowering cardiac output. Once bearing down ceases, the pressure is lessened, and a larger than normal amount of blood returns to the heart.

8. It is optimal to consume a high-fiber diet of _____ to _____ g of fiber daily.

9. Manipulation of the bowel during surgery and anesthesia can result in inhibition of peristalsis causing paralytic _____.

IDENTIFICATION

1. Locate the internal anal sphincter, the external anal sphincter, the anal canal, the rectum, and the anal valve on the figure below and write the appropriate body part on the lines provided.

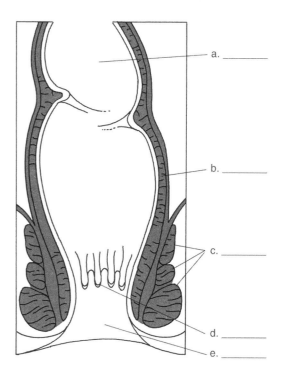

a. _____

b. _____

c. _____

d. _____

e. _____

2. Name the type of ostomy depicted in the figures below by writing your answers on the lines provided. Indicate the type of stool that would be expected with each ostomy.

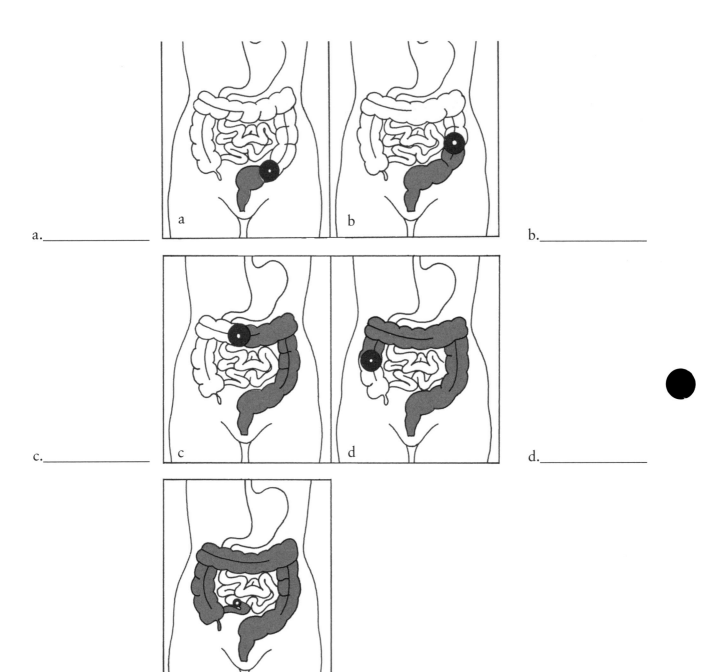

a._____

b._____

c._____

d._____

e._____

MATCHING EXERCISES

Matching Exercise 1

Match the bowel studies listed in Part A with their definition listed in Part B.

PART A

a. Endoscopy

b. Esophagogastroduodenoscopy

c. Colonoscopy

d. Sigmoidoscopy

e. Fecal occult blood test

f. Barium enema

PART B

____ **1.** Direct visualization of the lining of a hollow body organ using a long flexible tube containing glass fibers that transmit light into the organ, allowing the return of an image that can be viewed

____ **2.** Visual examination of the lining of the distal sigmoid colon, the rectum, and the anal canal using either a flexible or a rigid instrument

____ **3.** Visual examination of the lining of the large intestine with a flexible, fiber-optic endoscope

____ **4.** Visual examination of the lining of the esophagus, the stomach, and the upper duodenum with a flexible, fiber-optic endoscope

____ **5.** Use of a commercial tape, dipstick, or solution to test for blood in the stool

____ **6.** Barium sulfate is instilled into the large intestine through a rectal tube inserted through the anus

Matching Exercise 2

Match the type of enema in Part A with its use in Part B.

PART A

a. Oil-retention enemas

b. Carminative enemas

c. Medicated enemas

d. Anthelmintic enemas

PART B

____ **1.** Used to lubricate the stool and intestinal mucosa, making defecation easier

____ **2.** Administered to destroy intestinal parasites

____ **3.** Used to administer medications that are absorbed through the rectal mucosa

____ **4.** Used to help expel flatus from the rectum and provide relief from gaseous distention

Matching Exercise 3

Match the term in Part A with its definition listed in Part B.

PART A

a. Feces

b. Stool

c. Constipation

d. Diarrhea

e. Incontinence

f. Peristalsis

PART B

____ **1.** Passage of dry, hard stools

____ **2.** Solid waste products that have reached the distal end of the colon and are ready for excretion

____ **3.** Passage of excessively liquid and unformed stools

____ **4.** Inability of the anal sphincter to control the discharge of fecal and gaseous material

____ **5.** Contraction of circular and longitudinal muscles of the intestine

____ **6.** Once excreted, feces are called by this name

Anatomy Review

Match the organs of the gastrointestinal system listed in Part A with the illustration in Part B.

PART A

a. Splenic flexure

b. Sigmoid colon

c. Cecum

d. Hepatic flexure

e. Common bile duct

f. Stomach

g. Esophagus

h. Descending colon

i. Ileum

j. Hepatic duct

k. Gallbladder
 l. Duodenum
m. Jejunum
 n. Rectum

o. Ascending colon
p. Pancreatic duct
q. Ileocecal junction
 r. Transverse colon

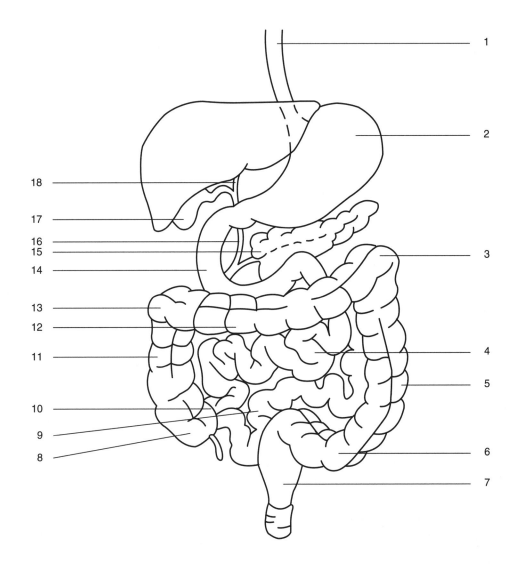

PART B

____ **1.**

____ **2.**

____ **3.**

____ **4.**

____ **5.**

____ **6.**

____ **7.**

____ **8.**

____ **9.**

____ **10.**

____ **11.**

____ **12.**

____ **13.**

____ **14.**

____ **15.**

____ **16.**

____ **17.**

____ **18.**

SHORT ANSWER

1. List four functions of the large intestine.

   a. _____

   b. _____

   c. _____

   d. _____

2. State how the two divisions of the autonomic nervous system affect peristalsis.

   a. _____

   b. _____

3. List observations the nurse makes during each step of abdominal assessment.

   a. Inspection: _____

   _____

   b. Auscultation: _____

   _____

   c. Percussion: _____

   _____

   d. Palpation: _____

   _____

4. Give an example of how the following factors might affect a patient's bowel elimination.

   a. Developmental considerations: _____

   _____

   b. Daily patterns: _____

   _____

   c. Food and fluids: _____

   _____

   d. Activity and muscle tone: _____

   _____

   e. Lifestyle: _____

   _____

   f. Psychological variables: _____

   _____

   g. Medications: _____

   _____

   h. Diagnostic studies: _____

   _____

5. When caring for patient with acute abdominal pain related to diverticular disease, list some questions you would ask about bowel elimination.

   _____

   _____

   _____

6. List four factors that promote healthy elimination patterns.

   a. _____

   b. _____

   c. _____

   d. _____

7. A postoperative patient reports painful defecation due to hard, dry stools. List three expected outcomes for this patient.

   a. _____

   b. _____

   c. _____

8. Specify dietary measures to alleviate the following gastrointestinal problems.

   a. Constipation: _____

   _____

   b. Diarrhea: _____

   _____

   c. Flatulence: _____

   _____

9. List four reasons for prescribing cleansing enemas.

   a. _____

   b. _____

   c. _____

   d. _____

10. Briefly describe the following types of ostomies and the characteristic of stool passed.

    a. Ileostomy: _____

    _____

    b. Colostomy: _____

    _____

11. Describe how the following factors help promote healthy bowel habits in patients.

   a. Timing: _____

   _____

   b. Positioning: _____

   _____

   c. Privacy: _____

   _____

   d. Nutrition: _____

   _____

   e. Exercise: _____

   _____

APPLYING YOUR KNOWLEDGE

CRITICAL THINKING QUESTIONS

1. Develop a list of preferred foods to ensure healthy bowel elimination for the following patients.

   a. Patient with constipation following a cesarean section

   b. 40-year-old male with job stress has frequent diarrhea

   c. Toddlers with hard, dry stools and frequent stomachaches

2. What other factors are likely to promote healthy bowel elimination in these patients?

REFLECTIVE PRACTICE: CULTIVATING QSEN COMPETENCIES

Use the following expanded scenario from Chapter 39 in your textbook to answer the questions below.

   Scenario: Leroy, newly diagnosed with cancer, is taking acetaminophen with codeine for pain. He comes to the outpatient health center with constipation. "Nobody told me I would get so constipated," he says. "It's been almost a week, and I'm still not moving my bowels normally. I didn't know anything could hurt so bad. I'll take my chances with the cancer pain in the future rather than take more pain meds and have this happen again."

1. Patient-centered care/evidence-based practice: What nursing interventions might the nurse implement for this patient?

   _____

   _____

2. Patient-centered care/evidence-based practice: What would be a successful outcome for this patient?

   _____

   _____

3. Evidence-based practice: What intellectual, technical, interpersonal, and ethical/legal competencies are most likely to bring about the desired outcome?

   _____

   _____

4. Teamwork and collaboration: What resources might be helpful for Leroy?

   _____

   _____

PATIENT CARE STUDY

Use this care study to apply your knowledge by completing the Nursing Process Worksheet found in Appendix A.

   Scenario: Ms. Elgaresta, age 54, a single woman, is being followed by a cardiologist who monitors her arrhythmia. Last month, she started taking a new heart medication. At this visit, she says to the nurse practitioner who works with the cardiologist: "Right after I started taking that medication, I got terribly constipated, and nothing seems to help. I'm desperate and about ready to try dynamite unless you can think of something else!" She reports a change in her bowel movements from one soft stool daily to straining to produce one or two hard stools weekly. Reluctant to suggest substituting another medication too quickly, she asks more questions and Ms. Elgaresta responds, "I've never been much of a drinker, 2 cups of coffee in the morning and maybe a glass of wine at night. Water? Almost never. And I don't drink juices or soft drinks." Analysis of her diet reveals a diet low in fiber: "I never was one much for vegetables, and they can just keep all this bran stuff that's out on the market! Coffee and a cigarette. That's for me!" Ms. Elgaresta is a workaholic computer programmer and spends what little spare time she has watching TV. She reports tiring after walking one flight of stairs and says she avoids all forms of vigorous exercise.

PRACTICING FOR NCLEX

MULTIPLE-CHOICE QUESTIONS

Circle the letter that corresponds to the best answer for each question.

1. A nurse is administering a large-volume cleansing enema to a patient. Which nursing action is performed correctly?
   a. Placing the patient on a bedpan in the supine position while receiving the enema
   b. Using cool tap water for the enema solution
   c. Elevating the solution to no higher than 10 inches above the level of the anus
   d. Administering the solution slowly over a period of 5 to 10 minutes

2. A nurse is changing a patient's ostomy appliance and observes that the peristomal skin is excoriated. What is the priority nursing intervention in this situation?
   a. Notifying the primary health care provider
   b. Suspecting ischemia and notifying the surgeon
   c. Cleaning the outside of the bag thoroughly when emptying
   d. Ensuring the opening in the appliance is not too large

3. A nurse is administering a large-volume enema preoperatively. Which nursing action is performed correctly in this procedure?
   a. Positioning the patient on their back and draping properly
   b. Slowly and gently inserting the enema tubing 2 to 3 inches (5 to 7 cm) for an adult
   c. Introducing the solution quickly over a period of 3 to 5 minutes
   d. Encouraging the patient to hold the solution for at least 20 minutes

4. A nurse irrigating a Salem sump nasogastric tube that has been attached to suction finds that the flush solution meets resistance during instillation. What action will the nurse take next?
   a. Inject 30 mL of air into the blue vent port to decrease pressure and reestablish ability to flush the tube.
   b. Check the suction canister to ensure that the suction is working appropriately.
   c. Assess for abdominal distention, nausea, or abdominal discomfort.
   d. Use warm water when attempting to flush the tube to ensure its patency.

5. A nurse is caring for a patient who is scheduled for an esophagogastroduodenoscopy (EGD). What action would the nurse take to prepare the patient for this procedure?
   a. Ensure that the patient ingests a gallon of bowel cleanser, such as GoLytely.
   b. Administer barium contrast mixture before the test.
   c. Administer two Fleet enemas and a light breakfast the day of the procedure.
   d. Reinforce to the patient they do not eat or drink for 6 to 12 hours before the test as per policy.

6. A nurse is teaching a patient about psyllium to relieve constipation. How does the nurse explain how this medication works?
   a. By chemically stimulating peristalsis
   b. By softening the fecal material
   c. By increasing intestinal bulk to promote peristalsis
   d. By drawing water into the intestines to stimulate peristalsis

7. 2. A nurse is scheduling a patient for the following diagnostic tests. In what order should the nurse schedule the tests for accurate results?
   a. Barium studies, endoscopic examination, fecal occult blood test
   b. Fecal occult blood test, barium studies, endoscopic examination
   c. Barium studies, fecal occult blood test, endoscopic examination
   d. Endoscopic examination, barium studies, fecal occult blood test

ALTERNATE-FORMAT QUESTIONS

MULTIPLE-RESPONSE QUESTIONS

Circle the letters that correspond to the best answers for each question.

1. A nurse is administering an oil-retention enema to a patient. Which nursing actions in this procedure are performed correctly? Select all that apply.
   a. Selecting a large rectal tube
   b. Slowly instilling the 500 mL of oil
   c. Administering the oil-retention enema at body temperature
   d. Instructing the patient to retain the oil for at least 30 minutes

e. Administering a cleansing enema prior to the oil-retention enema

f. Recommending a cleansing enema after the oil-retention enema if needed

2. A nurse in a family medical practice is assessing the bowel elimination of patients. What developmental factors affecting elimination should the nurse consider? Select all that apply.

a. Voluntary control of defecation occurs between ages 12 and 18 months.

b. The number of stools that infants pass varies greatly.

c. Some children have bowel movements only every 2 or 3 days.

d. A child who has not had a bowel movement daily is most likely constipated.

e. In an infant, a liquid stool signifies diarrhea.

f. Constipation is often a chronic problem for older adults.

3. A nurse in a long-term care facility assisting patients with menu selection takes into consideration the effects of foods and fluids on bowel elimination. Which examples correctly describe these effects? Select all that apply.

a. Patients with lactose intolerance may experience diarrhea or gas after eating starchy foods.

b. Patients who are constipated should eat eggs and pasta to relieve the condition.

c. Patients who are constipated should eat more fruits and vegetables.

d. Patients with flatulence should avoid gas-producing foods such as cauliflower and onions.

e. Alcohol and coffee tend to have a constipating effect on patients.

f. Patients with food intolerances may experience altered bowel elimination.

4. A nurse is assessing the bowel elimination patterns of hospitalized patients. Which nursing actions related to the assessment process are performed correctly? Select all that apply.

a. Auscultating the abdomen before inspection and palpation are performed

b. Placing the patient in the supine position with their abdomen exposed

c. Draping the patient's chest and pubic area and extending their legs flat against the bed

d. Encouraging the patient to drink fluids to fill the bladder before the assessment

e. Using a warmed stethoscope to listen for bowel sounds in all abdominal quadrants

f. Anticipating that normal bowel sounds will consist of gurgles and clicks

5. A nurse is collecting a stool specimen from a patient. Which measures are appropriate for this procedure? Select all that apply.

a. Asking the patient to void first to ensure accuracy of the test

b. Providing a clean bedpan or toilet for defecation, depending on the nature of the study

c. Teaching the patient not to place toilet tissue in the bedpan or specimen container

d. Following medical aseptic techniques

e. Handwashing before and after glove use when handling a stool specimen

f. Collecting 2 inches of formed stool or 20 to 30 mL of liquid stool for a stool specimen

6. A nurse on the GI unit is reviewing nursing implications of antidiarrheal medications with a group of nursing students. Which statements will the nurse include in the review? Select all that apply.

a. "Atropine is preferred in older adults as it does not affect level of consciousness."

b. "Diphenoxylate should be used in patients taking opioids to decrease constipation."

c. "Diphenoxylate should not be used if antibiotic-associated diarrhea is suspected."

d. "Avoid Pepto-Bismol in children under 12 without consulting a health care provider."

e. "Higher than recommended doses of loperamide may increase serious cardiac events."

f. "Loperamide has a shorter duration than diphenoxylate and atropine."

7. Which of the following commonly used enema solutions would the nurse recommend to distend the intestine and increase peristalsis? Select all that apply.

a. Tap water

b. Soap

c. Normal saline

d. Mineral oil

e. Hypertonic

f. Olive oil

8. A nurse is performing digital removal of a fecal impaction. Which nursing actions follow guidelines for this procedure? Select all that apply.

    a. Having the patient lie on their stomach and pie-folding top linens over them

    b. Placing the patient in a side-lying position

    c. Vigorously working the finger around and into the hardened mass to break it up

    d. Using nonsterile gloves for the procedure because the intestinal tract is not sterile

    e. Lubricating the index finger generously to reduce irritating the rectum and inserting it gently into the anal canal

Sequencing Question

1. Place the following steps for digital removal of stool in the order in which they would normally occur:

    a. Slowly and gently work the finger around and into the hardened mass to break it up and then remove pieces of it. Instruct the patient to bear down if possible while extracting feces to ease in removal.

    b. Place the patient in the left side-lying position and place a bedpan on the bed for depositing removed feces.

    c. Use an oil-retention enema if necessary.

    d. Remove the impaction at intervals if it is severe. This helps to avoid discomfort as well as irritation, which can injure intestinal mucosa.

    e. Wash and dry the patient's buttocks and anal area. Assist the patient to a comfortable position.

    f. Lubricate the forefinger generously to reduce irritation of the rectum and insert it gently into the anal canal. The presence of the finger added to the mass tends to cause discomfort for the patient if the work is not done slowly and gently.

    g. Use nonsterile gloves for the procedure because the intestinal tract is not sterile.

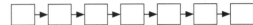

Prioritization Question

1. A nurse on the GI unit receives report on a group of patients. Which patient will the nurse assess first? Circle the letter that corresponds to the best answer.

    a. Patient who is NPO for surgery later that day

    b. Patient whose colostomy stoma is purple-blue

    c. Patient needing a large-volume cleansing enema

    d. Patient with 2.5-cm red blood on toilet tissue after wiping

40

Oxygenation and Perfusion

ASSESSING YOUR UNDERSTANDING

FILL IN THE BLANKS

1. Another word for pulmonary ventilation, the movement of air in and out of the lungs is _____.

2. Living cells require gas _____ of oxygen and carbon dioxide, a byproduct of oxidation.

3. Incomplete lung expansion or lung collapse of a portion of the lung is _____.

4. Any impediment or obstruction that air meets as it moves through the airway is termed airway _____.

5. _____ of the lungs refers to the ease with which the lungs can be inflated.

6. The nurse documents that a patient underwent aspiration of fluid from the pleural space in the electronic health record as a _____ was performed.

7. Infants born before 34 weeks may not have produced sufficient _____, leading to collapse of the alveoli and poor alveolar exchange.

8. The mass of tissue in the heart that initiates the transmission of cardiac impulse causing contraction of the heart is the _____ node. It is also called the pacemaker.

9. The nurse documents a disturbance of the rate and/or rhythm of the heart as a(n) _____.

10. The amount of blood pumped per minute, measured in liters per minute is the cardiac _____; this is expressed by the formula CO = SV × HR.

REVIEW

1. Identify the location of the organs of the respiratory tract listed here by writing the appropriate organ on the lines provided on the figure below.

Diaphragm
Epiglottis
Esophagus
Frontal sinus
Laryngeal pharynx
Larynx and vocal cords
Left lung
Mediastinum

Nasal cavity
Nasopharynx
Oropharynx
Right bronchus
Right lung
Sphenoidal sinus
Terminal bronchiole
Trachea

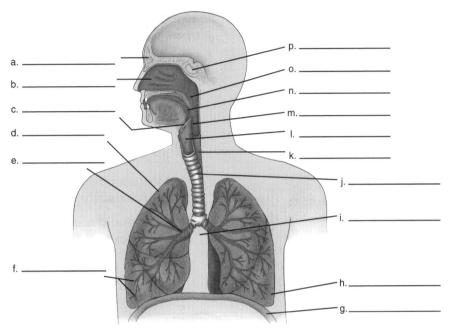

2. Identify the components of the airway device illustrated below. Place your answers on the lines provided.

a. _____
b. _____
c. _____
d. _____

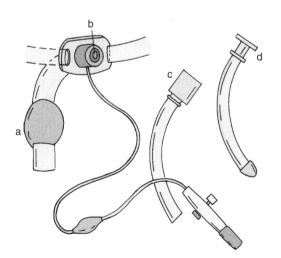

MATCHING EXERCISES

Matching Exercise 1

Match the definition in Part B with the term listed in Part A.

PART A

a. Ventilation
b. Inspiration
c. Hypoventilation
d. Hypoxia
e. Respiration or gas exchange
f. Perfusion

PART B

____ 1. Movement of muscles and thorax to bring air into the lungs

____ 2. Movement of oxygen and carbon dioxide between the air and the blood

____ 3. Inadequate amount of oxygen in the cells

____ 4. Movement of air in and out of the lungs

_____ **5.** Decreased rate of air movement into the lungs

_____ **6.** Process by which the oxygenated capillary blood passes through tissue

Matching Exercise 2

Match the type of oxygen delivery system in Part A with its description in Part B.

PART A

a. Nasal cannula

b. Simple facemask

c. Partial rebreather mask

d. Nonrebreather mask

e. Venturi mask

f. Oxygen tent

g. High-flow nasal cannula

PART B

_____ **1.** This is a face mask with side vents that permits room air to enter, diluting the oxygen concentration in the mask. It connects to oxygen tubing, using an oxygen flow rate greater than 5 L/min; it should be comfortably snug over face but not tight.

_____ **2.** High-flow/fixed performance devices produce oxygen flow outputs with a constant mix of air and oxygen as a result of the design of the device's exchangeable barrel to control the oxygen concentration, rather than the rate and depth of the patient's breathing.

_____ **3.** This consists of a disposable, plastic device with two protruding prongs for insertion into the nostrils; it is connected to an oxygen source with a humidifier and a flow meter.

_____ **4.** This mask provides the highest concentration of oxygen inhaled from a reservoir of 100% oxygen; exhaled air escapes through side vents.

_____ **5.** This mask provides a reservoir bag with 100% oxygen mixing with the patient's exhaled air; vents permit exhalation.

_____ **6.** This oxygen therapy delivers a continuous mixture of air/oxygen through a heater/humidifier to a wide-bore nasal cannula. It uses oxygen flow rates 30 L/min to 60 L/min, up to 100% humidified oxygen.

Matching Exercise 3

Match the auscultatory respiratory sounds in Part A to its definition in Part B.

PART A

a. Crackles

b. Bronchial

c. Wheezes

d. Adventitious

e. Vesicular

f. Bronchovesicular

PART B

_____ **1.** Low-pitched, soft sounds heard over peripheral lung fields

_____ **2.** Loud, high-pitched sounds heard primarily over the trachea and larynx

_____ **3.** Medium-pitched blowing sounds heard over the major bronchi sounds

_____ **4.** Continuous musical sounds, produced as air passes through airways constricted by swelling, narrowing, secretions, or tumors; often heard in patients with asthma or a buildup of secretions

_____ **5.** Inspiratory, soft, high-pitched intermittent popping sounds, produced by air passing through fluid in the airways or alveoli and opening of deflated small airways and alveoli

_____ **6.** Extra, abnormal sounds of breathing, such as wheezing or crackles

SHORT ANSWER

1. List three factors on which normal respiratory functioning depends.

a. _____

b. _____

c. _____

2. Briefly describe the functions of the upper and lower airways, listing their main components.

a. Upper airway: _____

_____

b. Lower airway: _____

_____

3. State the purpose of each of these laboratory studies used to assess cardiopulmonary function.

   a. ABG: _____

   _____

   b. Creatine kinase: _____

   _____

   c. Troponin: _____

   _____

   d. Cytologic study: _____

   _____

4. List four factors that influence the diffusion of gas in the lungs.

   a. _____

   _____

   b. _____

   _____

   c. _____

   _____

   d. _____

   _____

5. Describe the two ways that oxygen is carried in the body.

   a. _____

   b. _____

6. Briefly describe the variations in respiration experienced by the following age groups.

   a. Infant: _____

   _____

   b. Preschool- and school-aged child: _____

   _____

   c. Older adult: _____

   _____

7. Describe nursing responsibilities before, during, and after a thoracentesis.

   _____

   _____

   _____

8. Describe the effects of smoking and vaping on the body.

   _____

   _____

   _____

9. Briefly describe the following techniques designed to promote oxygenation and ventilation.

   a. Deep breathing: _____

   _____

   b. Incentive spirometry: _____

   _____

   c. Pursed-lip breathing: _____

   _____

   d. Diaphragmatic breathing: _____

   _____

   e. Voluntary coughing: _____

   _____

10. As the visiting nurse for a patient with emphysema who is receiving oxygen therapy, list five safety precautions you would initiate or confirm are in place.

    a. _____

    b. _____

    c. _____

    d. _____

    e. _____

11. Briefly describe the following types of airways and their uses.

    a. Oropharyngeal/nasopharyngeal airway:

    _____

    _____

    b. Endotracheal tube: _____

    _____

    c. Tracheostomy tube: _____

    _____

    _____

12. What is the nurse's responsibility when managing a patient's chest tube and drainage device?

_____

_____

_____

13. Describe six comfort measures for patients with impaired respiratory functioning.

    a. _____

    b. _____

    c. _____

    d. _____

    e. _____

    f. _____

14. Describe the nurse's role in providing tracheostomy care for a patient.

    _____

    _____

    _____

15. Define the following cardiopulmonary problems and their manifestations.

    a. Angina: _____

    _____

    b. Myocardial infarction: _____

    _____

    c. Dysrhythmia/arrhythmia: _____

    _____

    d. Heart failure: _____

    _____

APPLYING YOUR KNOWLEDGE

CRITICAL THINKING QUESTIONS

1. Develop a set of nursing strategies to promote adequate respiratory functioning in the following patients.

    a. Patient with lung cancer presents with blood in his sputum.

    b. Child with cystic fibrosis is having difficulty breathing.

    c. Female with asthma develops pneumonia.

    d. 48-year-old man who smokes a pack of cigarettes a day presents with emphysema.

2. When a nurse notes tachypnea in a patient with pulmonary disease, what additional assessments could be made?

REFLECTIVE PRACTICE: CULTIVATING QSEN COMPETENCIES

Use the following expanded scenario from Chapter 40 in your textbook to answer the questions below.

Scenario: Joan McIntyre, age 72, has been admitted to your medical unit with an acute exacerbation of chronic obstructive pulmonary disease (COPD). This is the fifth time she has been in the hospital this year. She is receiving supplemental oxygen and multiple medications to support her breathing. She is very weak, unable to perform activities of daily living (ADLs) for herself and becomes extremely short of breath with minimal exertion. She has verbalized feelings of despair and has asked the staff, "to let me go if I should stop breathing."

1. Patient-centered care/evidence-based practice/teamwork and collaboration: How would the nurse respond to Ms. McIntyre's request to not provide resuscitation if she stops breathing?

    _____

    _____

    _____

2. Patient-centered care: What would be a successful outcome for this patient?

    _____

    _____

    _____

3. Patient-centered care/evidence-based practice/teamwork and collaboration: What intellectual, technical, and ethical/legal competencies are most likely to bring about the desired outcome?

    _____

    _____

    _____

4. Teamwork and collaboration: What resources might be helpful for Ms. McIntyre?

    _____

    _____

    _____

PATIENT CARE STUDY

Use this care study to apply your knowledge by completing the Nursing Process Worksheet found in Appendix A.

Scenario: Toni is an adolescent in the mental health unit following a suicide attempt. Her health record reveals that on several occasions when her mother was visiting, she began hyperventilating with a respiratory rate of 42 and increased depth noted. Gasping for breath on these occasions, she nevertheless pushed away all who approached her to assist. Her mother confided that she and her husband are in the midst of a divorce and that it hasn't been easy for Toni at home: "I know she's been having a rough time at school, and I guess I've been too caught up in my own troubles to be there for her." When you attempt to discuss this with Toni and mention her mother's concern, she begins hyperventilating again.

PRACTICING FOR NCLEX

MULTIPLE-CHOICE QUESTIONS

Circle the letter that corresponds to the best answer for each question.

1. A school-aged child with a history of asthma is in the school nurse's office reporting shortness of breath. The nurse assesses what respiratory parameter to determine the severity of symptoms?
   a. Tidal volume (TV)
   b. Total lung capacity (TLC)
   c. Peak expiratory flow rate (peak flow)
   d. Residual volume (RV)

2. A nurse in the emergency department is caring for a group of patients. Which patient will the nurse assess first?
   a. Infant with a respiratory rate of 20 bpm
   b. Preschool-aged child with a respiratory rate of 22 bpm
   c. School-aged child with a respiratory rate of 20 bpm
   d. Older adult with a respiratory rate of 18 bpm

3. A nurse assesses a patient and detects dyspnea, tachypnea, tachycardia, and pallor with circumoral cyanosis. What action will the nurse take next?
   a. Count the respiratory rate
   b. Assess pulse oximetry
   c. Measure the apical pulse
   d. Recommend a chest x-ray

4. When inspecting a patient's chest to assess respiratory status, the nurse documents which of these abnormal findings in the electronic health record?
   a. Intercostal spaces are retracted.
   b. Skin on the thorax is warm and dry.
   c. Anteroposterior diameter is less than the transverse diameter.
   d. Chest is slightly convex with no sternal depression.

5. A nurse is following up on respiratory assessments with a new graduate nurse. Which finding will the preceptor expect the graduate to prioritize for follow-up?
   a. Vesicular breath sounds posteriorly
   b. Kyphosis of the dorsal spine
   c. Diminished breath sounds at bases
   d. Hyperresonance to percussion

6. A new graduate nurse seeks out the preceptor to validate findings of soft, inspiratory high-pitched, and discontinuous breath sounds in a patient with a cardiopulmonary problem. The preceptor states the graduate nurse is correct when documenting which breath sound?
   a. Vesicular
   b. Wheezes
   c. Crackles
   d. Bronchial

7. A nurse auscultates the lungs of a patient with asthma. Which lung sound does the nurse anticipate is present upon auscultation?
   a. Crackles
   b. Bronchial
   c. Wheezes
   d. Vesicular

8. A nurse notes a patient has decreased respiratory expansion during the assessment. What action is most appropriate for the nurse to take?
   a. Placing the patient in a high Fowler's position
   b. Documenting the presence of a barrel chest
   c. Initiating CPR
   d. Planning for transfer to the ICU

9. In which patient will the nurse prioritize use of the incentive spirometer?
   a. Patient with angina
   b. Patient with dysrhythmia
   c. Patient scheduled for heart catheterization
   d. Patient whose chest x-ray demonstrates atelectasis

10. A nurse is teaching an adolescent with asthma how to properly use a metered-dose inhaler. Which teaching point will the nurse include?
   a. "Inhale through the nose instead of the mouth."
   b. "Be sure to shake the canister before using it."
   c. "Inhale the medication rapidly."
   d. "Inhale two sprays with one breath for faster action."

11. A nursing student asks the primary nurse how pursed-lip breathing relieves symptoms of chronic obstructive pulmonary disease (COPD). Which response by the nurse is appropriate?
   a. It increases carbon dioxide, which stimulates breathing.
   b. It teaches the patient to prolong inspiration and shorten expiration.
   c. It helps liquefy secretions.
   d. It decreases the amount of air trapping and resistance.

12. A primary nurse reminds a nursing student who is suctioning a patient through a tracheostomy tube to avoid occluding the Y-port during insertion of the suction catheter to prevent what circumstance?
   a. Trauma to the tracheal mucosa
   b. Prevention of suctioning
   c. Loss of sterile field
   d. Suctioning of carbon dioxide

13. When caring for a patient with a tracheostomy, which action represents correct care?
   a. Cleaning the wound around the tube and inner cannula at least every 24 hours
   b. Assessing a newly inserted tracheostomy every 3 to 4 hours
   c. Using gauze dressings over the tracheostomy that are filled with cotton
   d. Suctioning the tracheostomy tube using sterile technique

14. A nurse is caring for a patient who had chest surgery and returns with a chest tube connected to a dry suction control chest drainage device providing –20 cm suction. Which finding indicates the chest drainage system is working properly?
   a. The fluid in the water seal is at 2 cm.
   b. The bellows on the device is not visible.
   c. There is no drainage in the chest tube or device.
   d. Intermittent bubbling is seen in the suction control chamber.

15. A nurse is teaching a parent and child to use a bronchodilating metered-dose inhaler. The nurse suggests use of which reservoir device to enhance delivery of a predictable amount of medication to the lungs?
   a. Nebulizer
   b. Spacer
   c. Resuscitation bag
   d. Atomizer

ALTERNATE-FORMAT QUESTIONS

Multiple-Response Questions

Circle the letters that correspond to the best answers for each question.

1. A nurse is reviewing the results of a patient's arterial blood gas and pH analysis. What are normal findings? Select all that apply.
   a. pH 7.45
   b. PCO_2 40 mm Hg
   c. PO_2 70 mm Hg
   d. HCO_3^- 30 mEq/L
   e. Base excess or deficit +2 mmol/L
   f. pH 7.52

2. A nurse is preparing a patient for a complete blood count. Which actions will the nurse perform? Select all that apply.

   a. Emphasize that there is no discomfort during the venipuncture.

   b. Inform the patient that this test can assist in evaluating the body's response to illness.

   c. Teach the patient that specimen collection takes approximately 5 to 10 minutes.

   d. Administer an analgesic to the patient prior to the test.

   e. Explain that, based on results, additional testing may be performed.

   f. Ensure that no food is consumed 6 hours prior to the test.

3. A nurse in a family practice clinic performs assessments of cardiopulmonary functioning and oxygenation during regular physical assessments. Based on developmental variations, which findings would the nurse consider normal? Select all that apply.

   a. Blood pressure increases over time until it reaches the adult level around age eight.

   b. Decreased strength of the respiratory and abdominal muscles in older adults causes the diaphragm to move less efficiently.

   c. The normal infant's chest is small, and the airways are short, making aspiration a potential problem.

   d. Changes of aging in older adults increase the risk for pneumonia and other chest infections.

   e. Infants' respiratory rates are rapid until the alveoli increase in number and size.

   f. The older adult's chest is unable to stretch resulting in an increase in maximum inspiration.

4. Which conditions would a nurse document as normal findings after performing a respiratory assessment? Select all that apply.

   a. Slightly contoured chest with no sternal depression

   b. Anteroposterior diameter of the chest less than the transverse diameter

   c. Quiet and nonlabored respiration occurring at a rate of 18 to 30 bpm

   d. Barrel chest appearance in older adults

   e. Bronchial, vesicular, and bronchovesicular breath sounds

   f. Crackles heard on inspiration

5. A nurse in the PACU inserts an oropharyngeal airway in a patient who is snoring after anesthesia. Which actions should a nurse perform when inserting an oropharyngeal airway? Select all that apply.

   a. Using an airway that reaches from the nose to the back angle of the jaw

   b. Washing hands and putting on PPE, as appropriate

   c. Placing the patient supine with their head turned to one side

   d. Inserting the airway with the curved tip pointing down toward the base of the mouth

   e. Rotating the airway 180 degrees as it passes the uvula

   f. Removing the airway for a brief period every 4 hours or according to facility policy

6. A nurse is teaching a patient the proper use of inhaled medications. What are appropriate teaching points to include? Select all that apply.

   a. "Bronchodilators are used to liquefy or loosen thick secretions or reduce inflammation in airways."

   b. "Using a spacer will allow more medication to be inhaled."

   c. "When using an MDI, the patient must activate the device before and after inhaling."

   d. "DPIs are actuated by the patient's inspiration, so there is no need to coordinate the delivery of puffs with inhalation."

   e. "Metered-dose inhalers deliver a controlled dose of medications with each compression of the canister."

   f. "Inhalers can be used safely without serious side effects whenever they are needed by the patient."

7. A nurse is preparing to suction a patient's endotracheal tube. Which actions are appropriate for the nurse to perform? Select all that apply.

   a. Hyperoxygenating prior to suctioning with 50% oxygen

   b. Selecting a suction catheter less than 50% of lumen of the tube

   c. Instilling saline into the tube prior to suctioning

   d. Using a suction pressure of 20 mm Hg

   e. Stopping the procedure if the patient develops bradycardia

   f. Requesting a chest x-ray after the procedure

Sequencing Questions

1. Place the following steps for teaching a patient to use an incentive spirometer in the order in which they should occur.

   a. Instruct the patient to exhale normally and then place lips securely around mouthpiece and not to breathe through his or her nose.

   b. Medicate with ordered pain medication if needed.

   c. Tell the patient to hold their breath and count to three when unable to inhale anymore. Check position of gauge to determine progress and level attained.

   d. Tell patient to complete breathing exercises about 5 to 10 times every 1 to 2 hours, if possible, and to rest between breaths as necessary.

   e. Assist patient to an upright or semi-Fowler's position if possible and remove dentures if they fit poorly.

   f. Demonstrate how to steady device with one hand and hold mouthpiece with other hand.

   g. Instruct the patient not to breathe through the nose and to inhale slowly and as deeply as possible through the mouthpiece.

   h. Instruct the patient to remove lips from mouthpiece and exhale normally.

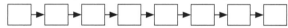

2. Place the following steps for inserting a nasopharyngeal airway in the order in which they should occur.

   a. Remove the airway, clean it, and place it in the other naris at least every 8 hours or according to facility policy. Assess for any evidence of skin breakdown.

   b. Wash your hands, put on PPE as indicated, and identify the patient.

   c. Explain what you are going to do and the reason for doing it, even though the patient does not appear to be alert.

   d. Gently insert the airway into the naris, narrow end first, pointing it down toward the back of the throat until the rim is touching the naris. If resistance is met, stop and try inserting in the other naris.

   e. Put on gloves; put on mask and goggles or face shield as indicated. Lubricate the airway with the water-soluble lubricant, covering the airway from the tip to the guard rim.

   f. Use an airway that is the correct size. Measure the nasopharyngeal airway for correct size. Measure the nasopharyngeal airway length by holding the airway on the side of the patient's face. The airway should reach from the tip of the nose to the earlobe. The airway with the largest outer diameter that fits the patient's nostril should be used.

   g. If the patient is awake and alert, position in semi-Fowler's position. If the patient is not conscious or alert, position in a side-lying position.

   h. Check placement by closing the patient's mouth and placing your fingers in front of the tube opening to check for air movement. Assess the pharynx to visualize the tip of the airway behind the uvula. Assess the nose for blanching or stretching of the skin.

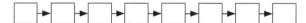

Prioritization Question

1. A patient brought to the emergency department with an opioid overdose who develops apnea. Which device will the nurse use to provide ventilation? Circle the letter that corresponds to the best answer.

   a. Manual resuscitation bag

   b. Nonrebreather mask

   c. Oropharyngeal airway

   d. Nasopharyngeal airway

CHAPTER 41

Fluid, Electrolyte, and Acid–Base Balance

ASSESSING YOUR UNDERSTANDING

FILL IN THE BLANK

1. The balance, or _____, of fluid, electrolytes, and acid–base is interrelated and maintained through the functions of almost every organ of the body.

2. _____ fluid is the fluid within cells, constituting about 70% of the total body water or about 40% of the adult's body weight.

3. _____ fluid is all the fluid outside the cells, accounting for about 30% of the total body water or about 20% of the adult's body weight.

4. _____ fluid losses cannot be measured or seen and include fluid lost from evaporation through the skin and as water vapor from the lungs during respiration.

5. _____ fluid losses can be measured and include fluid lost during urination, defecation, and wounds.

6. _____ are substances that can break down into particles called ions.

7. A(n) _____ is an atom or molecule carrying an electrical charge.

8. Ions with a positive charge are called _____.

9. Ions develop a negative charge and are called _____.

10. _____ are liquids that hold a substance in solution.

11. In _____, water passes from an area of lesser solute concentration to an area of greater solute concentration until equilibrium is established.

12. A solution that has about the same osmolality as plasma (280 mOsm/L) is considered a(n) _____ solution and remains in the intravascular compartment.

13. A(n) _____ solution has a greater osmolality than the plasma drawing water into the intravascular compartment, causing the cells to shrink.

14. A(n) _____ solution has a lower osmolality than plasma and moves out of the intravascular space and into ICF, causing cells to swell and possibly burst.

MATCHING EXERCISES

Matching Exercise 1

Match the cation in Part A with its function listed in Part B. Answers may be used more than once.

PART A

a. Sodium

b. Potassium

c. Calcium

d. Magnesium

PART B

_____ **1.** It is the chief regulator of cellular enzyme activity and cellular water content.

_____ **2.** It is necessary for nerve impulse transmission and blood clotting.

_____ **3.** It controls and regulates the volume of body fluids.

_____ **4.** It is the primary regulator of ECF volume.

_____ **5.** It is a catalyst for muscle contraction.

_____ **6.** It assists in the regulation of acid–base balance by cellular exchange with H^+.

_____ **7.** It acts on the cardiovascular system, producing vasodilation.

Matching Exercise 2

Match the anion in Part A with its function listed in Part B. Answers may be used more than once.

PART A

a. Chloride

b. Bicarbonate

c. Phosphate

PART B

_____ **1.** It acts with sodium to maintain the osmotic pressure of the blood.

_____ **2.** It promotes energy storage and is responsible for carbohydrate, protein, and fat metabolism.

_____ **3.** It is a major component of interstitial and lymph fluid; gastric and pancreatic juices; sweat, bile, and saliva.

_____ **4.** It is an anion that is the major chemical base buffer within the body.

_____ **5.** It has a role in acid–base balance as a hydrogen buffer.

_____ **6.** It combines with hydrogen ions to produce hydrochloric acid.

_____ **7.** It plays a role in muscle and red blood cell function.

Matching Exercise 3

Fill in the chart related to acid–base balance.

Name of Acid–Base Disturbance	Characteristics
1. Respiratory acidosis	Low pH, high $PaCO_2$, normal HCO_3^-
2.	Low pH, normal $PaCO_2$, low HCO_3^-
3.	High pH, normal $PaCO_2$, high HCO_3^-
4. Metabolic alkalosis	High pH, low $PaCO_2$, normal HCO_3^-

Matching Exercise 4

Match the term in Part A with its definition listed in Part B.

PART A

a. Filtration

b. Hydrostatic pressure

c. Diffusion

d. Active transport

e. Buffer

f. Intravascular fluid

g. Interstitial fluid

h. Oncotic pressure

PART B

_____ **1.** Fluid that surrounds tissue cells, including lymph

_____ **2.** Liquid constituent of blood

_____ **3.** Process that requires energy for the movement of substances through a cell membrane from an area of lesser concentration to an area of higher concentration

_____ **4.** Passage of a fluid through a permeable membrane

_____ **5.** Force exerted by a fluid against the container wall

_____ **6.** Substance that prevents body fluids from becoming overly acidic or alkaline

_____ **7.** Tendency of solutes to move freely throughout a solvent

_____ **8.** Concentration of particles in a solution, or its pulling power

CORRECT THE FALSE STATEMENTS

Mark the item "T" for true or "F" for false. If false, correct the underlined word or words to make the statement true in the space provided.

____ **1.** The human body is composed of <u>50% to 60%</u> water by weight. ____

____ **2.** Substances capable of breaking into electrically charged ions when dissolved in a solution are called <u>solutes</u>. ____

____ **3.** A <u>hypertonic solution</u> has a lower osmolarity than plasma. ____

____ **4.** <u>Ingested liquids</u> make up the largest amount of water normally taken into the body. ____

____ **5.** The acidity or alkalinity of a solution is determined by its concentration of <u>oxygen</u> ions. ____

____ **6.** An <u>acid</u> is a substance that can accept or trap hydrogen ions. ____

____ **7.** Normal blood plasma is slightly <u>acidic</u> and has a normal pH of 7.35 to 7.45. ____

____ **8.** The <u>kidneys</u> are the primary controller of the body's carbonic acid supply. ____

____ **9.** Excessive retention of sodium in ECF results in a condition termed fluid volume excess or <u>hypervolemia</u>. ____

____ **10.** <u>Hypokalemia</u> refers to a surplus of sodium in ECF that can result from excess water loss or an overall excess of sodium. ____

____ **11.** Acid–base imbalances occur when the ECF and ICF carbonic acid or bicarbonate levels become <u>equal</u>. ____

____ **12.** <u>Arterial blood gases</u> are most commonly used to assess and treat acid–base imbalances. ____

SHORT ANSWER

1. Fill in the normal values of the ABG.
   a. pH: _____
   b. pCO_2: _____
   c. HCO_3^-: _____
   d. PaO_2: _____
   e. SaO_2: _____

2. Briefly describe how the following processes transport materials to and from intracellular compartments.
   a. Osmosis: _____
   b. Diffusion: _____
   c. Active transport: _____

3. Give an example of how water is derived from the following sources.
   a. Ingested liquids: _____
   b. Food: _____
   c. Metabolic oxidation: _____

4. List three mechanisms for water loss in the body.
   a. _____
   b. _____
   c. _____

5. Explain how the following organs/systems of the body maintain fluid homeostasis.
   a. Kidneys: _____
   b. Cardiovascular system: _____
   c. Lungs: _____
   d. Thyroid: _____
   e. Gastrointestinal tract: _____
   f. Nervous system: _____

6. Give a brief description of the following conditions.
   a. Acidosis: _____
   b. Alkalosis: _____

7. Describe the following acid–base imbalances and their effect on the body.

   a. Respiratory acidosis: _____

   _____

   b. Respiratory alkalosis: _____

   _____

   c. Metabolic acidosis: _____

   _____

   d. Metabolic alkalosis: _____

   _____

8. Describe the causes of the following changes in hemoglobin and hematocrit.

   a. Increased hematocrit: _____

   _____

   b. Decreased hematocrit: _____

   _____

   c. Increased hemoglobin: _____

   _____

   d. Decreased hemoglobin: _____

   _____

9. Briefly describe the following screening tests and how they are performed.

   a. Urine pH and specific gravity: _____

   _____

   b. Serum electrolytes: _____

   _____

   c. Arterial blood gases: _____

   _____

10. List the important points a home health care nurse should address when caring for a patient on home infusion therapy.

   _____

   _____

   _____

APPLYING YOUR KNOWLEDGE

CRITICAL THINKING QUESTIONS

1. Assess the following patients for fluid, electrolyte, and acid–base balance. What knowledge of the factors that influence fluid and electrolyte and acid–base balance would you draw on to develop a plan to prevent recurrence of these patient problems?

   a. A long-distance runner who is practicing on a hot day experiences dizziness and shows signs of dehydration.

   b. An older adult with persistent heartburn ingests a large amount of sodium bicarbonate in 1 day.

   c. An infant is brought to the ER severely dehydrated after an extended bout of diarrhea.

2. Plan a low-sodium diet for a patient who has high blood pressure. List healthy foods that are low in salt, as well as foods that are high in salt and that should be avoided.

REFLECTIVE PRACTICE: CULTIVATING QSEN COMPETENCIES

Use the following expanded scenario from Chapter 41 in your textbook to answer the questions below.

Scenario: Jack Soo Park, a 78-year-old man receiving intravenous (IV) therapy with antibiotics, states, "I'm having trouble breathing. It just started a little while ago." Physical examination reveals a bounding pulse; distended neck veins; shallow, rapid respirations; and crackles and wheezes in the lungs. Excess fluid volume is suspected. Further checking reveals an IV fluid administration error that has resulted in overhydration.

1. Patient-centered care/ teamwork and collaboration: Based on the data in this scenario, what body systems are involved in Mr. Park's fluid volume excess? What interventions would be appropriate?

   _____

   _____

   _____

2. Patient-centered care/evidence-based practice: What would be a successful outcome for Mr. Park?

_____

_____

_____

3. Evidence-based practice/safety: What intellectual, technical, and ethical/legal competencies are most likely to bring about the desired outcome?

_____

_____

_____

4. Teamwork and collaboration: What resources might be helpful for Mr. Park?

_____

_____

_____

PATIENT CARE STUDY

Use this care study to apply your knowledge by completing the Nursing Process Worksheet found in Appendix A.

Scenario: Rebecca is a college freshman who had her wisdom teeth removed yesterday morning. She had a sore throat several days before the extraction but did not mention this to the oral surgeon. Because of her sore throat, she had greatly decreased her food and fluid intake. The night of the surgery, she had an oral temperature of 39.5°C (103.1°F). Friends gave her some Tylenol, which brought her temperature down, and encouraged her to drink more fluids. When they checked on her this morning, her temperature was elevated again, and she said she had felt too weak during the night to drink. They took her to the student health service, where the admitting nurse noticed her dry mucous membranes, decreased skin turgor, and rapid pulse. At 5 ft 2 inches and 98 lb, Rebecca had lost 4 lb in the past week.

PRACTICING FOR NCLEX

MULTIPLE-CHOICE QUESTIONS

Circle the letter that corresponds to the best answer for each question.

1. A nurse develops a health problem for a patient of "fluid overload." What etiology is most appropriate for the nurse to include?
   a. Excessive use of laxatives
   b. Diaphoresis
   c. Renal failure
   d. Increased cardiac output

2. A nurse is caring for a patient with a potassium level of 2.8 mEq/mL. When carrying out the prescription to provide potassium supplementation, which action by the nurse is essential?
   a. Explaining the purpose of the medication
   b. Observing for muscle cramping
   c. Infusing the medication with an infusion pump
   d. Anticipating decreased bowel sounds

3. A visiting nurse is caring for a patient who receives a daily diuretic and is reporting leg cramps and fatigue. What would the nurse recommend?
   a. "Take your pulse daily and notify the provider if it is irregular."
   b. "Eat foods higher in potassium such as bananas, citrus fruits, and melons."
   c. "Do not take the diuretic for a few days and see if the problem resolves."
   d. "Try increasing the sodium in your diet."

4. A nurse is caring for older adults in a long-term care facility. The nurse teaches the AP to encourage fluid intake in these patients because of what age-related alteration?
   a. Increased sense of thirst
   b. Increase in nephrons in the kidneys
   c. Increased renal blood flow
   d. Decreased sense of thirst

5. When caring for a patient admitted with dehydration, which finding indicates a positive outcome of care?
   a. Jugular vein distention
   b. Brisk skin turgor
   c. Dry oral mucus membranes
   d. Weight loss

6. A nurse is administering 20 mEQ of potassium chloride in 100 mL NSS to a patient with a potassium level of 2.8 mEq/dL. Which action by the nurse is essential?

    a. Teaching the patient why the medication is needed

    b. Explaining that muscle weakness will resolve after treatment

    c. Administering no more than 10 mEq/hr

    d. Anticipating diarrhea will develop after infusion

7. When caring for a patient with hypocalcemia, which food will the nurse recommend the patient consume?

    a. Chicken and fish

    b. Dairy and cheese

    c. Breads and pastas

    d. Bananas and citrus

8. A nurse is caring for a patient receiving TPN via a PICC line. Which nursing action is essential?

    a. Using clean technique when changing the dressing

    b. Flushing using normal saline and/or heparin solution according to facility policy

    c. Keeping the external portion of catheter coiled on top of dressing

    d. Changing the catheter caps every 10 days or as per facility policy

9. A nurse is administering 1,000-mL 0.9 normal saline over 10 hours (set delivers 60 gtt/1 mL). Using the formula below, what is the flow rate?

$$\text{gtt/min} = \frac{\text{milliliters per hour} \times \text{drop factor (gtt/mL)}}{\text{time (60 min)}}$$

    a. 60 gtt/min

    b. 100 gtt/min

    c. 160 gtt/min

    d. 600 gtt/min

10. A nurse is selecting a site for an IV infusion. What practice reflects safe care?

    a. Scalp veins should be selected for infants because of their accessibility.

    b. Antecubital veins should be used for long-term infusions.

    c. Leg veins should be used to keep the arms free for the patient's use.

    d. Using veins in surgical areas will increase potency of medication.

11. A nurse working in a trauma unit during a natural disaster is informed blood supplies are critically low. If necessary, what blood type will the nurse anticipate would be used if the patient's blood type is not available?

    a. A

    b. O

    c. B

    d. AB

12. A nurse is caring for a patient receiving a blood transfusion who develops hives and itching. What action will the nurse take first?

    a. Stop the transfusion.

    b. Notify the provider.

    c. Administer an antihistamine.

    d. Administer acetaminophen.

13. A nurse is caring for a patient with extreme respiratory distress. An ABG demonstrates respiratory acidosis, indicating which of these underlying problems?

    a. Increased levels of blood buffers

    b. Low oxygen levels

    c. Inadequate excretion of CO_2

    d. Loss of bicarbonate

14. When caring for patients whose SaO_2 is 89%, which intervention will the nurse perform immediately?

    a. Place the patient supine.

    b. Place the patient on their left side.

    c. Administer bicarbonate.

    d. Administer oxygen.

15. A nurse is administering a blood transfusion. Which response indicates a hemolytic reaction requiring immediate intervention?

    a. Dyspnea, dry cough, and pulmonary edema.

    b. Hives, itching, and anaphylaxis.

    c. Facial flushing, fever, chills, headache, low back pain, and shock

    d. Shortness of breath and auscultated crackles bilaterally in the bases

ALTERNATE-FORMAT QUESTIONS
Multiple-Response Questions
Circle the letters that correspond to the best answers for each question.

1. What nursing actions would be performed when preparing an IV solution and tubing when initiating an IV infusion? Select all that apply.
   a. Maintaining aseptic technique when opening sterile packages and IV solution
   b. Clamping the tubing, uncapping the spike, and inserting it into the entry site on the bag as manufacturer directs
   c. Squeezing the drip chamber and allowing it to fill a quarter full
   d. Removing the cap at the end of the tubing, releasing the clamp, and allowing fluid to move through the tubing
   e. Allowing fluid to flow and capping at the end of the tubing before all air bubbles have disappeared
   f. Applying a label to the tubing reflecting the day/date for the next set change, per facility guidelines

2. Following preparation of the IV solution and tubing, what actions will the nurse perform when selecting a site and palpating a vein to start an IV infusion? Select all that apply.
   a. Place the patient in a high Fowler's position in bed.
   b. Select an appropriate site and palpate accessible veins.
   c. Apply a tourniquet 6 inches above the venipuncture site to distend the vein.
   d. Direct the ends of the tourniquet away from the site and check that the radial pulse is still present.
   e. Ask the patient to keep a tightly closed fist while observing and palpating for a suitable vein.
   f. If a vein cannot be felt, release the tourniquet, and lower the arm below the level of the heart to fill the veins.

3. Which actions will the nurse perform after selecting a site and palpating accessible veins to start an IV infusion? Select all that apply.
   a. Clean the entry site with saline, followed by an alcohol swab according to facility policy.

   b. Place their dominant hand about 4 inches below the entry site to hold the patient's skin taut against the vein.
   c. Enter the skin gently, holding the catheter by the hub in their nondominant hand, bevel side down, at a 10- to 30-degree angle.
   d. Advance the needle or catheter into the vein. A sensation of "give" can be felt when the needle enters the vein.
   e. When blood returns through the lumen of the needle or the flashback chamber of the catheter, advance the catheter into the vein until the hub is at the venipuncture site.
   f. Release the tourniquet, quickly remove the protective cap from the IV tubing, and attach the tubing to the catheter or needle.

4. The nurse on a surgical unit is assessing patients receiving IV therapy. What signs of complications and their typical causes will the nurse identify? Select all that apply.
   a. Swelling, pain, coolness, or pallor at the insertion site may indicate infiltration of the IV.
   b. Redness, swelling, heat, and pain at the site may indicate phlebitis.
   c. Local or systemic manifestations may indicate an infection is present at the site.
   d. A pounding headache, fainting, rapid pulse rate, increased blood pressure, chills, back pains, and dyspnea are signs of an air embolus.
   e. Bleeding at the site when the IV is discontinued indicates an infection is present.
   f. Engorged neck veins, increased blood pressure, and dyspnea occur when a thrombus is present.

5. A nurse is teaching a patient about the function of sodium in the body. What teaching points would the nurse make? Select all that apply.
   a. "Sodium does not influence ICF volume."
   b. "Sodium is the primary regulator of ECF volume."
   c. "The daily value of sodium cited on nutrition facts labels is 1,200 mg."
   d. "Sodium is normally maintained in the body within a relatively narrow range, and deviations quickly result in serious health problems."

e. "The normal extracellular concentration of sodium is 85 to 95 mEq/L."

f. "Sodium participates in the generation and transmission of nerve impulses."

6. A nurse monitoring an IV infusion notes the signs and symptoms of a thrombus. What nursing interventions will the nurse perform? Select all that apply.

a. Stop the infusion immediately.

b. Apply warm compresses as ordered by the primary care provider.

c. Rub or massage the affected area.

d. Monitor vital signs and pulse oximetry.

e. Restart the IV at another site.

f. Place patient on their left side in the Trendelenburg position.

7. What IV solutions would the nurse expect to be ordered for a patient who has hypovolemia to increase vascular volume? Select all that apply.

a. 10% dextrose in water ($D_{10}W$)

b. 0.45% NaCl (½-strength normal saline)

c. 0.9% NaCl (normal saline)

d. Lactated Ringer's solution

e. 5% dextrose in 0.9% NaCl

f. 5% dextrose in water (D_5W)

8. A nurse is caring for a patient with renal failure who has a 1,500-mL fluid restriction. When measuring intake and output for this patient, what does the nurse document as intake? Select all that apply.

a. Fruit

b. Sips of water

c. Parenteral fluids

d. Ice chips

e. Chicken noodle soup

Chart/Exhibit Questions

Determine the acid–base imbalance in the cases in the following questions and circle the letter that corresponds to the best answer for each scenario. Refer to the Rules of ABG Interpretation table below for your answers.

Rules of ABG Interpretation		
pH	PaCO$_2$	HCO$_3$
<7.35 = acidosis	>45 mm Hg = respiratory acidosis	<22 mEq/L = metabolic acidosis
>7.45 = alkalosis	>35 mm Hg = respiratory alkalosis	>26 mEq/L = metabolic alkalosis

- It is OK to use what you know about your patient.
- The body responds to acid–base imbalances by activating compensatory mechanisms that minimize pH changes; a metabolic disturbance is compensated by the lungs, and a respiratory system disturbance is compensated by the kidneys.
- Any pH less than 7.35 = state of acidosis. Any pH greater than 7.45 = state of alkalosis.
- CO$_2$ is an acid; HCO$_3$ is a base. Any change in CO$_2$ reflects a respiratory change. Any change in HCO$_3$ reflects a metabolic change.
- If the pH has returned to *normal*, compensation has taken place.
- If the primary event is a *fall* in pH, whether respiratory or metabolic in origin, the arterial pH stays on the *acid* side after compensation.
- If the primary event is an *increase* in pH, whether respiratory or metabolic in origin, the arterial pH stays on the *base* side after compensation.

1. Patient with vomiting:

   ABGs: pH = 7.55; $PaCO_2$ = 45; HCO_3 = 36

   a. Respiratory acidosis
   b. Metabolic acidosis
   c. Metabolic alkalosis
   d. Respiratory alkalosis

2. Patient with a history of COPD:

   ABGs: pH = 7.36; $PaCO_2$ = 60; HCO_3 = 35

   a. Respiratory acidosis with renal compensation
   b. Metabolic acidosis with partial respiratory compensation
   c. Respiratory alkalosis
   d. Respiratory acidosis

3. Patient admitted with chronic kidney failure who is weak and tired:

   ABGs: pH = 7.24; $PaCO_2$ = 30; HCO_3 = 12

   a. Respiratory acidosis
   b. Respiratory alkalosis
   c. Metabolic alkalosis with partial respiratory compensation
   d. Metabolic acidosis with partial respiratory compensation

4. Patient with heart failure and dyspnea:

   ABGs: pH = 7.48; $PaCO_2$ = 22; HCO_3 = 24

   a. Respiratory alkalosis
   b. Respiratory acidosis
   c. Metabolic acidosis
   d. Metabolic alkalosis

5. Patient found "out of it" by friends on the floor of their room:

   ABGs: pH = 7.18; $PaCO_2$ = 79; HCO_3 = 26

   a. Respiratory alkalosis
   b. Respiratory acidosis
   c. Metabolic alkalosis with partial respiratory compensation
   d. Metabolic acidosis with partial respiratory compensation

6. Place an X in the appropriate boxes below.

   Determine if the ABG shown on the left side of the chart demonstrates acidosis or alkalosis; respiratory or metabolic. Determine whether compensation is present or not: Yes or No. If compensation is present, determine whether compensation is partial (P) or complete (C).

pH	$PaCO_2$	HCO_3^-	Acidosis or Alkalosis	Respiratory or	Metabolic	Comp Y/N	Complete (C) or Partial (P)
7.28	63	25					
7.20	40	14					
7.52	40	35					
7.16	82	30					
7.36	68	35					
7.56	23	26					
7.40	40	26					
7.56	23	26					
7.26	70	25					
7.52	44	38					
7.32	30	18					
7.49	34	26					

Hint: Compensation occurs in the unaffected system. Complete compensation returns the pH to normal; partial compensation occurs when the pH remains outside the normal range.

Hot Spot Questions

1. Place an "X" on the figure to indicate the spot where the insertion site of a peripherally inserted central catheter (PICC) would be found.

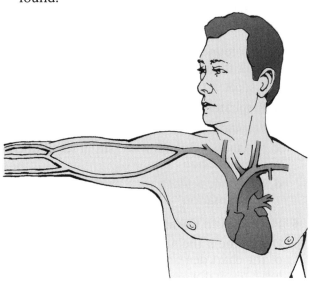

2. Indicate the insertion site of a triple-lumen nontunneled percutaneous central venous catheter by placing an "X" on the figure below where it would be inserted.

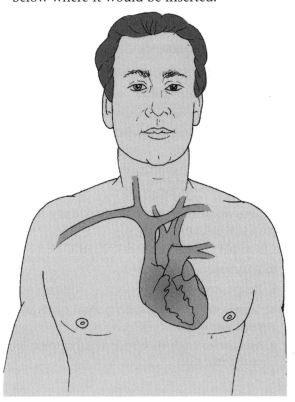

CHAPTER 42

Self-Concept

ASSESSING YOUR UNDERSTANDING

FILL IN THE BLANKS

1. A person who is a talented musician strives to reach full potential with consistent study and practice. This human need is termed self- _____.

2. All of the feelings, beliefs, and values associated with "I" or "me" comprise a person's self- _____.

3. The composite of all the basic facts, qualities, traits, images, and feelings one holds about oneself is known as the _____ self.

4. The self that one wants to be that developed in childhood and was based on the image of role models is known as the _____ self.

5. When a nursing student agrees to enroll in a nursing education program to please their parents or be denied money for their education, the student is displaying their _____ self.

6. Personal _____ describes a person's conscious sense of who they are.

7. Any impairment of the body or mind that makes it more difficult for that person to do certain activities and interact with the world around them is referred to as a(n) _____.

8. How _____ one felt as a child is a great predictor of how you manage all sorts of difficult situations later in life.

9. The stage of development of self-concept occurs at ages _____ to _____ years.

10. Adverse child experiences (ACEs) can lead to the development of chronic health problems, mental illness, and _____ abuse.

MATCHING EXERCISES

Matching Exercise 1

Match the definition in Part A with the term listed in Part B.

PART A

a. Self-esteem
b. Self-evaluation
c. Self-concept
d. Body image
e. Self-knowledge
f. Self-expectations

PART B

_____ 1. Need to feel good about oneself and believe others also hold one in high regard

_____ 2. Person's subjective view of their physical appearance

_____ 3. Includes basic characteristics (sex, age, race, occupation, cultural background, sexual orientation); a person's position within social groups; and qualities or traits that describe typical behaviors, feelings, moods

_____ **4.** These flow from the ideal self, the self that one wants to be or thinks one should be

_____ **5.** Mental image or picture of self

_____ **6.** Assessment of how well I like myself

Matching Exercise 2

Match the examples of risk factors for self-concept disturbances in Part A with the factors listed in Part B. Answers may be used more than once.

PART A

a. Personal identity disturbances

b. Body image disturbances

c. Self-esteem disturbances

d. Altered role performance

PART B

_____ **1.** An executive is laid off from their job due to cutbacks.

_____ **2.** A woman undergoes a radical mastectomy.

_____ **3.** A person finds themselves in an abusive relationship with their partner.

_____ **4.** A new parent discovers they are terrified of taking care of their newborn on her own.

_____ **5.** A school-aged child starts menstruating and developing earlier than her peers.

_____ **6.** A foreign exchange student attends school in the United States to learn a new language and customs.

_____ **7.** A recently divorced individual is lost without their partner.

SHORT ANSWER

1. What measures could you, as a nurse, employ to promote self-esteem in older adults?

_____

_____

_____

2. Reflect on your personal self-concept and how it affects the way you live your life. Keeping this in mind, answer the following questions.

a. Who am I? _____

_____

b. Who or what do I want to be? _____

_____

c. How well do I like me? _____

_____

3. Give an example of a question you might use to assess a patient for the following concepts.

a. Significance: _____

_____

b. Competence: _____

_____

c. Virtue: _____

_____

d. Power: _____

_____

4. Give an example of how each of the following factors might influence a person's self-concept.

a. Developmental considerations: _____

_____

b. Culture: _____

_____

c. Internal and external resources: _____

_____

d. History of success or failure: _____

_____

e. Stressors: _____

_____

f. Aging, illness, or trauma: _____

_____

5. List one example from your experience as a nurse that exemplifies the use of the following strategies for developing self-esteem in your practice.

a. Dispel the myth that it is necessary to know all there is to know about nursing to be a good nurse: _____

_____

b. Realistically evaluate strengths and weaknesses: _____

c. Accentuate the positive: _____

d. Develop a conscious plan for changing weaknesses into strengths: _____

e. Work to develop team self-esteem: _____

f. Actively demonstrate your commitment to nursing and concern about the nursing profession's public image: _____

6. Describe how you would record a self-concept assessment using your own personal strengths as an example.

_____

7. Give an example of an interview question you could use to assess self-concept in the following areas.

a. Personal identity: _____

b. Patient strengths: _____

c. Body image: _____

d. Self-esteem: _____

e. Role performance: _____

8. Describe three strategies nurses can use to help patients identify and use personal strengths.

a. _____

b. _____

c. _____

9. Give three examples of how nurses can help patients experiencing illness or life crisis maintain a sense of self-worth.

a. _____

b. _____

c. _____

10. Describe nursing strategies to develop self-esteem that you might use to meet the needs of the following older adult patients with disturbances in self-concept.

a. Older adult, newly admitted to a long-term care facility, states they have lost all sense of self (Self-Identity Disturbance): _____

b. Patient with deformities related to arthritis tells you they no longer recognize themselves when looking in the mirror (Body Image Disturbance): _____

c. Individual recovering from a stroke that has paralyzed their right side says, "I don't know if I can live like this" (Self-Esteem Disturbance): _____

d. Person complains that she no longer has the patience to babysit for their grandchildren whom they love (Role Performance Disturbance): _____

APPLYING YOUR KNOWLEDGE

CRITICAL THINKING QUESTIONS

1. There are many factors that influence the self-concept of patients, including developmental considerations, culture, internal or external resources, history of success or failure, stressors, and aging, illness, or trauma. Interview several patients to find out how these factors have influenced their self-concept. Reflect on their similarities and differences.

2. Would you describe yourself as having high or low self-concept? Ask your peers or friends if they agree with your assessment. How might your self-concept influence the relationships you establish with patients and colleagues?

REFLECTIVE PRACTICE: CULTIVATING QSEN COMPETENCIES

Use the following expanded scenario from Chapter 42 in your textbook to answer the questions below.

Scenario: Anthony is a middle-aged male with a history of diabetes. He recently underwent a below-the-knee amputation because of complications resulting from poor glucose control. One morning, he states, "I feel like damaged goods. I'm not a whole man anymore."

1. Patient-centered care: What interventions might the nurse employ to try to resolve Anthony's self-image disturbance?

_____

_____

_____

2. Patient-centered care: What would be a successful outcome for this patient?

_____

_____

_____

3. Patient-centered care/teamwork and collaboration/safety: What intellectual, technical, and ethical/legal competencies are most likely to bring about the desired outcome?

_____

_____

_____

4. Teamwork and collaboration: What resources might be helpful for this patient?

_____

_____

_____

PATIENT CARE STUDY

Use this care study to apply your knowledge by completing the Nursing Process Worksheet found in Appendix A.

Scenario: An English teacher asks you, the school nurse, to see one of her students, Julie, whose grades have recently dropped and who no longer seems to be interested in school or anything else. "She was one of my best students, and I can't figure out what's going on," the teacher says. "She seems reluctant to talk about this change." When Julie, a 16-year-old junior, walks into your office, you are immediately struck by her stooped posture, unkempt hair, and sloppy appearance. Julie is attractive, but at 5 ft 3 inches and 150 lb, she is overweight. Julie is initially reluctant to talk, but she breaks down at one point and confides that for the first time in her life she feels "absolutely awful" about herself. "I've always concentrated on getting good grades and achieved this easily. But now, this doesn't seem so important. I don't have any friends. All I hear the girls talking about is boys, and I was never even asked out by a boy, which I guess isn't surprising. Look at me!" After a few questions, it becomes clear that Julie has new expectations for herself based on what she observes in her peers, and she finds herself falling far short of her new, ideal self. Julie admits that, in the past, once she set a goal for herself, she was always able to achieve it because she is strongly self-motivated. Although she has withdrawn from her parents and teachers, she admits that she does know adults she can trust who have been a big support to her in the past. She says, "If only I could become the kind of teenager other kids like and have lots of friends!"

PRACTICING FOR NCLEX

MULTIPLE-CHOICE QUESTIONS

Circle the letter that corresponds to the best choice for each question.

1. A child in the hospital lists his favorite sports figures and tells the nurse he is going to be just like them. What human need is this patient demonstrating?
   a. Self-knowledge
   b. Self-expectations
   c. Self-evaluation
   d. Self-actualization

2. A nurse encourages a young patient whose leg was amputated to continue to pursue their dream to become a dancer with unique gifts and talents. What human need is the nurse is assisting the patient to reach?
   a. Self-actualization
   b. Self-concept
   c. Self-esteem
   d. Ideal self

3. A nurse assessing children in a pediatrician's office would expect a child to achieve self-recognition at what age?
   a. At birth
   b. By 18 months
   c. By 3 years
   d. By 6 years

4. A nursing student is concerned that one of their peers who has not maintained healthy relationships with other students would be at risk for what self-concept disturbance?
   a. Personal identity disturbance
   b. Body image disturbance
   c. Self-esteem disturbance
   d. Altered role performance

5. When a nurse asks a patient to describe her personal characteristics and traits, the nurse is most likely assessing the patient for what self-concept factors?
   a. Body image
   b. Role performance
   c. Self-esteem
   d. Personal identity

6. Which question would the nurse include on a self-concept assessment related to body image?
   a. "Do you like who you are?"
   b. "Who influenced you the most growing up?"
   c. "How do you feel about recent physical changes?"
   d. "Who would you most like to be?"

7. Which question would the nurse ask to assess a patient's self-identity during a focused self-concept assessment?
   a. "Who would you like to be?"
   b. "What do you like most about your body?"
   c. "What are your personal strengths?"
   d. "Do you like being a teacher?"

8. Which question would provide the nurse with the information needed first when assessing self-concept?
   a. "How would you describe yourself to others?"
   b. "Do you like yourself?"
   c. "What do you see yourself doing 5 years from now?"
   d. "What are some of your personal strengths?"

9. A nurse is caring for a patient who is beginning chemotherapy for cancer treatment. The nurse recognizes the patient's self-concept is positive and they are coping with potential changes in body image when they make which statement?
   a. "I won't be able to go to work if all my hair falls out."
   b. "I'm glad my friend gave me a beautiful scarf for my head."
   c. "I worry that the side effects of my treatment will scare second-graders."
   d. "My son asked if he'll still recognize me when I lose my hair."

10. A psychiatric nurse is discussing maintaining positive self-esteem in children. Which nursing action best promotes a positive self-concept?
   a. Suggesting parents tell children about their positive and negative qualities

b. Giving the child frequent opportunities to try risky activities

c. Trying to focus on what the child's behavior is trying to convey

d. Discouraging unusual personal styles and preferences in dress

11. When caring for a patient with diabetes who is experiencing complications of poor glycemic control, what question related to the patient's self-concept would the nurse use?

a. "Does the patient know how to measure their blood glucose?"

b. "Is the patient able to afford a glucometer?"

c. "Does the patient value themselves sufficiently to manage their health?"

d. "Can the patient state the relationship between diabetes and blindness?"

ALTERNATE-FORMAT QUESTIONS

Multiple-Response Questions

Circle the letters that correspond to the best answers for each question.

1. A nurse is preparing a focused assessment guide to assess patients for self-esteem. Which questions address personal identity? Select all that apply.

a. "Is there anything about your body that you would change?"

b. "How would you describe yourself?"

c. "What would you list as your strengths?"

d. "How satisfied are you with yourself?"

e. "What are your relationships with others like?"

f. "What are your fears in life?"

2. A school nurse is teaching parents how to build self-esteem in children. Which strategies would the nurse include? Select all that apply.

a. "Point out examples of your child's ability in many different circumstances."

b. "Listen to what your child says about their behavior and try to fix the problem."

c. "Address your child's negative qualities including their taste, preferences, or personal style."

d. "Find occasions to frequently and honestly praise your child."

e. "Explore the need being expressed by the negative behavior and address that behavior."

f. "Make your expectations clear; let your child practice the necessary skills; and make it safe to fail."

3. A nurse is counseling adolescents in a group-home setting. What aspect of self-esteem is developed in this age group? Select all that apply.

a. Sense of self is consolidated.

b. The emphasis is on sexual identity.

c. It is important to meet role expectations well.

d. Parental influences on self-concept are often rejected.

e. A sense of being trusted and loved, of being competent and trustworthy develops.

f. Differentiation of self and nonself is beginning.

Prioritization Question

1. A school nurse is assessing school-aged children for adverse child experiences (ACEs). Which child will the nurse prioritize for follow-up first? Circle the letter that corresponds to the best answer.

a. Child whose parent had a heart attack last year

b. One who fractured their wrist roller skating

c. Child whose parent recently attempted suicide

d. One whose parents set a strict bedtime

CHAPTER 43

Stress and Adaptation

ASSESSING YOUR UNDERSTANDING

FILL IN THE BLANKS

1. _____ is a condition in which the human system responds to changes in its normal balanced state; a _____ is something perceived as challenging, threatening, or demanding, triggering a stress reaction.

2. Physiologic mechanisms within the body respond to internal changes to maintain _____, a relative constancy in the internal environment.

3. The reflex pain response is an example of the local _____ syndrome.

4. The _____ response is a local response to injury or infection; it serves to localize and prevent the spread of infection and promote wound healing.

5. The _____ or _____ response is the body's method of preparing the body to either fight off a stressor or run away from it.

6. A person who develops diarrhea while under prolonged stress is said to be experiencing psychosomatic, or a(n) _____– _____ interaction.

7. The most common human response to stress is _____, a vague, uneasy feeling of discomfort or dread, the source of which is often unknown or nonspecific.

8. Behaviors used to decrease stress and anxiety, often without conscious thought are called _____ mechanisms.

9. The prolonged stress experienced by family members caring for a loved one at home for long periods is known as caregiver _____.

10. Unconscious reactions to stressors, called _____ mechanisms, are used to protect a person's self-esteem during times of mild to moderate anxiety.

11. A _____ is a disturbance caused by a precipitating event, such as a perceived loss, a threat of loss, or a challenge, that is perceived as a threat to self. In a crisis, the person's usual methods of coping are ineffective.

MATCHING EXERCISES

Matching Exercise 1

Match the type of defense mechanism in Part A with its example listed in Part B.

PART A

a. Compensation

b. Denial

c. Displacement

d. Introjection

e. Projection

f. Rationalization

PART B

____ 1. A patient bangs his hand on the bed tray in frustration over his rehabilitation progress.

____ 2. A patient who has sexual feelings for a nurse accuses her of sexual harassment.

____ 3. A patient who cannot stop smoking becomes a fitness fanatic.

____ **4.** A patient adopts his spiritual director's philosophy of life.

____ **5.** A patient refuses to accept their diagnosis of cancer.

____ **6.** A patient who continually forgets to take his medications complains, "There are too many pills to take."

Matching Exercise 2

Match the type of coping mechanism in Part A with its example listed in Part B.

PART A

a. Regression

b. Repression

c. Sublimation

d. Reaction formation

e. Undoing

f. Dissociation

PART B

____ **1.** A patient doesn't remember striking a nurse during a painful procedure.

____ **2.** A patient who screamed at a nurse in anger over a lack of privacy gives the nurse a box of candy.

____ **3.** A patient who actually admires her doctor's medical ability questions his competency.

____ **4.** A long-term care facility patient who is depressed becomes incontinent.

____ **5.** A wheelchair-bound patient becomes involved in wheelchair races.

____ **6.** An adult cannot recall memories of a car accident occurring in his childhood, that killed his mother.

Matching Exercise 3

Match the homeostatic regulators of the body listed in Part A with their action listed in Part B.

PART A

a. Parasympathetic

b. Sympathetic

c. Pituitary

d. Adrenals

e. Thyroid

f. Cardiovascular

g. Renal

PART B

____ **1.** Secretes adrenocorticotropic hormone and thyroid-stimulating hormone

____ **2.** Functions under stress conditions to bring about the fight-or-flight response

____ **3.** Functions under normal conditions and at rest

____ **4.** Secretes thyroid hormone and calcitonin

____ **5.** Serves as a transport system and pump

____ **6.** Filters, excretes, and reabsorbs metabolic products and water

____ **7.** Produces epinephrine and norepinephrine; supports the sympathetic nervous system

SHORT ANSWER

1. Briefly describe the following adaptive responses to stress and give an example of each response.

   a. Mind–body interaction: _____

   _____

   b. Local adaptation syndrome: _____

   _____

   c. General adaptation syndrome: _____

   _____

2. Describe the inflammatory response.

   _____

   _____

3. List three variables affecting the length of the alarm stage of the GAS.

   a. _____

   _____

   b. _____

   _____

   c. _____

   _____

4. Describe the following levels of anxiety. In your practice, have you experienced any of these levels of anxiety?

   a. Mild anxiety: _____

   _____

   _____

b. Moderate anxiety: _____
_____
_____

c. Severe anxiety: _____
_____
_____

d. Panic: _____
_____
_____

5. Define the following coping mechanisms and give an example that you witnessed in a patient, friend, relative, or used yourself.

a. Attack behavior: _____
_____

b. Withdrawal behavior: _____
_____

c. Compromise behavior: _____
_____

6. List three examples of situations in which stress may have a positive impact on a person.

a. _____
b. _____
c. _____

7. Give three examples of the following sources of stress.

a. Developmental stress: _____
_____
_____

b. Situational stress: _____
_____
_____

8. An adolescent is admitted to your unit with a fractured leg and facial lacerations from a motor vehicle accident. List two remarks a nurse might make during the nursing history to assess this patient for anxiety.

a. _____
b. _____

9. You are a visiting nurse for a patient recovering from a stroke who is being taken care of by their daughter-in-law, who is also the parent of 2-year-old twins. During your

visit, you notice that the caregiver is unfocused, restless, and states they have resumed smoking. You suspect caregiver burden. How would you plan and implement care to help relieve their stress?

_____
_____
_____
_____

10. Briefly describe how the following can help reduce stress.

a. Exercise: _____
_____

b. Rest and sleep: _____
_____

c. Nutrition: _____
_____

11. List the five steps of the problem-solving technique used in crisis intervention.

a. _____
b. _____
c. _____
d. _____
e. _____

12. List four personal factors that affect stress.

a. _____
b. _____
c. _____
d. _____

13. Give three examples of how a family can help a patient manage stress.

a. _____
b. _____
c. _____

14. When caring for a patient experiencing extreme stress related to a family crisis briefly discuss the following:

a. Physical manifestations of stress
_____
_____

b. Steps of crisis intervention
_____
_____

c. Stress-reduction techniques

_____

_____

d. Positive outcome measures

_____

_____

APPLYING YOUR KNOWLEDGE

CRITICAL THINKING QUESTIONS

1. Describe the nursing interventions you would use to relieve the stress of the following patients.

   a. A family breadwinner with a partner and three children is being treated for an ulcer. They recently lost their job and are having a hard time finding a new one. They don't know if they can make the mortgage and school payments.

   b. An adolescent is admitted to a unit for drug rehabilitation. They put pressure on themselves to be "the best" in sports and academic work and says that they couldn't handle the stress without getting high.

2. Recall a period in your life when you were under a considerable amount of stress, such as during exams, following a death, or during an illness. How did the stress affect you physically? Did it alter your health state? What did you do to compensate for the effects of stress on your body? How can you use this information in caring for patients?

REFLECTIVE PRACTICE: CULTIVATING QSEN COMPETENCIES

Use the following expanded scenario from Chapter 43 in your textbook to answer the questions below.

Scenario: Joan, a 46-year-old woman with a history of inflammatory bowel disease, comes to the outpatient clinic with reports of increasing episodes of diarrhea. She says, "I think my bowel disease is flaring up again." Further assessment reveals she started a new job a month ago after being out of the workforce for the past 15 years. "Since the children are in school most of the day, my spouse and I decided it was time for me to go back to work to help out financially," she says.

1. Patient-centered care: What might be the cause of the flare-up of this patient's inflammatory bowel disease? What nursing interventions would be beneficial for this patient?

_____

_____

_____

2. Patient-centered care: What would be a successful outcome for this patient?

_____

_____

_____

3. Patient-centered care: What intellectual, interpersonal, and ethical/legal competencies are most likely to bring about the desired outcome?

_____

_____

_____

4. Teamwork and collaboration: What resources might be helpful for this patient?

_____

_____

_____

PATIENT CARE STUDY

Use this care study to apply your knowledge by completing the Nursing Process Worksheet found in Appendix A.

Scenario: Tisha Brent, age 52, comes to the clinic complaining of feelings of nervousness and an inability to sleep. During the health history, she says, "This past year has been almost more than I could stand." She tells you that in 1 year, her grandmother and father died, her husband was diagnosed with cancer, her daughter got a divorce, and her son became depressed and unable to work. She believes herself to be "the strong person in the family; the one who always takes care of everyone else."

Mrs. Brent works full time as a social worker but is finding it more and more difficult to help others because of her own worries. She tells you that she rarely sees her friends anymore because she must care for her husband. She also says that she has no appetite, cries often, and sometimes has trouble catching her breath. Findings from the physical assessment included a weight loss of 10 lb in the past 3 months (with weight 5% below normal for height), tachycardia, slightly elevated blood pressure, and hand tremors.

PRACTICING FOR NCLEX

MULTIPLE-CHOICE QUESTIONS

Circle the letter that corresponds to the best answer for each question.

1. A nurse assesses patients in a long-term care facility for diseases that are associated with stress. Which is an autoimmune disease that is related to stress?
   a. Graves' disease
   b. Asthma
   c. Hypertension
   d. Esophageal reflux

2. A visiting nurse is caring for a patient with cancer who is not responding well to treatment. What is an example of the patient's use of displacement as a defense mechanism?
   a. Concentrating on body-building instead
   b. Refusing to see their doctor
   c. Shouting at their dog to keep quiet
   d. Blaming their spouse for the treatment outcome

3. A nurse is assessing a patient who was involved in a shooting. The patient's vital signs show that his body is attempting to adapt to the stressor. In what stage of the general adaptation syndrome does the nurse identify this occurs?
   a. Alarm reaction
   b. Resistance
   c. Exhaustion
   d. Homeostasis

4. A nurse notes a patient who responds to bad news concerning his lab reports by crying uncontrollably is handling stress by using which response?
   a. Adaptation technique
   b. Coping mechanism
   c. Withdrawal behavior
   d. Defense mechanism

5. Which statement correctly explains the effects of stress on a person's basic human needs?
   a. As a person strives to meet basic human needs at each level, stress can serve as either a stimulus or a barrier.
   b. Basic human needs and responses to stress are generalized.
   c. Basic human needs and responses to stress are unaffected by sociocultural backgrounds, priorities, and past experiences.
   d. Stress affects all people in their attainment of basic human needs in the same manner.

6. A nurse plans care based on basic human needs. The nurse plans to help the patient meet which need in a withdrawn and isolated patient?
   a. Physiologic
   b. Safety and security
   c. Self-esteem
   d. Love and belonging

7. A patient's body uses what physiologic mechanism when reacting to blood loss to maintain an essential balance?
   a. Stress
   b. Self-regulation
   c. Homeostasis
   d. Fight-or-flight response

8. A patient responds to an approaching diagnostic test with a rapidly beating heart and shaking hands. The nurse correlates this response to which response?
   a. Sympathetic nervous system
   b. Parasympathetic nervous system
   c. Pituitary gland
   d. Renal system

9. The nurse on a psychiatric unit cares for multiple patients experiencing anxiety. Which patient response does the nurse document as the panic level of anxiety?
   a. Losing control and expressing irrational thinking
   b. Experiencing increased alertness and motivated learning
   c. Focusing narrowly on specific detail
   d. Displaying a narrow perception field

10. Nurses on a telemetry unit have traditionally enjoyed their work, colleagues, and coped with demands of the job effectively. A nurse becomes concerned that a colleague who recently began displaying anxiety and stress, may be experiencing what condition?

    a. Culture shock

    b. Adaptation syndrome

    c. Ineffective coping

    d. Burnout

11. What illness-related task for a patient adapting to a chronic illness would a nurse help the patient work toward?

    a. Maintaining self-esteem

    b. Maintaining personal relationships

    c. Carrying out medical treatment

    d. Confronting family problems

12. A nurse stops in a patient's room the night before their surgery and finds the patient unable to sleep and full of uncertainty of the outcome of the procedure. Which of these statements would be most helpful to the patient at this time?

    a. "It is okay to become angry before a surgical procedure."

    b. "It is common for people awaiting surgery to feel anxious. I could sit with you a bit."

    c. "Don't be concerned about the outcome of the surgery; you have the best surgeon."

    d. "Many people develop depression until the outcome of surgery is known."

13. A nurse's neighbor has lost their spouse of 40 years. The nurse becomes concerned when the neighbor demonstrates which of these coping mechanisms?

    a. Walking in the evening as they used to do

    b. Visiting with their children on Sundays

    c. Drinking alcohol each night to fall asleep

    d. Baking the neighbors cakes and cookies

ALTERNATE-FORMAT QUESTIONS

Multiple-Response Questions

Circle the letters that correspond to the best answers for each question.

1. Nursing students in a psychiatric nursing course are studying the four levels of anxiety that can develop. Which of these would the students select as correct? Select all that apply.

    a. Moderate anxiety is present in day-to-day living, and it increases alertness and perceptual fields.

    b. Although mild anxiety may interfere with sleep, it also facilitates problem solving.

    c. Mild anxiety is manifested by a quivering voice, tremors, increased muscle tension, and a slight increase in pulse.

    d. Severe anxiety creates a very narrow focus on specific detail, causing all behavior to be geared toward getting relief.

    e. Severe anxiety causes a person to lose control and experience dread and terror.

    f. During the panic stage, there is increased physical activity, concentration only on the present, and feelings of impending doom.

2. A nurse is caring for a group of patients who are experiencing various stressors. Which statements accurately describe the individual's use of defense mechanisms against stressors? Select all that apply.

    a. Withdrawal behavior involves physical withdrawal from the threat or emotional reactions such as admitting defeat, becoming apathetic, or feeling guilty and isolated.

    b. Defense mechanisms are conscious reactions to stressors.

    c. Displacement occurs when a person refuses to acknowledge the presence of a condition that is disturbing.

    d. Projection occurs when a person's thoughts or impulses are attributed to another person.

    e. Repression occurs when a person consciously excludes an anxiety-producing event from conscious awareness.

    f. Reaction formation occurs when a person tries to give questionable behavior a logical or socially acceptable explanation.

3. A nurse is describing the effect of stress on the body to a group of health practitioners. Which statements accurately describe the role of stress on the health and illness of patients? Select all that apply.

    a. Stress has a negative impact on a person as they strive to meet basic human needs at each level.

    b. People react to stress in a consistent and predictable manner.

c. The health–illness continuum is affected by stress.

d. The effects of stress on a sick or injured person are usually positive.

e. As the duration, intensity, or number of stressors increases, the ability to adapt is lessened.

f. Recovery from illness and return to normal function are compromised by prolonged stress.

4. A psychiatric nurse practitioner is discussing stress with students in postconference. What example best describes examples of situational stress? Select all that apply.

a. Toddler learning to control elimination

b. School-aged child attending her first party

c. Adult getting married to his high school sweetheart

d. Patient recovering from a car accident

e. Teenager being offered a cigarette by a friend

f. High school graduate enrolling in the armed services

5. A nurse is discussing psychosocial stressors discussed in the nightly news. Which will the nurse include? Select all that apply.

a. News reports on television about a war

b. Being caught in a blizzard

c. Acquiring a nosocomial infection

d. Being diagnosed with HIV

e. Fearing a terrorist attack

f. Being involved in an accident

Sequencing Question

1. Place the following steps of the general adaptation syndrome (GAS) in the order in which they would normally occur.

a. Rest and recovery or death occur.

b. Alarm reaction begins.

c. Fight-or-flight response occurs.

d. Neuroendocrine activity increases vital signs.

e. Stage of resistance begins.

f. Panic, crisis, and exhaustion occur.

g. Neuroendocrine activity returns to normal.

h. Stage of exhaustion begins.

i. Threat occurs.

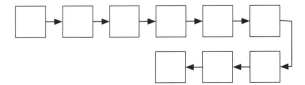

CHAPTER 44

Loss, Grief, and Dying

ASSESSING YOUR UNDERSTANDING

FILL IN THE BLANKS

1. When an older adult grieves for the loss of their youth, this type of loss that is intangible to others is known as _____ loss.

2. _____ is a state of grieving due to loss of a loved one; _____ is the actions and expressions of grief, including the symbols and ceremonies (e.g., a funeral or final celebration of life).

3. According to Engel, _____ is the final resolution of the grief process.

4. Abnormal or distorted grief that may be unresolved or inhibited is known as _____ grief.

5. According to the Uniform Definition of Death Act (1981), death is defined as present when a person has sustained either irreversible cessation of circulation and respiratory functions or cessation of _____ function.

6. The goal of _____ care is to give patients with life-threatening illnesses the best quality of life using aggressive management of symptoms and care of the whole person—body, mind, and spirit; heart and soul.

7. _____ is the ingredient in life that enables a person both to consider a future and to actively bring that future into being.

8. _____ care is care provided for people with limited life expectancy, often in the home.

9. A good death is one that allows a person to die on their own terms, relatively free of pain, and with _____.

10. Some facilities use the term "allow _____ death" instead of Do Not Resuscitate because it is stated in the positive, rather than negative.

MATCHING EXERCISES

Matching Exercise 1

Match the term in Part A with the appropriate definition listed in Part B.

PART A

a. Actual loss

b. Inhibited dysfunctional grief

c. Physical loss

d. Psychological loss

e. Anticipatory loss

f. Grief

PART B

____ 1. Type of loss in which a person displays grief behaviors for a loss that has yet to take place

____ 2. Type of loss that can be recognized by others as well as by the person sustaining the loss

____ 3. Type of loss that may be caused by an altered self-image and inability to return to work

____ 4. Type of loss that is tangible, such as the loss of a limb or organ

____ 5. Internal emotional reaction to loss such as it occurs with separation or death

_____ **6.** Person suppresses feelings of grief and may instead manifest somatic symptoms, such as abdominal pain or heart palpitations

Matching Exercise 2

Match Engel's six stages of grief listed in Part A with the appropriate definition listed in Part B.

PART A

a. Shock and disbelief

b. Developing awareness

c. Restitution

d. Resolving the loss

e. Idealization

f. Outcome

PART B

_____ **1.** "I know I won't be having Sunday dinner with my mother anymore. Maybe my husband and I can eat out this Sunday."

_____ **2.** "I can't believe my mother died of breast cancer! She was never seriously ill in her life."

_____ **3.** "My mother was the perfect parent. I wish I could be more like her with my kids."

_____ **4.** "Every time I think of my mother, I can't help but cry."

_____ **5.** "I've been attending Mass every morning to pray for my mother's soul and to help me get over her death."

_____ **6.** "I miss my mother, but at least now I can accept her death and try to get on with my life."

CORRECT THE FALSE STATEMENTS

Mark the item "T" for true or "F" for false. If false, correct the underlined word or words to make the statement true in the space provided.

_____ **1.** A person experiencing abbreviated grief may have trouble expressing feelings of loss or may deny them. _____

_____ **2.** In the denial and isolation stage of dying, the patient expresses rage and hostility and adopts a "why me?" attitude. _____

_____ **3.** In the case of a terminal illness, the health care provider is usually responsible for deciding what and how much the patient should be told. _____

_____ **4.** In a living will, the patient appoints an agent they trust to make decisions if they become incapacitated. _____

_____ **5.** The Patient Self-Determination Act of 1990 requires all hospitals to inform their patients of advance directives. _____

_____ **6.** A slow-code order may be written on the chart of a terminally ill patient if the patient or family has expressed a wish that there be no attempts to resuscitate the patient in the event of cardiopulmonary failure. _____

_____ **7.** Terminal weaning is the gradual withdrawal of mechanical ventilation from a patient with a terminal illness or an irreversible condition with a poor prognosis. _____

_____ **8.** The nurse assumes responsibility for handling and filing the death certificate with proper authorities. _____

_____ **9.** After the patient has been pronounced dead, the health care provider is responsible for preparing the body for discharge. _____

SHORT ANSWER

1. Describe two nursing responsibilities that should be carried out after the death of a patient in each of the following areas.

a. Care of the body: _____

_____

b. Care of the family: _____

_____

c. Discharging legal responsibilities: _____

_____

2. Briefly describe behaviors that occur in the following stages of dying, according to Kübler-Ross.

a. Denial and isolation: _____

_____

b. Anger: _____

_____

c. Bargaining: _____

_____

d. Depression: _____

_____

e. Acceptance: _____
_____

3. Your patient is a 50-year-old woman newly diagnosed with terminal uterine cancer. What information should be provided to her regarding her condition?

_____
_____

4. How would you respond to a patient dying of AIDS who says: "Nurse, please help me die"? Incorporate the ANA's Position Statement on Euthanasia, Assisted Suicide, and Aid in Dying.

_____
_____

5. Describe the role of the nurse in caring for patients and their families during terminal weaning from mechanical ventilation.

_____
_____

6. List three goals for nurses who wish to become effective in caring for patients experiencing loss, grief, or dying and death.

a. _____
_____

b. _____
_____

c. _____
_____

7. Your patient is a middle-aged patient dying of liver cancer at home with his family. List three patient goals or outcomes for this patient and his family.

a. _____

b. _____

c. _____

8. As a nursing student planning to participate in a debate in a bioethics class, list three arguments in favor of (pro) and against (con) assisted suicide and direct voluntary euthanasia.

a. Pro: _____
_____

b. Con: _____
_____

9. What is the role of the nurse during the following code situations?

a. No-code: _____
_____
_____

b. Comfort measures only: _____
_____
_____

c. Do-not-hospitalize order: _____
_____

d. Terminal weaning: _____
_____
_____

10. Explain the differences in these documents used in end-of-life care, including the nurse's role.

a. Durable power of attorney: _____
_____

b. Living will: _____
_____

c. POLST form: _____
_____

APPLYING YOUR KNOWLEDGE

CRITICAL THINKING QUESTIONS

1. Discuss nursing care to help the following patients deal with their grief.

a. A young athlete has their left leg amputated after it was crushed in a car accident.

b. You find a young adult woman crying softly in her bed after undergoing a hysterectomy.

c. A middle-aged patient has just been told that she has an inoperable brain tumor.

2. Think of a time when you lost someone dear to you. How did you cope with your loss? Were you aware of going through Engel's six stages of grief? How long did it take you to resolve the loss and get back to normal life activities? Interview some friends about coping with losing a loved one and compare their experiences to yours. How can you use this knowledge in your care of patients?

REFLECTIVE PRACTICE: CULTIVATING QSEN COMPETENCIES

Use the following expanded scenario from Chapter 44 in your textbook to answer the questions below.

Scenario: Yvonne, a 20-year-old single woman, has just given birth to a baby, 11 weeks premature. The newborn weighs 2 lb 2 oz (1,021 g) and is immediately admitted to the neonatal intensive care unit because of severe respiratory distress. Up until this point, Yvonne had a normal pregnancy and was expecting a healthy baby girl. "I was so happy to be pregnant and I wanted to be a mother so much. But my baby is so tiny! And now the doctors are telling me that she has less than a 50% chance of surviving the next 24 hours."

1. Patient-centered care/evidence-based practice: How might the nurse react to Yvonne in a manner that respects her right to privacy while at the same time helping her through the grief process?

_____

_____

_____

2. Patient-centered care/evidence-based practice: What would be a successful outcome for this patient?

_____

_____

_____

3. Patient-centered care/teamwork and collaboration: What intellectual, interpersonal, and/or ethical/legal competencies are most likely to bring about the desired outcome?

_____

_____

_____

4. Teamwork and collaboration: What resources might be helpful for Yvonne?

_____

_____

_____

PATIENT CARE STUDY

Use this care study to apply your knowledge by completing the Nursing Process Worksheet found in Appendix A.

Scenario: LeRoy is a 40-year-old architect whose life partner, Michael, is dying of AIDS. Although both LeRoy and Michael "did the bathhouse scene" in the early 1980s and had multiple unprotected sexual encounters, they have been in a monogamous relationship for the past 14 years. Michael has been in and out of the hospital during the past 3 years and is now dying of end-stage AIDS at home. He is enrolled in a hospice program. LeRoy has been very supportive of Michael throughout the different phases of his illness but at present seems to be "losing it." Michael noticed that LeRoy is sleeping at odd times and seems to be losing weight. He suspects that LeRoy may be drinking more than usual and using recreational drugs. He also says that LeRoy is "acting strangely"; he seems emotionally withdrawn and unusually uncommunicative. "I don't think he's able to deal with the fact that I'm dying," Michael tells you. "He won't let me talk about it at all." The hospice nurse notes that LeRoy is now rarely home when he comes to visit. When the hospice nurse calls to arrange a meeting with LeRoy, LeRoy informs him that he is "managing quite well, thank you" and that he has no concerns or problems to discuss.

PRACTICING FOR NCLEX

MULTIPLE-CHOICE QUESTIONS

Circle the letter that corresponds to the best answer for each question.

1. With the support of the nurse, parents of an infant who died shortly after birth arrange for a funeral service. What stage of grief, according to Engel, involves the rituals surrounding loss, including funeral services?
   a. Shock and disbelief
   b. Developing awareness
   c. Restitution
   d. Resolving the loss

2. A patient who was brought to the emergency room for gunshot wounds dies in the intensive care unit a few hours later. The nurse anticipates what action related to the need for an autopsy will apply to this patient?
   a. The closest surviving family member must give consent for the autopsy to be performed.
   b. This death may be an accident, suicide, or homicide; the coroner determines the need for an autopsy.
   c. The health care provider should be present to prepare the patient for an autopsy.
   d. Because the nature of death has been established an autopsy should not be performed.

3. A nurse is caring for an older adult with severe pneumonia who has a no-code order entered in the electronic health record. Which nursing action will best help establish a trusting nurse–patient relationship?
   a. Discussing the patient's fears and doubts openly and serving as a nonjudgmental listener
   b. Reducing verbal and nonverbal contact with the patient to avoid confusing them
   c. Avoiding providing death education because it is outside the scope of professional nursing practice
   d. Arranging a visit from a spiritual advisor, regardless of the patient's wishes, to provide hope in the face of death

4. A nurse in the intensive care unit is caring for a patient who has been declared brain dead. What is the nurse's priority?
   a. Providing care to the patient and family
   b. Contacting the organ-sharing network
   c. Assisting the family with contacting relatives
   d. Preparing the patient for unresolved grief

5. The wife of a man who is dying tells the nurse: "Harold was so good to me. He was like a saint with his patience. I will miss him terribly." Which stage of grief is this woman experiencing, according to Engel?
   a. Restitution
   b. Awareness
   c. Outcome
   d. Idealization

6. After the death of their spouse, the surviving spouse reported frequent headaches and loss of appetite. No medical cause was found. The remaining spouse would likely be experiencing which type of grief?
   a. Abbreviated
   b. Anticipatory
   c. Unresolved
   d. Inhibited

7. Which health problem specifically addresses human response to loss and impending death in the problem statement?
   a. Complicated grieving related to loss of partner
   b. Anxiety related to unknown reaction to stages of death
   c. Dressing self-care deficit related to weakness
   d. Impaired comfort related to complications of chemotherapy

8. The health care provider and nurse tell a patient's adult son that the patient has died. The son states, "You are mistaken, they are not gone. Check again." What behavior is the patient's son displaying?
   a. Anger
   b. Denial
   c. Acceptance
   d. Bargaining

9. A hospice nurse is helping to coordinate end-of-life care for a patient with a progressive neuromuscular disease. Which question will best help the nurse develop a plan of care?
   a. "What is important to you to accomplish in your remaining time?"
   b. "How do you typically cope with challenges?"
   c. "What resources do you think you'll need?"
   d. "What hobbies or activities do you want to do?"

10. As individuals approach death, the nurse focuses on which of these most common needs?
    a. They remain at home.
    b. Their families are taken care of.
    c. Their life has meaning and purpose.
    d. They receive adequate nutrition.

11. A family member of a patient with kidney failure asks the nurse what their parent's do not resuscitate order means. How does the nurse respond?
    a. "If your parent's heart stops, we will not perform CPR."
    b. "If your loved one is receiving dialysis, it will be discontinued."
    c. "Antibiotics for infections will be withheld."
    d. "Your parent will be ineligible to receive a blood transfusion."

12. Nurses in an intensive care unit discuss incorporating a practice called "The Pause" on their unit. How do the nurses explain this practice to other health care team members?
    a. "Before a surgical procedure, the team members stop to verify the patient's identification and site of surgery."
    b. "After opening the airway in a witnessed cardiac arrest, the nurse obtains the defibrillator and directs someone to call the code team."
    c. "Following a failed resuscitation or patient death, the health care team stops to reflect and honors their life."
    d. "After signing an advance directive, the person must wait 24 hours for it to become valid."

ALTERNATE-FORMAT QUESTIONS
Multiple-Response Questions
Circle the letters that correspond to the best answers for each question.

1. A nurse is assessing a dying patient for realism of expectations and perception of condition. Which interview questions address this concern? Select all that apply.
   a. "What are your expectations related to your condition?"
   b. "Do you know how to contact your doctor and get answers to your questions?"
   c. "How do you see the next few weeks playing out?"
   d. "What have you been told about your condition?"
   e. "How well do you think those around you are coping?"
   f. "What good do you think may happen in the midst of all of this?"

2. A nurse receives in shift report that a patient is demonstrating signs of imminent death. Which signs does the nurse anticipate are present? Select all that apply.
   a. Increased body temperature
   b. Restlessness and agitation
   c. Weak irregular pulse
   d. Cheyne–Stokes respirations
   e. Mottling of extremities
   f. Increased blood pressure

3. A nurse is conducting grief resolution for a patient who lost his wife in a motor vehicle accident in which he was the driver. Which interventions best accomplish this goal? Select all that apply.
   a. Encouraging the patient's desire to keep silent about the event
   b. Avoiding noticing or focusing on the patient's grief
   c. Avoiding identification of fears regarding the loss
   d. Listening to the spouse's expressions of grief
   e. Including significant others in discussions and decisions as appropriate
   f. Communicating acceptance of discussing loss

4. A nurse is discussing end-of-life decisions with a patient who has terminal cancer. Which statements describe tools available to the patient regarding their wishes? Select all that apply.

   a. Living wills provide specific instructions about the kinds of health care that should be provided in specific situations.

   b. In a living will, a patient appoints an agent that they trust to make decisions if they become incapacitated.

   c. The Patient Self-Determination Act of 1990 requires all hospitals to inform their patients about advance directives.

   d. The status of advance directives varies from state to state.

   e. Nurses are legally responsible for arranging for a durable power of attorney for all terminal patients.

   f. Legally, all attempts must be made by the health care team to resuscitate a terminal patient.

5. A nurse is explaining the preparation of a death certificate to a student nurse. Which statements accurately describe this process? Select all that apply.

   a. "U.S. law requires that a death certificate be prepared for each person who dies."

   b. "Death certificates are sent to a national health department, which compiles many statistics from the information."

   c. "The nurse assumes responsibility for handling and filing the death certificate with the proper authorities."

   d. "A health care provider's signature is required on a death certificate."

   e. "The nurse is responsible to ensure that the health care provider has signed a death certificate."

   f. "A death certificate is signed by the health care provider and others in special cases."

6. Which actions are performed by the nurse when a patient dies? Select all that apply.

   a. Washing the patient's body

   b. Removing all tubes according to facility policy, unless an autopsy is to be performed

   c. Placing identification on the shroud or garment and wrist

   d. Placing identification tags on the patient's dentures or other prostheses

   e. Arranging for family members to view the body before it is discharged to the mortician

   f. Attending the funeral of a deceased patient and making follow-up visits to the family

Prioritization Question

1. A nurse in inpatient hospice facility is caring for a group of patients. Which patient does the nurse identify as close to death and will visit first?

   a. Patient with BP 102/48

   b. Patient with dysphagia

   c. Patient with flushed skin

   d. Patient with Cheyne–Stoke breathing

CHAPTER 45

Sensory Functioning

ASSESSING YOUR UNDERSTANDING

FILL IN THE BLANKS

1. Sensory _____ is the conscious process of selecting, organizing, and interpreting data from the senses into meaningful information.

2. Sensory _____ is the process of receiving data about the internal or external environment through the senses.

3. _____ refers to awareness of positioning of body parts and body movement; _____ describes the subconscious sense of the movements and position of the body and especially its limbs, independent of vision.

4. _____ is the sense that perceives the solidity of objects and their size, shape, and texture.

5. The body quickly becomes accustomed to constant stimuli. For example, the repeated stimulus of a continuing noise, such as city traffic, or a noxious odor eventually goes unnoticed. This phenomenon is termed _____.

6. Sensory _____ occurs when a person experiences decreased sensory input or input that is monotonous, unpatterned, or meaningless.

7. Hospitalized patients who experience noise, lights, frequent touch and procedures, strange sights or odors may experience sensory _____.

8. A sensory- _____ disorder is difficulty in the way the brain takes in, organizes, and uses sensory information, causing a person to have problems interacting effectively in the everyday environment.

9. Age-related loss of hearing is referred to as _____.

MATCHING EXERCISES

Matching Exercise 1

Match the senses listed in Part A with their definition in Part B. You may not need all answers.

PART A

a. Visual

b. Auditory

c. Olfactory

d. Gustatory

e. Tactile

f. Kinesthesia

g. Visceral

PART B

____ 1. Sense of taste

____ 2. Sense of sight

____ 3. Sense of smell

____ 4. Sense of hearing

____ 5. Sense of touch

____ 6. Awareness of positioning of body parts and body movement

Matching Exercise 2

Match the type of stimulation in Part A with the example listed in Part B. Some answers may be used more than once.

PART A

a. Visual

b. Auditory

c. Gustatory/olfactory

d. Tactile

PART B

____ **1.** A nurse wears a brightly colored top when caring for patients confined to bed.

____ **2.** A nurse collaborates with the hospital nutritionist to prepare meals with varied seasonings and textures.

____ **3.** Soft music plays in a patient's room who has eye patches following ophthalmic surgery.

____ **4.** A nurse hugs a depressed patient who has made the effort to bathe and dress themselves.

____ **5.** A nurse explains a procedure to a comatose patient.

____ **6.** A nurse arranges a patient's cards in a heart shape on her wall.

SHORT ANSWER

1. List four conditions that must be present for a person to receive data necessary to experience the world.

a. _____

b. _____

c. _____

d. _____

2. Give an example of how the following factors may place a patient at high risk for sensory deprivation.

a. Environment: _____

_____

b. Impaired ability to receive environmental stimuli: _____

_____

c. Inability to process environmental stimuli:

_____

_____

3. Briefly describe the following effects of sensory deprivation:

a. Perceptual responses: _____

_____

b. Cognitive responses: _____

_____

c. Emotional responses: _____

_____

4. List three examples of sensory overload you could observe when providing care for patients.

a. _____

b. _____

c. _____

5. Give an example of sensory stimulation that could be provided for each of the following age groups.

a. Infant: _____

_____

b. Adult: _____

_____

c. Older adult: _____

_____

6. Give an example of two goals for patients with impaired sensory functioning.

a. _____

b. _____

7. A home health nurse is visiting an older adult with diabetes living at home with their spouse. You notice that the drapes are shut; the room is dark and, there are no pictures, flowers, or visually stimulating objects. The patient appears in good physical health but seems slightly disoriented and confused about the date and time of day. Develop a nursing care plan for this patient with emphasis on the need for sensory stimulation.

_____

_____

_____

_____

8. List four kinds of education for a patient to prevent eye injury at home or in the community.

    a. _____

    b. _____

    c. _____

    d. _____

9. Give two suggestions for increasing environmental stimulation and role model appropriate interactional behaviors for children in the following areas.

    a. Visual: _____

    _____

    b. Auditory: _____

    _____

    c. Olfactory: _____

    _____

    d. Gustatory: _____

    _____

    e. Tactile: _____

    _____

10. Give three examples of how a nurse might communicate with the following patients.

    a. Visually impaired patients: _____

    _____

    b. Hearing-impaired patients: _____

    _____

    c. Unconscious patients: _____

    _____

APPLYING YOUR KNOWLEDGE

CRITICAL THINKING QUESTIONS

1. Test your friends' senses by trying out these tactile, gustatory, and olfactory exercises.

    a. Gather several items from your home/ work area such as a key, a cotton ball, a toothpick, a tongue depressor, etc., and place them in a paper bag. Have your peers take turns identifying the objects in the bag without looking at them. As an item is identified, remove it from the bag. What is being assessed? Discuss the importance of tactile experiences to the vision-impaired patient.

    b. Gather several foods such as pudding, gelatin, mints, chocolate, etc. Blindfold your peers and give them a taste of each food. See how many they can identify correctly.

    c. Reflect on the role different senses play. Do you believe that using only one sense at a time heightens the awareness of that sense? Relate the exercises above to the special needs of hearing-impaired and vision-impaired patients.

2. Walk down a busy street and try to pick out individual sounds. How many noises became indistinct due to sensory overload? Relate this experience to a patient in a critical care unit.

REFLECTIVE PRACTICE: CULTIVATING QSEN COMPETENCIES

Use the following expanded scenario from Chapter 45 in your textbook to answer the questions below.

Scenario: Dolores, a 74-year-old woman, comes to the older adult clinic with her 77-year-old husband who was diagnosed with macular degeneration and progressive vision loss. She states, "Now I've noticed he's also having difficulty hearing me. I'm worried because he doesn't want to leave the house and we hardly see any of our friends anymore. We used to go out to the movies or dinner at least once a week. Lately, if we get out once a month, that's a lot!"

1. Patient-centered care/safety: What nursing interventions might be appropriate for Dolores' spouse?

    _____

    _____

    _____

2. Patient-centered care/safety: What would be a successful outcome for this patient?

    _____

    _____

    _____

3. Patient-centered care: What intellectual and interpersonal competencies are most likely to bring about the desired outcome?

    _____

    _____

    _____

4. Teamwork and collaboration: What resources might be helpful for the patient and partner?

_____

_____

_____

PATIENT CARE STUDY

Use this care study to apply your knowledge by completing the Nursing Process Worksheet found in Appendix A.

Scenario: George, an 81-year-old, married, African American man, reports, at his wife's prodding, that he is not hearing as well as he used to. "More and more, people just seem to be mumbling instead of talking." You notice that he is seated on the edge of his chair and bends toward you when you speak to him. His wife reports that he has stopped going out and stays in another room when they have visitors because he is embarrassed by his inability to hear. "This is a shame, because George was always the life of the party," she says. You ask George if he has ever had his hearing evaluated, he says no, he's been trying to convince himself that nothing's wrong.

PRACTICING FOR NCLEX

MULTIPLE-CHOICE QUESTIONS

Circle the letter that corresponds to the best answer for each question.

1. A patient in the intensive care unit is displaying new onset of confusion, agitation, and disorientation as a result of a medication toxicity. The nurse documents that the patient is experiencing which problem?
   a. Somnolence
   b. Dementia
   c. Delirium
   d. Hallucinations

2. A nurse takes into consideration factors that affect sensory stimulation in hospitalized patients when planning patient care. Which statement will the nurse use as the basis for care?
   a. Different personality types demand the same level of stimulation.
   b. Decreased sensory stimulation may be sought during periods of low stress.
   c. Illness does not affect the reception of sensory stimuli.
   d. A person's culture may dictate the amount of sensory stimulation considered normal.

3. A nurse providing care for an unconscious person bases their care on which rationale?
   a. Hearing is the first sense lost, so verbal communication is unnecessary.
   b. Assume the patient can hear you and converse with them in a normal tone of voice.
   c. Do not touch the unconscious patient unnecessarily because it may confuse them.
   d. Keep the environmental noise level high in the patient's room to help stimulate the patient.

4. Nursing students learn about the care of patients in a variety of settings. Which patient would the students place at highest risk for sensory deprivation?
   a. Patient in an isolation room
   b. Patient visiting a health care provider's office
   c. Patient in the emergency department
   d. Patient in a long-term care facility

5. A nurse teaches a patient with diabetic neuropathy to avoid which of these actions commonly used to relieve pain?
   a. Placing a heating pad on the foot or legs
   b. Attending physical therapy
   c. Using acetaminophen for a headache
   d. Using lavender aromatherapy

6. A patient receiving mechanical ventilation cannot speak. What would be most helpful to keep the patient from becoming confused and isolated?
   a. Speaking loudly to overcome the sound of the ventilator while providing care
   b. Having the patient's family remain at the bedside
   c. Offering pen and paper or a magic slate for the patient to write questions and answers
   d. Suggesting the family visit once daily to avoid excess sensory stimulation

7. When caring for a patient who lost their sight in an accident, the nurse documents in the assessment that the patient is experiencing which condition?

   a. Sensory overload

   b. Sensory deficit

   c. Sensory deprivation

   d. Sensory overstimulation

8. Which action by the nurse would be most helpful for a patient whose family has to shout to be heard, yet the patient maintains that their hearing is fine?

   a. Telling the patient that new hearing aids are practically invisible and should not draw attention to their hearing deficit

   b. Explaining that many patients with hearing loss isolate themselves to avoid embarrassment of giving wrong answers in conversations

   c. Asking the patient if they have recently had a vision screening

   d. Teaching the patient that their family is frustrated and becoming isolated

9. An older adult in a long-term care facility states that their food does not taste good as it used to. Which action can the nurse use to stimulate taste and appetite?

   a. Provide oral hygiene before meals

   b. Serve food of similar textures

   c. Avoid aromatic foods

   d. Perform a neurologic assessment

ALTERNATE-FORMAT QUESTIONS

Multiple-Response Questions

Circle the letters that correspond to the best answers for each question.

1. For which conditions would the nurse assess a patient to determine if they are able to adequately receive the data necessary to experience the world? Select all that apply.

   a. Response

   b. Stimulus

   c. Receptor or sense organ

   d. Arousal mechanism

   e. Intact nerve pathway

   f. Functioning brain

2. A nurse is caring for a group of patients on a neurology unit with vision and hearing deficits. Which actions are appropriate for the nurse to perform? Select all that apply.

   a. Reducing the tone of their voice

   b. Providing for safe ambulation

   c. Encouraging patients to consume a low-fat diet

   d. Cleaning patients' eyeglasses daily

   e. Standing to the patients' side when speaking

   f. Offering menus and teaching materials in large print

3. A nurse working on a neurology unit assesses patients for negative effects of sensory deprivation. For which will the nurse observe? Select all that apply.

   a. Inaccurate perception of sights, sounds, tastes, and smells

   b. Increased coordination and equilibrium

   c. Inability to control the direction of thought content

   d. Increased attention span and ability to concentrate

   e. Difficulty with memory, problem solving, and task performance

   f. Emotionally caring attitude and stable moods

4. A nurse is planning strategies to increase sensory stimulation for patients in isolation. Which considerations should the nurse keep in mind? Select all that apply.

   a. The amount of stimuli different people consider optimal is constant.

   b. Sensory functioning is established at birth and is independent of stimulation received during childhood.

   c. It is recommended that medically fragile infants have greater light and visual and vestibular stimulation.

   d. Sensory functioning tends to decline progressively throughout adulthood.

   e. A person's culture may dictate the amount of sensory stimulation considered normal.

   f. Different personality types demand different levels of stimulation.

5. Which actions are performed according to guidelines for caring for visually impaired patients? Select all that apply.

   a. Waiting for the person to sense your presence in the room before identifying yourself

   b. Speaking in a normal tone of voice

   c. Explaining the reason for touching the person after doing so

   d. Orienting the person to the arrangement of the room and its furnishings

   e. Assisting with ambulation by walking slightly behind the person

   f. Sitting in the person's field of vision if partial or reduced peripheral vision is present

6. Which actions are performed according to guidelines for caring for patients with hearing impairments? Select all that apply.

   a. Increasing the noise level in the room

   b. Cleaning ears on a daily basis

   c. Positioning yourself so that the light is on your face when you speak

   d. Talking to the person from a distance so that they may read your lips

   e. Demonstrating or pantomiming ideas you wish to express

   f. Writing down any ideas that you cannot convey to the person in another manner

CHAPTER 46

Sexuality

ASSESSING YOUR UNDERSTANDING

FILL IN THE BLANKS

1. _____ is the degree to which a person exhibits and experiences maleness or femaleness physically, emotionally, and mentally.

2. _____ identity refers to romantic, emotional, affectionate, or sexual attraction to other people.

3. Sexual _____ refers to the preferred biologic sex of the partner of an individual.

4. A woman who experiences menstrual cycle–related distress is said to have _____ syndrome.

5. Areas that when stimulated cause sexual arousal and desire are called _____.

6. The _____ contraceptive patch supplies continuous daily circulating levels of ethinylestradiol and norelgestromin to prevent conception.

7. _____ is motivated by a need to dominate and humiliate the victim; it is an act of violence.

8. Human _____ is a form of modern-day slavery in which victims are subjected to force, fraud, or coercion for the purpose of commercial sex, debt bondage, or involuntary labor.

9. The outcome of teaching about sexuality is a change in _____, a change in patient attitude, and a change in _____.

MATCHING EXERCISES

Matching Exercise 1

Match the terms listed in Part A with their definitions in Part B.

PART A

a. Gender identity

b. Transgender

c. Gender diverse

d. Biologic sex

e. Gay or lesbian

f. Gender dysphoria

PART B

_____ 1. Clinically significant distress or impairment because biologic sex or sex assigned at birth is not congruent with gender identity

_____ 2. Term used to denote chromosomal sexual development

_____ 3. People who live full-time as members of a biologic sex that differs from the sex and gender they were assigned at birth

_____ 4. Inner sense a person has of being male, female, or nonbinary

_____ 5. A wide range of gender identities that may vary from expected developmental norms; it includes nonbinary, genderqueer, and gender fluid

_____ 6. Person who experiences sexual fulfillment with a person of the same biologic sex

Matching Exercise 2

Match the terms listed in Part A with their definitions in Part B.

PART A

a. HPV

b. Trichomoniasis

c. Syphilis

d. Chlamydia

e. Genital herpes

f. Gonorrhea

PART B

____ **1.** Gram-negative bacteria causing purulent penile discharge, dysuria

____ **2.** Infection from a protozoan with flagella identified on Pap smear; males typically asymptomatic

____ **3.** Women acquiring this problem are at risk for cervical and other cancers

____ **4.** May cause a chronic lifelong infection of the genitals, rectum, or mouth

____ **5.** Single painless genital lesion; when untreated can affect organ systems

____ **6.** Bacterial infection causing vaginal discharge, burning on urination, urinary frequency, dysuria, and urethral soreness

SHORT ANSWER

1. Give an example of teaching or an intervention that could improve sexual relations for patients with the following health problems.

a. Chronic pain: _____

_____

b. Diabetes: _____

_____

c. Cardiovascular disease: _____

_____

d. Loss of body part: _____

_____

e. Spinal cord injury: _____

_____

f. Mental illness: _____

_____

g. Sexually transmitted infections (STIs): ____

_____

2. Briefly describe interventions for patients with HIV.

_____

_____

3. List three general categories of patients who should have a sexual history recorded by the nurse.

a. _____

b. _____

c. _____

4. List three interview questions a nurse may use during a sexual history when assessing a male for impotence.

a. _____

b. _____

c. _____

5. Complete the following table, listing the advantages and disadvantages associated with contraceptive methods.

Method	Advantages	Disadvantages
a. Behavioral		
b. Barrier methods		
c. Intrauterine devices		
d. Hormonal methods		
e. Sterilization		

APPLYING YOUR KNOWLEDGE

CRITICAL THINKING QUESTIONS

1. List interview questions you would use to obtain a sexual history from the following patients. Consider how comfortable would you be asking these patients the necessary questions and how you might develop the skills necessary to perform the interview.

   a. An 18-year-old female victim of date rape who is brought to the emergency room for testing and treatment: _____

   _____

   b. A 5-year-old girl who presents with soreness and redness in the genital area: _____

   _____

2. List interview questions you would use to care for patients experiencing the following sexual dysfunctions.

   a. Male undergoing radiation treatment for colon cancer reports of impotence: _____

   _____

   b. Menopausal female reports vaginal dryness and pain during intercourse: _____

   _____

   c. Sexually active teenager reports a burning sensation during urination: _____

   _____

REFLECTIVE PRACTICE: CULTIVATING QSEN COMPETENCIES

Use the following expanded scenario from Chapter 46 in your textbook to answer the questions below.

   Scenario: Jefferson, a middle-aged man with a history of diabetes and hypertension, is receiving numerous medications as treatment. During a routine visit to his primary care provider, Jefferson confides that he has been having problems "in the bedroom." He reports difficulty attaining and maintaining an erection.

1. Patient-centered care/interprofessional collaboration: What issues might the nurse address in the plan of care for Jefferson? What patient teaching should be incorporated into the plan of care?

2. Patient-centered care: What would be a successful outcome for this patient?

3. Patient-centered care/safety: What intellectual and interpersonal competencies are most likely to bring about the desired outcome?

4. Teamwork and collaboration: What resources might be helpful for Jefferson?

PATIENT CARE STUDY

Use this care study to apply your knowledge by completing the Nursing Process Worksheet found in Appendix A.

   Scenario: Anthony, a muscular, healthy 19-year-old college freshman in the School of Nursing, confides to his nursing advisor that "everything is great" about college life, with one exception: "I find myself questioning the values I learned at home about sex and marriage. My mom taught her sons to respect women and that sex is something you saved until marriage. Problem is that no one here seems to subscribe to this philosophy. I feel like I'm abnormal in some way to even think like this. Everyone in the dorms is having sex, and no one even thinks you're serious if you talk about virginity positively. Did my mom sell me a bill of goods? Is it true that if you take the proper precautions, no one gets hurt and everyone has a good time?" Anthony reports that he is a virgin and that he really misses his close family back home: "I do get lonely at times and would love to just cuddle with someone or hug, but no one seems to understand this."

PRACTICING FOR NCLEX

MULTIPLE-CHOICE QUESTIONS

Circle the letter that corresponds to the best answer for each question.

1. A nurse is teaching patients about sexually transmitted infections (STIs). What would the nurse include as a teaching point?

   a. "Most of the time, STIs cause no symptoms."

   b. "Health problems from STIs tend to be more severe in males."

   c. "Reported STIs are at an all-time low due to targeted education about STIs."

   d. "STIs are most prevalent among the adult population."

2. A community health nurse is planning a round table discussion with the health department on health issues in the LGBTQIA+ population. Which statistics would the nurse include to support the need for additional funding for health centers serving this population?

   a. Lesbians and bisexual females are more likely to be underweight or anorexic.

   b. LGBTQIA+ populations have lower rates of tobacco, alcohol, and other drug use.

   c. LGBTQIA+ youth are two to three times more likely to attempt suicide.

   d. Lesbians are more likely to get preventive services for cancer.

3. A nurse in a long-term care facility implements care that advocate for patient sexual needs. Which action best demonstrates this advocacy?

   a. Anticipating potentially shaming situations for the patient

   b. Avoiding discussing the patient's sexuality with the health care provider to maintain privacy

   c. Ensuring the patient wears a hospital gown to protect personal clothing

   d. Addressing the patient using pronouns typically associated with their name

4. A nurse caring for patients in a health care provider's office takes developmental stage into consideration when assessing sexuality. What is an example of a developmentally appropriate intervention?

   a. Teaching parents of an 18-month-old to discourage self-manipulation of genitals

   b. Teaching parents of a 4-year-old that they may cause anxiety in the child by intolerance of inconsistency of sex-role behavior

   c. Warning parents of a 2-year-old that toilet training should be initiated immediately to prevent compulsive behaviors later

   d. Stating that same-sex preference for relationships in the school-aged child may be related to heterosexual or homosexual tendencies

5. A nurse in the gynecology clinic is assessing a patient diagnosed with human papillomavirus (HPV). What symptom(s) of this STI does the nurse anticipate?

   a. Foul-smelling, thin, grayish white vaginal discharge

   b. Possible vaginal bleeding or spotting

   c. Single painless genital lesion 10 days to 3 months after exposure

   d. Profuse watery vaginal discharge

6. A patient visits a community clinic with complaints of foul-smelling vaginal discharge that is thin, foamy, and green in color; itching of their vulva and vagina; and burning on urination. What STI would the nurse suspect?

   a. Acquired immunodeficiency syndrome (AIDS)

   b. Chlamydia

   c. *Trichomoniasis*

   d. *Gonorrhea*

7. A nurse is discussing contraception with an adolescent patient who asks the nurse: "What if I can't have an orgasm?" What is the nurse's best response?

   a. "Women who have multiple orgasms are promiscuous."

   b. "There are many ways to give and receive sexual pleasure."

   c. "The larger the penis, the greater the potential for achieving orgasm."

   d. "The ability to achieve orgasm is the only indicator of a person's sexual responsiveness."

8. Which example best supports the diagnosis of impaired sexual functioning related to dyspareunia?

   a. A patient with a colostomy believes they cannot have a sexual relationship with their partner who will be repulsed by their stoma.

   b. An adult patient with a history of stroke is afraid to have sex with their partner fearing it will elevate their blood pressure.

   c. A woman in the process of menopause has pain and burning during intercourse.

   d. An adult with alcoholism is no longer interested in having sex with their partner.

ALTERNATE-FORMAT QUESTIONS

Multiple-Response Questions

Circle the letters that correspond to the best answers for each question.

1. A nurse is counseling a young rape victim in the emergency department and recommends emergency contraception. Which statements describe this process? Select all that apply.

   a. A vaginal sponge will be prescribed to be worn daily for 7 days.

   b. The health care provider will prescribe increased doses of oral contraceptives.

   c. The health care provider will insert a copper IUD within 5 to 7 days of the unprotected sex.

   d. An emergency D&C will be performed within 24 hours of unprotected sex.

   e. A vaginal ring will be inserted within 36 hours of unprotected sex.

   f. Plan B One-Step may be obtained without a prescription at a drugstore or family planning clinic.

2. A nurse is teaching a male adolescent how to use a condom. Which teaching points would the nurse include? Select all that apply.

   a. "Roll the condom onto the penis before it becomes erect."

   b. "If the condom has no nipple receptacle, leave a space at the end for semen to collect."

   c. "Use a condom with every act of intercourse."

   d. "Immediately after ejaculation remove the condom and discard it."

   e. "Avoid use of a spermicide with the latex condom."

   f. "If using a lambskin condom, the condom may be reused a second time."

3. The nurse is advising an adolescent male about sexual myths that have him concerned. Which statements describe accurate patient teaching regarding these concerns? Select all that apply.

   a. "A larger penis allows for a more satisfying sexual experience."

   b. "Nocturnal emissions indicate the existence of a sexual disorder."

   c. "Nocturnal emissions are signs of a sexually transmitted infection."

   d. "Masturbation or self-stimulation is a natural and healthy outlet for sexual urges."

   e. "No male or female should feel pressured into sexual activity at any age."

   f. "Nocturnal emissions are normal in males of all ages."

4. Which patients would be more likely to experience sexual dysfunction? Select all that apply.

   a. Young adult patient in traction

   b. Adult male with a history of hypertension

   c. Adolescent who is still a virgin

   d. Postmenopausal female patient

   e. Middle-aged male with an enlarged prostate (BPH)

   f. Young adult female experiencing PMS

5. A nurse is providing education at a senior center addressing factors that affect sexual dysfunction in older adults. Which interventions would be appropriate? Select all that apply.

   a. Reminding them that sexual intercourse and similar forms of sexual expression are considered dangerous for older adults with cardiovascular disease

   b. Actively seeking a new partner for patients who have lost a spouse and are not sexually active

   c. Educating them, their intimate partners, and their family about the sexual side effects of specific medications

   d. Assisting in attitude and value clarification about substance use, sexuality, and sexual behavior

   e. Encouraging them to have a thorough physical evaluation by a health care provider

   f. Providing open, nonjudgmental response when they display a need for warmth, close contact, and companionship

6. Which statements describe sexual dysfunction in males or females? Select all that apply.

   a. Premature ejaculation is a condition in which a male consistently reaches ejaculation or orgasm before or soon after entering the vagina.

   b. Delayed ejaculation refers to the male's inability to ejaculate into the vagina or delayed intravaginal ejaculation.

c. Vaginismus is painful intercourse.

d. Dyspareunia is a condition in which the vaginal opening closes tightly and prevents penile penetration.

e. Vulvodynia is a chronic vulvar discomfort or pain characterized by burning, stinging, irritation, or rawness of the female genitalia that interferes with sexual activity.

f. Inhibited sexual desire refers to a female's inability to reach orgasm.

Sequencing Question

1. Place the following series of reactions that control the menstrual cycle in the order in which they occur.

a. The leftover empty follicle fills up with a yellow pigment and is then called the corpus luteum.

b. A number of follicles mature, but only one produces a mature ovum.

c. Ovulation occurs.

d. If fertilization does not occur, the body sheds the lining of the uterus.

e. Menstrual flow begins.

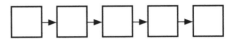

Prioritization Question

1. A nurse at a family practice must assess four patients. For which patient will the nurse prioritize the assessment? Circle the letter that corresponds to the best answer.

a. A 3-year-old whose parent is concerned they like to be without clothes

b. A preteen whose parent believes they are pregnant

c. Adult male with penile discharge

d. An adolescent requesting contraceptives

CHAPTER 47

Spirituality

ASSESSING YOUR UNDERSTANDING

FILL IN THE BLANKS

1. A patient recently diagnosed with prostate cancer tells the nurse that he believes God is far away and could not care less about his condition. This patient may be suffering from spiritual _____.

2. Spiritual _____ is the impaired ability to experience and integrate meaning and purpose in life through connectedness with self, others, art, music, literature, nature, or a higher power.

3. A nurse who asks a patient how his religious beliefs help or hinder him to feel at peace is assessing the patient for the spiritual need for _____.

4. A patient who tells a nurse that she no longer goes to church on Sunday may be experiencing the form of spiritual distress known as spiritual _____.

5. A mother who refuses to sign a consent form for a blood transfusion for her daughter due to religious reasons is most likely practicing the Christian Scientist or Jehovah's _____ faith.

6. An _____ is a person who denies the existence of a higher power; an _____ holds that nothing can be known about the existence of a higher power.

7. The role of the _____ nurse is that of health educator, health counselor, developer of support groups, and integrator of faith and health.

8. A child's _____ play a key role in the development of their spirituality.

9. _____ describes a specific state of distress that occurs when the intactness or integrity of the person is threatened or disrupted.

MATCHING EXERCISES

Matching Exercise 1

Match the type of spiritual distress listed in Part A with the appropriate example listed in Part B.

PART A

a. Spiritual pain

b. Spiritual alienation

c. Spiritual anxiety

d. Spiritual guilt

e. Spiritual anger

f. Spiritual despair

PART B

____ 1. A parent cannot accept the death of their newborn and says, "How long will it hurt this badly?"

____ 2. A patient with a terminal illness cannot accept their eventual death and asks, "What kind of God are you?"

____ 3. A Roman Catholic college student stops going to Mass on Sundays and moves in with their partner, tells you, "I really want to do this, but it still feels wrong."

____ 4. An older adult with a hip replacement is confined to home and cannot get to usual daily religious services.

_____ **5.** A patient dying of AIDS has no friends or support system and believes that God and humanity have abandoned them.

_____ **6.** A young adult challenges their faith and their belief in God.

Matching Exercise 2

Match the examples of a nurse's supportive presence listed in Part A with the appropriate example listed in Part B. Answers may be used more than once.

PART A

a. Facilitating the practice of religion

b. Promoting meaning and purpose

c. Promoting love and relatedness

d. Promoting forgiveness

PART B

_____ **1.** A nurse attempts to meet a patient's religious dietary restrictions.

_____ **2.** A nurse explores with a patient the importance of learning to accept themselves, even with their faults.

_____ **3.** A nurse treats their patient with respect, empathy, and genuine caring.

_____ **4.** A nurse explores with a patient spiritual practices from which they might derive strength and hope.

_____ **5.** A nurse encourages a patient to explore their relationship with their family and identify the origin of negative beliefs about people.

_____ **6.** A nurse helps a patient explore their self-expectations and determine how realistic they are.

SHORT ANSWER

1. List three spiritual needs underlying all religious traditions that are common to all people.

a. _____

b. _____

c. _____

2. List four methods nurses can use to assist patients in meeting their spiritual needs.

a. _____

b. _____

c. _____

d. _____

3. Explain how the following religious influences may affect a person.

a. Life-affirming influences: _____

_____

b. Life-denying influences: _____

_____

4. Give two examples of religious practices associated with health care that may have significant impact on a patient.

a. _____

b. _____

5. Briefly describe how religious faith may affect a patient in the following areas.

a. As a guide to daily living: _____

_____

b. As a source of support: _____

_____

c. As a source of strength and healing: _____

_____

d. As a source of conflict: _____

_____

6. Give an example of how the following factors may influence a person's spirituality.

a. Developmental considerations: _____

_____

b. Family: _____

_____

c. Ethnic background: _____

_____

d. Life events: _____

_____

7. Describe how you would communicate to patients and families in the following situations.

a. A family who insists on continuing care deemed medically futile for a terminally ill patient because they believe that God is going to work a miracle: _____

_____

_____

_____

b. Christian scientist parents of a child needing an appendectomy who refuse to sign a consent form for surgery: _____

_____

_____

_____

8. List six common characteristics of the religions discussed in this chapter.

a. _____
b. _____
c. _____
d. _____
e. _____
f. _____

9. Give an example of an interview question or statement you could use when assessing a patient for the following types of spiritual distress.

a. Spiritual pain: _____

_____

b. Spiritual alienation: _____

_____

c. Spiritual anxiety: _____

_____

d. Spiritual anger: _____

_____

e. Spiritual loss: _____

_____

f. Spiritual despair: _____

_____

10. You are visiting a patient at home who was paralyzed in a car accident. The patient tells you that they believe God has abandoned them and their family, which includes two small children. Suggest a health problem for this patient and develop a nursing care plan that includes at least two interventions to help her with her spiritual needs.

Health Problem: _____

Interventions: _____

_____

_____

11. Briefly suggest two to four guidelines for preparing a patient's room to receive a spiritual counselor.

_____

_____

_____

APPLYING YOUR KNOWLEDGE

CRITICAL THINKING QUESTIONS

1. How would you respond to parents who ask you to pray with them for their child's recovery from surgery? Would you feel comfortable praying with them? Do you believe nurses should pray aloud with patients and families? Write down a prayer for the sick that you can use in these situations.

2. Identify your own spiritual beliefs. How do these beliefs influence the way you carry on your daily routine in life? Do these beliefs affect the way you relate to others? In what ways might they affect the way you react to patients of different faiths?

REFLECTIVE PRACTICE: CULTIVATING QSEN COMPETENCIES

Use the following expanded scenario from Chapter 47 in your textbook to answer the questions below.

Scenario: Margot, a 75-year-old woman, is taking care of her 80-year-old husband with advanced Alzheimer's disease, who was just discharged from the hospital and requires constant supervision. When visited at home, she says, "I really miss going to church and seeing everyone. They're so supportive. That was the one thing that helped to keep me going."

1. Patient-centered care/safety: How might the nurse use blended nursing skills to provide holistic, competent nursing care for Margot and her husband?

_____

_____

_____

2. Patient-centered care: What would be a successful outcome for this patient/family?

_____

_____

_____

3. Patient-centered care/safety/evidence-based practice: What intellectual and interpersonal competencies are most likely to bring about the desired outcome?

_____

_____

_____

4. Teamwork and collaboration/safety: What resources might be helpful to Margot and her husband?

_____

_____

_____

PATIENT CARE STUDY

Use this care study to apply your knowledge by completing the Nursing Process Worksheet found in Appendix A.

Scenario: Jeffrey, a 31-year-old attorney, has been transferred to a step-down from the cardiac care unit after a massive heart attack. "Bad hearts run in my family, but I never thought it would happen to me," he says. "I jog regularly, work out at the gym, eat a low-fat diet, and I don't smoke." Jeffrey is 5 ft 7 inches tall, weighs 150 lb, and is well built. He tells the nurse, "I've really got a lot on my mind tonight. I can't stop thinking about how close I was to death. If I wasn't with someone who knew CPR, I probably wouldn't be here today." Gentle questioning reveals that Jeffrey is worried about what would have happened had he died. "I don't think I've ever thought seriously about my mortality, and I sure don't think much about God. My parents were semiobservant Jews, but I don't go to synagogue myself. I celebrate holidays, but that's about all. If there is a God, I wonder what He thinks about me." He asks if there is a rabbi he could talk with. "For the last few years, all I've been concerned about is paying off my school debts and making money. I guess there's a whole lot more to life, and maybe this was my invitation to sort out my priorities."

PRACTICING FOR NCLEX

MULTIPLE-CHOICE QUESTIONS

Circle the letter that corresponds to the best answer for each question.

1. A nurse is caring for a patient with a life-threatening illness and would like to offer a healing presence. What demonstrates that the nurse is providing a healing presence?

a. Assisting the patient with needed care

b. Suggesting the patient turn to organized religion

c. Offering empathy and caring

d. Telling the patient about someone with a similar problem

2. A terminally ill patient tells a nurse that they do not belong to an organized religion. What patient knowledge would the nurse gain from this statement?

a. This person is an atheist.

b. The patient has no belief system.

c. This individual is an agnostic.

d. They may still be deeply spiritual.

3. A nurse is differentiating beliefs of atheists from agnostics. Which statement is accurate?

a. Both deny the existence of God.

b. Nurses offer religious counseling to change the beliefs of both groups.

c. Both are guided by a philosophy of living that does not include a religious faith.

d. Both have religious influences that are life denying.

4. When planning care for patients on a surgical gynecology unit, a nurse will base care on the understanding that a patient from which faith will most likely defer to her husband when making health care decisions?

a. Islam

b. Judaism

c. Roman Catholicism

d. Protestantism

5. A nurse working in a diverse community appreciates that members of which religion are encouraged to obtain health care provided by members of the Black community?

a. Baha'i International Community

b. American Muslim Mission

c. Native American Religion

d. Islam

6. A nurse providing care includes plans to support the spiritual needs of patients of all religious and spiritual traditions. Which point remains consistent for all people?
   a. Attending formal ceremonies or services
   b. Finding power in relationship with God
   c. Supporting the rights of all people for justice
   d. Needing meaning and purpose

7. When assessing a child's spiritual dimension, a nurse should be aware of which basic tenet?
   a. Children do not have a definite perception of God.
   b. God has tremendous and expansive power.
   c. Children do not experience spiritual distress.
   d. God is punitive.

ALTERNATE-FORMAT QUESTIONS

Multiple-Response Questions

Circle the letters that correspond to the best answers for each question.

1. A nurse determining the effects of religion on the diet and lifestyle of patients considers that which religions prohibit the use of alcohol? Select all that apply.
   a. Christian Scientist
   b. Church of Jesus Christ of Latter-Day Saints
   c. Roman Catholicism
   d. American Muslim Mission
   e. Islam
   f. Judaism

2. A nurse is caring for a patient who practices Daoism. Which religious beliefs would the nurse keep in mind when planning care for this patient? Select all that apply.
   a. Allah, who is all-seeing, all-hearing, all-speaking, all-knowing, all-willing, and all-powerful, is their one God.
   b. They oppose the "false teachings" of other sects.
   c. They worship one God revealed to the world through Jesus Christ.
   d. They believe that health is a manifestation of the harmony of the universe, obtained through the proper balancing of internal and external forces.
   e. The universal principle is the mysterious biologic and spiritual life rhythm or order of nature.

f. Inherent in Daoism is the appreciation of life and the desire to keep the body from untimely or unnecessary death.

3. Which nursing actions are appropriate when caring for a patient who participates in Hindu religion? Select all that apply.
   a. Accommodating the practice of obligatory prayers and fasting on holy days
   b. Considering the patient to be open to new ideas in health care practices
   c. Accepting that women are not allowed to make independent decisions
   d. Anticipating many dietary restrictions, conforming to individual sect doctrine
   e. Accommodating certain rites to be practiced following death
   f. Learning about rituals marking life changes, birth, puberty, initiation rites, and death

4. A nurse works in a hospital with a diverse population. Which religious groups would the nurse anticipate to regard Saturday as the Sabbath? Select all that apply.
   a. Roman Catholicism
   b. Buddhism
   c. Adventist
   d. Judaism
   e. Islam
   f. Hinduism

Prioritization Question

1. A nurse is caring for a patient who presents in the emergency department 28 weeks' pregnant and displaying profuse vaginal bleeding. Her blood pressure is 86/48. The patient and partner state, "No matter what happens, our religion prohibits accepting blood products. We will refuse blood transfusions!" What is the nurse's priority? Circle the letter that corresponds to the best answer.
   a. Asking the patient and partner if they would like to speak to their religious leader
   b. Drawing blood for a type and crossmatch in case a blood transfusion is needed
   c. Acknowledging their beliefs and initiating intravenous saline to increase the blood pressure
   d. Asking the health care provider to discuss the effect of blood loss on the pregnant patient and fetus

Answer Key

CHAPTER 1

ASSESSING YOUR UNDERSTANDING

FILL IN THE BLANKS

1. science
2. International Council of Nurses (ICN)
3. American Nurses Association (ANA)
4. *Scope and Standards of Practice*
5. Nurse practice acts
6. nursing process
7. continuing
8. Licensure
9. health, illness, health, coping with disability or death
10. Doctor
11. communities
12. health literacy
13. Burnout

CORRECT THE UNDERLINED WORDS

1. member
2. Florence Nightingale's
3. Licensed Practical Nurse (LPN)
4. the nation
5. Resilience

SHORT ANSWER: THINKING LIKE A NURSE

1. In thoughtful, person-centered care, the patient and their needs are the focus of the nursing process and of the nurse's clinical reasoning, judgment, and decision-making skills. The nurse integrates the human dimensions—the physical, intellectual, emotional, sociocultural, spiritual, and environmental aspects of each person—into nursing care to promote wellness, prevent illness, restore health, and facilitate coping with altered function or death.

2. Examples of nursing roles requiring graduate level education include: nurse practitioner, nurse midwife, nurse anesthetist, clinical nurse specialist, clinical nurse leader, nurse educator, and others.

3. In-service education is organization specific, providing education and training designed to increase the knowledge and skills of the staff. Formal education programs such as professional or practical nursing and advanced degrees lead to a degree or credential and are typically more labor intensive.

4. The National Student Nurses' Association (NSNA) prepares students to participate in professional nursing organizations. Professional organizations focus on current issues in nursing and health care, health care policy, and legislation. Nurses belonging to these organizations network with colleagues, have a voice in legislation, and keep current with trends and issues in nursing.

5. The nurse functions as part of an interprofessional group, advocating for patient care, communicating with team members in a professional, confident, and assertive manner, making recommendations based on current evidence. Collaborative practice facilitates the functions of all members of the health care team in provision of patient care. This function is supported by the QSEN competency of teamwork and collaboration.

6. State laws protect the public through a regulatory body (board of nursing), which makes and enforces rules and regulations concerning the nursing profession. They define the legal scope of nursing practice at all levels and exclude unlicensed people from practicing nursing. They establish criteria for the education and licensure of nurses and maintaining the license, or they can revoke or suspend a license for professional misconduct.

7. The nursing process, including assessment, analyzing/diagnosing, planning, intervening, and evaluating, is a framework for critical thinking and clinical reasoning, culminating in sound nursing judgment.

8. Sample answers:
   a. Promoting health: The nurse prepares the patient for tests, explaining each test thoroughly to the patient and focusing on any questions the patient may have. The nurse also identifies the patient's strengths (e.g., healthy diet, daily exercise routine) and weaknesses (e.g., inability to quit smoking).
   b. Preventing illness: The nurse refers the patient to a smoking cessation program and, if necessary, educates the patient about the nature and treatment of lung cancer.
   c. Restoring health: The nurse provides direct care for the patient, administers medications, and carries out procedures and treatments for the patient.

d. Facilitating coping: The nurse facilitates patient and family coping by helping the patient to live with altered functioning or prepare for death.

9. Nursing is a well-defined body of specific and unique knowledge, has a strong service orientation, has recognized authority by a professional group, has a code of ethics, is a professional organization that sets standards, conducts ongoing research, and has autonomy and self-regulation.

10. Sample answers:
   a. Cost of health care: Nursing education programs must prepare students at all levels for roles in case management and employment in the managed care environment.
   b. Growing population of patients who are older and more acutely ill: Greater life expectancy of people with chronic and acute conditions will challenge the health care system's ability to provide efficient and effective continuing care.
   c. Changing demographics and increasing diversity: Increases in diversity will affect the nature and prevalence of illness and disease requiring changes in practice that reflect and respect diverse values and beliefs.
   d. Current nursing shortage: Nursing shortages have a negative impact on patient care and are costly to the health care industry.
   e. Opportunities for lifelong learning and workforce development: Rapidly evolving technology, increasing clinical complexity in many patient care settings, advances in treatment, and the emergence of new diseases are all factors contributing to the increased need for a strong emphasis on critical thinking and lifelong learning among professional nurses.
   f. Growing need for interdisciplinary education for collaborative practice: Teaching methods that incorporate opportunities for interdisciplinary education and collaborative practice are required to prepare nurses for their unique professional role and to understand the role of other disciplines in the care of patients.

11. Sample answers:
   a. Technologic explosion: Dramatic improvements in the accessibility of clinical data across settings and time have improved both outcomes and care management. Nurses in the 21st century need to be skilled in the use of computer technology.
   b. Significant advances in nursing science and research: Nursing research is an integral part of the scientific enterprise of improving the nation's health. The growing body of nursing research provides a scientific basis for patient care and should be regularly used by the nation's nurses.
   c. Impact of health policy and regulation: Nursing schools, scholars, executives, and professional nursing organizations must more actively contribute to the development of health policy and regulation.

d. Globalization of the world's economy and society: Nursing science needs to address health care issues, such as emerging and reemerging infections, that result from globalization. Nursing education and research must become more internationally focused to disseminate information and benefit from the multicultural experience.
e. Shift to population-based care and the increasing complexity of patient care: Providing services for defined groups "covered" by managed care will demand skills and knowledge in clinical epidemiology, biostatistics, behavioral science, and their application to specific populations.
f. Era of the educated consumer, alternative therapies and genomics, and palliative care: Despite some information gaps, today's patient is a well-informed consumer who expects to participate in decisions affecting personal and family health care. Nursing education and practice must expand to include the implications of the emerging therapies from both genetic research and alternative medicine while managing ethical conflicts and questions. A significant gap in the body of scientific knowledge and clinical education with regard to palliative and end-of-life care remains, and nursing education must prepare graduates for a significant role in these areas.

12. Sample answers:
   a. Cognitive skills: Selecting nursing interventions to promote wound healing
   b. Technical skills: Correctly administering medication to a patient via an IV infusion
   c. Interpersonal skills: Displaying a caring attitude when interacting with a patient
   d. Ethical/legal skills: Explaining an advance directives form to a patient

13. Compassion fatigue results in a loss of satisfaction from providing good patient care; burnout causes a cumulative state of frustration with the work environment that develops over a long time; secondary traumatic stress causes feelings of despair caused by the transfer of emotion distress from a victim to a caregiver, which often develops suddenly. Healthy self-care practices include stress reduction training, the use of relaxation techniques, time management, assertiveness training, work–life balance measures, and meditation or mindfulness-based practices.

APPLYING YOUR KNOWLEDGE
CRITICAL THINKING QUESTIONS

1. Sample answers:
   a. Promoting health: Provided education on "my plate" healthful eating
   b. Preventing illness: Performed blood pressure screening and explained consequences of untreated high blood pressure
   c. Restoring health: Changed surgical dressings; ambulated a postoperative patient

  d. Facilitating coping: Honestly answered questions about mastectomy and recovery
  e. Answers will vary with student experiences.
2. A nurse cannot practice nursing without a license. Permitting this nurse to function on the unit in a professional capacity is fraudulent and could jeopardize the organization in terms of accreditation, state approval, or other consequence.

REFLECTIVE PRACTICE: CULTIVATING QSEN COMPETENCIES
Sample Answers

1. What basic human needs should be addressed by the nurse to provide individualized, holistic care for Roberto?
   Patient-centered care: The nurse should provide holistic care, beginning with his physiologic needs including nutrition and hydration via central venous catheter. After this, the nurse can focus on Roberto's needs for a safe environment due to his weakness from radiation and chemotherapy as well as treatment for and protection from additional pressure injuries. Prevention of and freedom from infection with a central venous catheter are essential. Finally, address self-actualization needs for acceptance of himself and his current situation.
2. Patient-centered care: What would be a successful outcome for this patient?
   Roberto expresses relief from symptoms of chemotherapy and radiation and demonstrates wound healing of his pressure injuries. He is able to state what community resources available to help with wound care, IV fluids, and care of the CVC as well as resources for home nursing, rehabilitation, and/or hospice care upon discharge.
3. Patient-centered care: What intellectual, technical, interpersonal, and ethical/legal competencies are most likely to bring about the desired outcome?
   Intellectual: knowledge of nursing actions to alleviate symptoms of chemotherapy and radiation, and properly care for a colostomy
   Technical: ability to properly administer fluids or medications via a central venous catheter, CVC site care and assessment for infection, assess and provide wound care for pressure injuries, and care for a colostomy, assess and encourage nutrition
   Interpersonal: ability to establish a trusting relationship with Mr. Pecorini and his wife that demonstrates respect for their human dignity throughout the patient care plan
   Ethical/legal: empathy for the patient with commitment to getting him the help he needs to achieve health goals; honest answers to questions related to his health and prognosis in collaboration with the interprofessional team
4. Teamwork and collaboration: What resources might be helpful for Roberto?
   Print, audiovisual, teaching aids, and demo-redemo of colostomy care and other procedures as he gains strength, social services, support groups; home

nursing care including AP for assistance with ADL and emptying colostomy
5. Informatics/teamwork and collaboration: Which information in the scenario above will the nurse enter in the electronic health record as a means of sharing information with the interprofessional team. Presence of CVC, appearance of dressing and site, catheter care and flushing; side effects of radiation therapy and chemotherapy where present; patient weight, IV fluids administered; I & O, wound assessment, and dressings (can photograph wound), wound care provided; nature of colostomy drainage, appliance change and teaching; discussions on after hospital care

PRACTICING FOR NCLEX
MULTIPLE-CHOICE QUESTIONS

1. a	**2.** d	**3.** c	**4.** b	**5.** b
6. a	**7.** c	**8.** b	**9.** d	**10.** d
11. b				

ALTERNATE-FORMAT QUESTIONS
Multiple-Response Questions

1. a, c, e
2. c, d, f
3. a, c, d, f
4. a, c, d

Sequencing Question

1.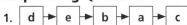

CHAPTER 2

ASSESSING YOUR UNDERSTANDING
FILL IN THE BLANKS

1. Traditional
2. Evidence-based practice
3. Concepts
4. theory
5. conceptual framework
6. systems
7. Developmental theory
8. Informed consent
9. psychosocial development
10. Maslow
11. Evidence-based practice
12. patient, family

MATCHING EXERCISES
Matching Exercise 1

1. d	**2.** c	**3.** a	**4.** b	**5.** e

Matching Exercise 2

1. f	**2.** a	**3.** d	**4.** c	**5.** e
6. b				

Matching Exercise 3

1. a	**2.** b

Matching Exercise 4

1. c   **2.** d   **3.** a   **4.** b

Matching Exercise 5

1. b   **2.** c   **3.** d   **4.** e   **5.** f
6. a

SHORT ANSWER

1. Four concepts that influence and determine nursing practice: (a) person (patient), (b) environment, (c) health, and (d) nursing.
2. Quality improvement: systematic and continuous actions leading to measurable improvement in health care services and the health status of targeted patient groups.
3. Sample answers:
   a. General systems theory: This theory explains breaking whole things into parts and then learning how these parts work together in systems. It includes the relationship between the whole and the parts and defines concepts about how the parts will function and behave.
   b. Adaptation theory: This theory defines adaptation as the adjustment of living matter to other living things and to environmental conditions. Adaptation is a dynamic or continuously changing process that effects change and involves interaction and response. Human adaptation occurs on three levels—internal, social, and physical.
   c. Developmental theory: Outlines the process of growth and development of humans as orderly and predictable, beginning with conception and ending with death. The growth and development of a person are influenced by heredity, temperament, emotional and physical environment, life experiences, and health status.
4. Sample answers:
   a. Nursing theories identify and define interrelated concepts specific to nursing and clearly state the relation between these concepts.
   b. Nursing theories must be logical and use orderly reasoning and identify relations that are developed using a logical sequence.
   c. Nursing theories must be consistent with the basic assumptions used in their development. They should be simple and general.
   d. Nursing theories should increase the nursing profession's body of knowledge by generating research and should guide and improve practice.
5. Sample answers:
   a. Cultural influences on nursing: Until the past two decades, nursing essentially had been considered "women's work," and women were considered inferior to men. After Nightingale established an acceptable occupation for educated women and facilitated improved attitudes toward nursing, the role of the woman as nurse became more favorably accepted.
   b. Educational influences on nursing: The service orientation of nursing was the strongest influence on nursing practice until the 1950s. After

World War II, women increasingly entered the workforce, became more independent, and sought higher education. Nursing education began to focus more on education instead of just training. In the 1960s, college- and university-based baccalaureate programs in nursing increased in number and enrollment, and master's and doctoral programs in nursing were established.
   c. Research and publishing in nursing: Beginning in the 1950s, great advances were made in technology and medical research; nursing leaders realized that research about the practice of nursing was necessary to meet the health needs of modern society.
   d. Improved communication in nursing: Nursing is based on communication with others—patients, other health care team members, community members, as well as with nurses practicing in a variety of specialty settings. Nurses need a knowledge base and common terminology to use in communicating with other professionals.
   e. Improved autonomy of nursing: Nursing can define its independent functions and contributions to health care. The development and use of nursing diagnosis, theory and research provide autonomy in the practice of nursing.
6. Four goals of nursing research according to the National Institute of Nursing Research (NINR):
   a. Build the scientific foundation for clinical practice
   b. Prevent disease and disability
   c. Manage and eliminate symptoms caused by illness
   d. Enhance end-of-life and palliative care
7. Answers will vary based on student experience.
8. Perceived barriers to EBP: inadequate knowledge and skills, a lack of experienced mentors to facilitate the process, and the perception that implementing EBP is too time consuming.
9. Bring a questioning attitude to these situations. "I notice that your technique is different from what I learned. Can explain this to me?"

APPLYING YOUR KNOWLEDGE
CRITICAL THINKING QUESTIONS

1. Answers will vary based on theorist and student experience.
2. Nurses share outcomes of their studies through presentations, grand rounds, or publications linking them to the existing body of knowledge.

REFLECTIVE PRACTICE: CULTIVATING QSEN COMPETENCIES
Sample Answers

1. Patient-centered care/evidence-based practice: How might the nurse respond to Rachel's concerns regarding the care of her mother?

The nurse should provide Rachel with information and practical tips for validating placement of the nasogastric tube and how to maintain its patency. The nurse demonstrates the procedure, then has the daughter a return demonstration. The nurse reassures Rachel that assistance will be available if any problems occur and provides her with the appropriate resources for help and information.

2. Patient-centered care: What would be a successful outcome for this patient?
Rachel accurately re-demonstrates the procedure for nasogastric tube feedings, has time to ask clarifying questions, then states confidence in her ability to take care of her mother. The patient is free from aspiration and complications, and she maintains/gains weight.

3. Patient-centered care/safety: What intellectual, technical, interpersonal, and ethical/legal competencies are most likely to bring about the desired outcome? The patient will maintain their weight and remain free from aspiration of the tube feeding formula.
Intellectual: knowledge of nasogastric tube feedings and associated care
Technical: individualizes teaching to meet Rachel's learning needs; explains and demonstrates proper verification of tube placement, irrigation, performing feedings and preventing aspiration based on sound scientific rationales
Interpersonal: ability to demonstrate empathy and respect for Rachel and her situation
Ethical/legal: ability to provide patient education consistent with the nursing code of ethics and within the scope of legal practice, with a focus on safety

4. Teamwork and collaboration: What resources might be helpful for Rachel?
Reference materials, including audiovisual aids for teaching the procedure for nasogastric tube feedings, what to do for problems or suspected aspiration, home health care services, nutritionist if applicable

PRACTICING FOR NCLEX
MULTIPLE-CHOICE QUESTIONS

1. a	**2.** a	**3.** c	**4.** b	**5.** a
6. b	**7.** c	**8.** b	**9.** d	

ALTERNATE-FORMAT QUESTIONS
Multiple-Response Questions

1. b, c, d
2. a, c
3. a, b, e
4. b, c, d, f

Sequencing Questions

1. e → a → f → g → b → h → i → d → c
2. d → b → a → c → e

CHAPTER 3

ASSESSING YOUR UNDERSTANDING
FILL IN THE BLANKS

1. Disease
2. chronic
3. acute
4. exacerbation
5. environmental
6. disease, infirmity
7. social determinant
8. morbidity, mortality
9. Health equity
10. Diversity, inclusion

MATCHING EXERCISES
Matching Exercise 1

1. f, Modifiable
2. a, Non-modifiable
3. e, Modifiable
4. b, Non-modifiable
5. c, Modifiable
6. e, Modifiable
7. b, Non-modifiable
8. d, Modifiable
9. a, Modifiable
10. c, Modifiable
11. b, Non-modifiable
12. a, Modifiable

Matching Exercise 2

1. c	**2.** d	**3.** a	**4.** b	**5.** e

Matching Exercise 3

1. d	**2.** a	**3.** e	**4.** e	**5.** b
6. c				

SHORT ANSWER

1. Examples of vulnerable populations include racial and ethnic minorities, those living in poverty, women, children, older adults, rural and inner-city residents, and people with disabilities and special health care needs.
2. To ensure that individuals are provided with the resources they need to have access to the same opportunities, individualized types, and degrees of support are needed.
3. Answers will vary with student experiences.
4. Acute illness has a rapid onset of symptoms, is temporary, and does not usually require medical treatment. Patients go through the following phases: (1) has symptoms, (2) assumes sick role, (3) dependent role; accepts diagnosis and follows the treatment plan, and (4) recovery and rehabilitation; gives up dependent role and resumes normal activities and responsibilities. Chronic illness has a slower onset; exhibits permanent, irreversible alterations in normal anatomy and physiology; requires special patient education for rehabilitation; has a long period of care or support; and goes through remissions and exacerbations.

Acute and chronic illnesses may occur at the same time, such as a patient with COPD who develops pneumonia.

5. Sample answers:
   a. Primary: Administering immunizations, teaching proper dental and oral care
   b. Secondary: Applying a tuberculosis test (PPD), giving medications
   c. Tertiary: Facilitating a support system, performing diabetic teaching
6. a. Being: recognizing self as separate and individual
   b. Belonging: being part of a whole
   c. Becoming: growing and developing
   d. Befitting: making personal choices to benefit oneself for the future
7. Answers will vary.

APPLYING YOUR KNOWLEDGE
CRITICAL THINKING QUESTIONS

1. Discussion: provide support and concern for potential loss of pregnancy, grief, and loss for both patients and their families. Physiologic repercussions of cocaine on mother's blood pressure and baby's response to sympathomimetic substance. The nurse answers questions regarding possible loss of pregnancy honestly, monitors vital signs of mothers and fetuses, carries out prescriptions for patient 2 to terminate contractions if prescribed, discusses consequences of cocaine use on blood pressure blood flow to fetus. The nurse remains nonjudgmental and supportive if either pregnancy was unwanted. Additional answers will vary.
2. Responses will vary based on individual discussions.

REFLECTIVE PRACTICE: CULTIVATING QSEN COMPETENCIES
Sample Answers

1. Patient-centered care/evidence-based practice: How might the nurse respond to Ruth's stated desire for a higher level of wellness?
   The nurse uses this opportunity to reinforce patient teaching and provide discharge education. The nurse presents information regarding a "heart healthy diet," the need for exercise, and reinforcement for smoking cessation.
2. Patient-centered care: What would be a successful outcome for this patient?
   Ruth describes a mini-stroke and identifies lifestyle factors (smoking, diet, exercise) that can be modified for stroke prevention.
3. Patient-centered care: What intellectual, interpersonal, and ethical/legal competencies are most likely to bring about the desired outcome?
   Intellectual: ability to integrate knowledge of preventive measures into the patient care plan; able to state signs and symptoms of stroke, state uses of prescribed medications
   Interpersonal: ability to assess health-related beliefs, goals, and practices

Ethical/legal: ability to participate as a trusted and effective patient advocate, including a commitment to securing the best possible care for Ms. Jacobi
4. Teamwork and collaboration: What resources might be helpful for this patient?
   Blood pressure monitoring, audiovisual teaching aids on post TIA ("mini-stroke"), recognizing signs and symptoms of stroke and when to seek help, suggestions for cardiovascular prudent diet/ menu plans, support groups, smoking cessation materials where applicable

PRACTICING FOR NCLEX
MULTIPLE-CHOICE QUESTIONS

1. a   **2.** a   **3.** c   **4.** d   **5.** a
6. b

ALTERNATE-FORMAT QUESTIONS
Multiple-Response Questions

1. b, c, e
2. a, d, e
3. a, c, f

Sequencing Question

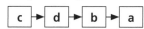

CHAPTER 4

ASSESSING YOUR UNDERSTANDING
FILL IN THE BLANKS

1. oxygen
2. safety, security
3. unrelated
4. values, interests
5. Environmental
6. infectious diseases, shortages
7. lonely, isolated
8. self-esteem
9. Holistic
10. support systems

MATCHING EXERCISES
Matching Exercise 1

1. e   **2.** d   **3.** a   **4.** b   **5.** c

Matching Exercise 2

1. e   **2.** a   **3.** b   **4.** d   **5.** c

SHORT ANSWER

1. Community health nursing focuses on whole populations within a community; community-based nursing is centered on the health care needs of individuals and families.
2. What is the family's structure? What is the family's socioeconomic status? What are family members' cultural background and religious affiliation? Who cares for the children if both parents work? What

are the family's health practices (e.g., types of foods eaten, mealtimes, immunizations, bedtime, exercise)? How does the family define health? What habits are present in the family (e.g., do any family members smoke, drink to excess, or use drugs)? How does the family cope with stress? Is any family member the primary caregiver for another family member? Do close friends or family members live nearby, and can they help if necessary?

3. The PPACA aims to provide improved health security and access to health care for all Americans. In addition to the major provisions that provide a right to coverage for Americans with preexisting conditions, allow young adults up to the age of 26 years to continue to be covered under their parents' plan, and end lifetime limits on coverage, this law expands Medicaid coverage to millions of low-income Americans and makes numerous improvements to the Children's Health Insurance Program (CHIP) (Affordable Care Act, 2012).

4. Nurses can develop environmental awareness by attending to environmental risk factors: air and water quality/pollution, aging infrastructure, global warming, climate change/crisis causing environmental degradation, natural disasters, weather extremes, food and water insecurity, economic disruption, and conflict and terrorism. Social inequalities exacerbate these consequences.

5. Sample answers:
   a. Physical: A family lives in a comfortable home located in a safe neighborhood. This meets the family needs of safety and comfort and enhances growth and development of the children.
   b. Economic: A family is able to afford adequate housing, food, clothing, and community demands. This meets the family's need for nourishment, shelter, and acceptance in society.
   c. Reproductive: The reproductive function of many families is to have and raise children or seeks family planning to limit their offspring. This meets society's need for more members without putting too heavy a demand on the family to care for their children.
   d. Affective and coping: Parents counsel their children to avoid drinking alcohol, smoking cigarettes, and using drugs. This meets the children's needs to be productive members of society and to avoid the pitfalls surrounding adolescence.
   e. Socialization: Through socialization, the family teaches; transmits beliefs, values, attitudes, and coping mechanisms; provides feedback; and guides problem solving, such as seeking expert counseling for a child having difficulty adjusting to school and relating to other children. This meets the child's need to fit in with other schoolmates and helps correct a problem before it gets out of hand.

6. Sample answers:
   a. Physiologic needs: The nurse helps to prepare the mother for her cesarean birth and administers any medications prescribed.
   b. Safety and security needs: The nurse monitors the mother's and baby's vital signs during and after the procedure.
   c. Love and belonging needs: The nurse helps the partner to cope with his fears, encourages him to support his partner, participate in the birth of his child.
   d. Self-esteem needs: The nurse reassures the mother that having a cesarean birth is a common procedure and that she should not feel guilty for not being able to have the baby vaginally.
   e. Self-actualization needs: The nurse helps the mother after surgery to continue with her original plan to breastfeed her infant.

APPLYING YOUR KNOWLEDGE
CRITICAL THINKING QUESTIONS
1. Answers will vary with student experience.
2. Nurses support a culture of health and can remain educated and active regarding legislation to support affordable care, regardless of name. The nurse can collaborate with the health care provider to obtain free sample medications or suggest the patient enroll in Medicaid if they are eligible. The nurse can assist the patient in finding a free clinic. Additional answers will vary with experience.

REFLECTIVE PRACTICE: CULTIVATING QSEN COMPETENCIES
Sample Answers
1. Patient-centered care/safety: What basic human needs should be addressed by the nurse to provide individualized, holistic care for Samuel?
   The nurse provides holistic, family-centered care, considering all the dimensions of basic human needs. For Samuel, these needs include physiologic needs related to his and his wife's health condition; safety and security needs for a safe environment for older adults, one with Alzheimer disease; love and belonging needs related to his desire to remain with and care for his wife; self-esteem needs based on his pride in taking care of himself and his wife; and self-actualization needs or acceptance of himself and his adaptation to the current situation.
2. Safety: What would a successful outcome be for this patient?
   Samuel verbalizes reasons he is unable to care for his wife at home and acknowledges a plan to provide a safe environment for himself and his wife.
3. Patient-centered care/evidence-based practice: What intellectual, interpersonal, and ethical/legal competencies are most likely to bring about the desired outcome?
   Intellectual: knowledge of Alzheimer disease and its effect on the family
   Interpersonal: using strong interpersonal skills to establish a trusting relationship with Samuel demonstrating respect for human dignity and autonomy

Ethical/legal: skill in working collaboratively with colleagues and community members to advocate for the health care needs of Samuel and his wife

4. Teamwork and collaboration: What resources might be helpful for Samuel?
Teaching aids for family members with Alzheimer disease, counseling services, community services, skilled nursing care or home care, respite care for Samuel or social work services to facilitate transition Samuel's wife to a memory care facility

PRACTICING FOR NCLEX

MULTIPLE-CHOICE QUESTIONS

1. d **2.** a **3.** d **4.** c **5.** d

ALTERNATE-FORMAT QUESTIONS

Multiple-Response Questions

1. c, d, e
2. b, c, e, f
3. b, d, e
4. b, c
5. a, b, c

Prioritization Questions

1. 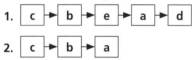 c → b → e → a → d

2. c → b → a

CHAPTER 5

ASSESSING YOUR UNDERSTANDING

FILL IN THE BLANKS

1. beliefs, behavioral expectations
2. subculture
3. ethnicity
4. Cultural assimilation
5. Culture conflict
6. Cultural blindness
7. shock
8. stereotyping
9. open-ended
10. adherence/compliance

MATCHING EXERCISE

1. e **2.** a **3.** b **4.** d **5.** c
6. f

SHORT ANSWER

1. Changes occurring in the U.S. population over the last several decades that may affect nursing care include: increased population, older population, more Hispanic and Asian individuals, fewer marriages, and fewer traditional families.
2. Nursing concerns include: lack of financial resources affects how individuals and families meet their basic needs and maintain their health.

Poverty often leads to lack of health insurance and access to wellness or illness care, inadequate care of infants and children, lack of access to basic health care services, and homelessness.

3. Sample answers:
   a. Encourage the patient to investigate bus routes to the office; check if medical services are available within walking distance; see if insurance will cover transportation to and from medical services.
   b. Boil water before using it; check with social services to see if they can provide any necessary services for patient.
   c. Research the community for free or low-cost medical clinics and services and make appropriate referrals.
4. Sample answers:
   a. Higher number of female-headed households from divorce, abandonment, unmarried motherhood, and changes in abortion laws place the household at a financial disadvantage.
   b. Most older adults live on fixed incomes, which often do not keep up with inflation. Many, particularly widows, are on the borderline of poverty or have already slipped into poverty.
   c. In some cases, poverty is passed from generation to generation. This is true in groups such as migrant farm workers, families living on welfare, and people who live in isolated areas such as Appalachia.
5. Sample answers:
   a. Feelings of despair, resignation, and fatalism
   b. "Day-to-day" attitude toward life, with no hope for the future
   c. Unemployment and need for financial or government aid
   d. Unstable family structure, possibly characterized by abusiveness and abandonment
   e. Decline in self-respect and retreat from community involvement

APPLYING YOUR KNOWLEDGE

1. Sample responses (answers will vary with student experience):
   a. Attempt to locate a male nurse; explain there is no one else but that you will provide for his dignity and cultural observances by carefully draping him and examining only what is necessary.
   b. Support her as a new mother, assess her support systems and if the father of the baby is in their lives, encourage childcare classes, and, depending on answers, consider human trafficking and rape as possible antecedents to the pregnancy.
   c. Attempt to obtain a translator, translation phone or use a phone or computer translation program or ask/pantomime for them to call someone who speaks English; carefully assess, using non-verbal cues, follow the hospital protocol for MI.
2. Answers will vary with student experience.

REFLECTIVE PRACTICE: CULTIVATING QSEN COMPETENCIES
Sample Answers

1. Patient-centered care/safety: How might the nurse respond to Danielle's request for a Haitian folk healer?
   To provide culturally competent, thoughtful, patient-centered care, the nurse assesses what the folk healer may do, explaining that only health care personnel may touch or manipulated the traction and equipment in the room. The nurse may research Haitian culture to properly prepare the room and patient for the visit. After the visit, the nurse reassesses the patient and skeletal traction, and documents the findings in the patient record.
2. Patient-centered care: What would be a successful outcome for this patient?
   The patient verbalizes that the folk healer relieved her anxiety related to hospitalization, pain, and/or healing of the fracture. She states her desire to continue with the nursing care plan.
3. Patient-centered care/evidence-based practice: What intellectual, interpersonal, and ethical/legal competencies are most likely to bring about the desired outcome?
   Intellectual: knowledge of Haitian cultural health care practices gained from research
   Interpersonal: formation of a caring relationship with the patient that encompasses the patient's beliefs and values
   Ethical/legal: careful documentation of patient goals and outcomes
4. Teamwork and collaboration: What resources might be helpful for Danielle's care?
   Research materials on the Haitian culture, community services; teaching regarding interactions of herbal/folk remedies with western medications, follow-up for assessment of fracture and possible physical therapy

PRACTICING FOR NCLEX
MULTIPLE-CHOICE QUESTIONS

1. b
2. d
3. b
4. c
5. d
6. c
7. b

ALTERNATE-FORMAT QUESTIONS
Multiple-Response Questions

1. a, d, e
2. a, d, f
3. a, b, e
4. a, c, d, e

CHAPTER 6

ASSESSING YOUR UNDERSTANDING
FILL IN THE BLANKS

1. laissez-faire
2. code of ethics
3. values clarification
4. prizing
5. values system
6. advocacy
7. Moral injury
8. whistle blowing
9. more
10. social justice

MATCHING EXERCISES
Matching Exercise 1

1. f
2. c
3. d
4. e
5. b
6. a

Matching Exercise 2

1. b
2. d
3. c
4. a
5. e

SHORT ANSWER

1. Sample answers:
   a. Values clarification: Have the mother state the three most important things in her life. Explore her answers with her and find out why she chose them and how her choices may affect her situation.
   b. Choosing: After exploring the mother's values, have her choose her key values freely. She may choose her child or profession.
   c. Prizing: Reinforce the mother's choices and, if possible, involve the husband and child in decision making.
   d. Acting: Assist the mother to plan new behaviors consistent with the values she has chosen and incorporate them into her life. For example, if she values her child, she may reduce the number of classes she takes at night and spend more time with her.
2. Sample answers (answers to part 2 of the question will vary):
   a. Cost-effectiveness and allocation
   b. Issues of cultural and/or religious variation
   c. Consideration of power
   d. Relationship between health care providers and patients
3. Sample answers (answers to part 2 of the question will vary):
   a. Autonomy: Respect the decision-making capacity of autonomous persons (e.g., patients have the right to refuse treatment they do not feel would be helpful to their condition).
   b. Nonmaleficence: Avoid causing harm (e.g., be sure you are fully knowledgeable about a procedure before performing it).
   c. Beneficence: Provide benefits and balance these benefits against risks and harms (e.g., securing

a patient with restraints who is at high risk for falls).

   d. Justice: Distribute benefits, risks, and costs fairly (e.g., give service to all patients regardless of their life circumstances).
   e. Fidelity: Be faithful to promises you made to the public to be competent and willing to use your competence to benefit patients entrusted to your care (e.g., not abandoning a patient entrusted to your care without first seeing to their needs).
4. Answers will vary with student experiences.
5. Answers will vary with student experiences.
6. Sample answers:
   a. Gather as much data as possible to support your recommendation.
   b. Identify the ethical problem and explore solutions to the problem.
   c. Plan a course of action you can justify (e.g., seeking assistance for the patient at a higher level).
   d. Implement your decision by speaking to your superiors and presenting your case in a competent manner.
   e. Evaluate your decision: What was the outcome? How does this make me feel? Did I make the right decision?
7. Sample answers:
   a. Breach of confidentiality, incompetent practice
   b. Covering for another nurse who is not performing her job competently, short staffing
   c. Health care provider incompetence, conflicts concerning the role of the nurse in certain situations
   d. Cost-containment versus hospitalization, health care rationing

APPLYING YOUR KNOWLEDGE
CRITICAL THINKING QUESTIONS

1. Sample answers
   a. While the adolescent is still a minor, the nurse can encourage the father to speak to the son and support him.
   b. The nurse assures the patient that all information is confidential, offer resources.
2. Sample answers
   a. The nurse's code of ethics requires fidelity, veracity, and accurate documentation and reporting.
   b. Education for the coworker may be needed or the nurse is neglecting their duties.
   c. The nurse advocates for safety by communicating through the shortage through the chain of command, documenting what was done, continuing the communication over a period of time. Some nurses "go public" or encourage unionization.
Additional answers will vary based on experience.

REFLECTIVE PRACTICE: CULTIVATING QSEN COMPETENCIES
Sample Answers

1. Patient-centered care: How might the nurse react to Mr. Raines's response to filling his prescriptions?
   The nurse should protect and support Mr. Raines's rights by being a strong patient advocate. This could be accomplished by investigating available social services and community services for Mr. Raines. The nurse could also check with the drug manufacturer to see if the company has a discount or free programs for needy patients.
2. Patient-centered care: What would be a successful outcome for this patient?
   Mr. Raines vocalizes the health benefits of taking his blood pressure medication and lists three reasons for seeking social services and other available assistance.
3. Safety: What intellectual, technical, interpersonal, and ethical/legal competencies are most likely to bring about the desired outcome?
   Intellectual: ability to integrate ethical principles and use an ethical framework and decision-making process to resolve ethical problems
   Technical: ability to integrate moral facility to provide the technical nursing assistance necessary to meet the needs of Mr. Raines
   Interpersonal: ability to advocate for patients whose values may be different from personal ones
   Ethical/legal: ability to identify and develop the essential elements of moral facility, cultivate the virtues of nursing, and understand ethical theories that dictate and justify professional conduct
4. Teamwork and collaboration: What resources might be helpful for Mr. Raines?
   Social services, communication of problem with clinic provider, community mental health services, government assistance, community services, drug-assistance programs

PRACTICING FOR NCLEX
MULTIPLE-CHOICE QUESTIONS

1. b   2. a   3. b   4. c   5. a
6. b   7. b   8. d

ALTERNATE-FORMAT QUESTIONS
Multiple-Response Questions

1. c, e
2. d, e
3. a, b, d, e
4. b, c, e, f
5. a, b, d

CHAPTER 7

ASSESSING YOUR UNDERSTANDING
FILL IN THE BLANKS
1. public
2. Nurse Practice Act
3. Licensure
4. expert witness
5. collective bargaining
6. incident
7. sentinel
8. incident report
9. Licensure (or certification)
10. revocable privilege

MATCHING EXERCISES
Matching Exercise 1
1. b **2.** f **3.** a **4.** e **5.** d
6. c

Matching Exercise 2
1. e **2.** a **3.** b **4.** f **5.** c
6. d

Matching Exercise 3
1. a **2.** d **3.** b **4.** d **5.** e
6. c

Matching Exercise 4
1. b **2.** e **3.** d **4.** a **5.** c

SHORT ANSWER
1. Sample answers:
   a. Failure to ensure patient safety: Hourly nursing rounds, fall reduction strategies, use the "rights" of medication administration, obtain education prior to using unfamiliar equipment, update knowledge on patient safety, new interventions to prevent and reduce injury
   b. Improper treatment or performance of treatment: Follow organization policies when performing procedures, use proper technique and evidence-based guidelines when performing procedures
   c. Failure to monitor, report, and rescue: Adhere to postprocedure guidelines, add additional monitoring based on changes in patient status, collaborate on changes in condition with health care provider; report need for changes in plan of care to health care provider and document interaction and orders
   d. Medication errors and reactions: Investigate patient's concerns regarding medication and prior to administering the medication; document an error and notify appropriate parties per organization's policy (do not document incident report in electronic health record)
   e. Failure to follow facility procedure: Adhere to facility procedures, advise the appropriate person of procedures that need to be revised rather than devise "work arounds"
   f. Adverse incidents: Do not assume, voice, or record any blame for an incident
2. Sample answers:
   a. Voluntary standards: Developed and implemented by the nursing profession itself; not mandatory; used for peer review; examples include professional nursing organizations, certifications.
   b. Legal standards: Developed by legislative action; implemented by authority granted by the state (or province) to determine minimum standards for the education of nurses, set requirements for licensure or registration, and decide when to revoke or suspend nurse's licenses; examples include licensure
3. Sample answers:
   a. Specialized diagnostic procedures or surgeries
   b. Experimental treatment or procedures
   c. On admission for routine treatment
4. Sample answers:
   a. Talking with patients in rooms that are not soundproof
   b. Pressing the patient for information not necessary for care planning
   c. Using tape recorders, dictation machines, computer banks, etc. without taking precautions to ensure patient confidentiality
5. Sample answers:
   a. Solid educational background and strong clinical experience
   b. Understanding of the legal aspects of nursing and malpractice liability
   c. Knowledge of the appropriate state (or provincial) Nurse Practice Act and standard of nursing care
6. Sample answer:
   Limit telephone orders to true emergency situations; repeat a telephone order back to the health care provider; document the order, its time and date, situation necessitating order, health care provider prescribing, reconfirming the order as it is read back, and signing name; and VO or TO. If possible, two nurses should listen to a questionable telephone order, with both nurses countersigning the order.
7. Sample answers:
   a. Contraindicated by normal practice
   b. Contraindicated by patient's present condition
8. Sample answers:
   a. The nurse is liable for their actions; the nurse must file an incident report.
   b. The incident report should contain the name of the patient; all witnesses; a complete factual account of the incident; the date, time, and place of the incident; pertinent characteristics of the person involved (e.g., alert, ambulatory, asleep) and of any equipment or resources being used; medications administered, and other relevant variables believed important to the incident.
   c. Answers will vary with student experiences.

9. Sample answers:
Full legal responsibility and accountability for these nursing actions rest with the nurse. Liability insurance protects the nurse's best interest if there is a conflict with the nurse and organization, typically covers the nurse beyond the limitations of employer's coverage and covers the nurse for care or advice given outside of work. The employer's policy provides coverage in the work setting.

APPLYING YOUR KNOWLEDGE
CRITICAL THINKING QUESTIONS

1. Sample answers:
   a. Remind the student that professional behavior involves nonmaleficence as a tenet of professional nursing. Ask how they would feel if harm came to the patient, or if the error was discovered and found to be covered up.
   b. Battery is an intentional tort and punishable by law. By not reporting this the patient and others may be further abused. Reporting this may escalate their actions. The nurse uses the ethical framework to arrive at the best decision.
   c. You can offer to replace items on the sterile field or as a student, defer to the scrub nurse. An incident report can be filed.
2. Risk managers are helpful resources for nurses with legal questions. Many risk managers encourage nurses and other clinicians to report "near misses" to better identify factors contributing to errors. The risk manager will likely review an event report and may ask the nurse questions. Answers will vary.

REFLECTIVE PRACTICE: CULTIVATING QSEN COMPETENCIES
Sample Answers

1. Teamwork and collaboration: How might the nurses involved in this scenario respond to Meredith' disclosure that she plans to press charges against the hospital?
The nurse continues to develop trusting nurse–patient relationships (satisfied patients rarely sue), practice within the scope of their competence, and identify potential liabilities in their practice and work to prevent them. The nurse should notify the nurse manager and seek advice from legal counsel. The nurse should not volunteer information regarding the case and should consider responses to the mother carefully as they may be named as a defendant. Nurses called must base testimony on only firsthand knowledge of the incident and not on assumptions. When in doubt about facts, the nurses should simply testify, "I do not remember that."
2. Safety/teamwork and collaboration: What intellectual, technical, interpersonal, and ethical/legal competencies are most likely to be used in this situation?
Intellectual: knowledge of brain tumor and end of life care in children; law and sources of law and ability to identify potential areas of liability in nursing
Technical: provide technical nursing care in a competent, legally appropriate manner
Interpersonal: ability to work collaboratively with other members of the health care team and legal department
Ethical/legal: ability to identify errors in personal action, complete and truthful documentation of care in electronic health record
3. Teamwork and collaboration: What resources might be helpful for the nurses in this case?
Risk manager/ organization's legal department if indicated, liability insurance, malpractice arbitration panel, nurse practice act

PRACTICING FOR NCLEX
MULTIPLE-CHOICE QUESTIONS

1. a	**2.** c	**3.** a	**4.** d	**5.** d
6. d	**7.** a	**8.** d	**9.** c	

ALTERNATE-FORMAT QUESTIONS
Multiple-Response Questions

1. a, b, d
2. b, d, e
3. a, e
4. a, c, e
5. c, d, e
6. a, c, d
7. a, c, e

Sequencing Question

1.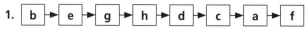

CHAPTER 8

ASSESSING YOUR UNDERSTANDING
FILL IN THE BLANKS

1. stimulus
2. auditory, visual, kinesthetic
3. face
4. safety
5. feedback
6. nonverbal
7. helping
8. orientation
9. validating
10. horizontal violence
11. State Board

MATCHING EXERCISES
Matching Exercise 1

1. a	**2.** b	**3.** c	**4.** d

Matching Exercise 2

1. a	**2.** b	**3.** f	**4.** c	**5.** d
6. e				

Matching Exercise 3

1. b   **2.** c   **3.** a

Matching Exercise 4

1. b   **2.** c   **3.** e   **4.** d   **5.** a

SHORT ANSWER

1. Sample Answers:
   a. You're trying so hard to control your weight. How do you think you did today?
   b. You look uncomfortable; are you in pain?
   c. I see you're upset. Would you like to talk about it?
   d. You seem frustrated. Is there something I can help with?
   e. You seem concerned about the surgery/procedure.

2. Sample answers:
   a. Touch: The nurse gently squeezes a patient's hand before surgery. The patient's response to this touch may express fear, gratitude, acceptance, etc. and the nurse can assess the temperature of the patient's skin.
   b. Eye contact: A patient avoids eye contact. The patient may be expressing defenselessness, avoidance of communication, or an expression of their culture.
   c. Facial expressions: A patient grimaces when looking at his surgical incision. The patient may be experiencing anxiety over the alteration in their physical appearance.
   d. Posture: A patient stands erect with good body alignment. The patient may be experiencing good health. Slouching may indicate sadness.
   e. Gait: A patient walks slightly bent over. The patient may be in pain or accommodating an illness.
   f. Gestures: A patient gives you a thumbs-up sign after receiving test results. The patient is most likely happy with the results.
   g. General physical appearance: A patient is sweating and having difficulty breathing. The patient may be experiencing a life-threatening condition.
   h. Mode of dress and grooming: A patient who has been bedridden for a week asks to take a shower and get dressed. The patient is likely feeling better.
   i. Sounds: A patient sighs whenever you mention their significant other. The patient may be experiencing difficulty with this relationship.
   j. Silence: A patient who has undergone a mastectomy remains silent when asked how she is feeling. The patient may angry or not yet able to express her feelings.

3. Sample answers:
   a. School-aged child: An 8-year-old boy has limited understanding of surgical procedures. Therefore, the nurse must explain the procedure in simple terms so that the child will cooperate without being frightened.
   b. Adolescent: Adolescents are developing their ability to think abstractly and can understand fairly detailed descriptions of clinical procedures.
   c. Older adult with a hearing impairment: The nurse should speak directly to the patient while facing them. When necessary, use nonverbal communication (e.g., sign language or finger spelling, or by writing any ideas that cannot be conveyed in another manner).

4. Occupation may give insight into a person's literacy, abilities, talents, interests, and economic status.

5. Sample answers:
   a. Assessing: Verbal and nonverbal communication are essential nursing tools used when gathering information. The nurse clearly communicates what will happen, asks permission to perform the physical assessment and conveys dignity and respect during the interaction. The nurse may refer to the electronic health record or team members for additional assessment information.
   b. Diagnosing: Once formulated, the nurse communicates the diagnosis through the written care plan, through oral communication to team members (such as in report), and to the patient.
   c. Planning: The patient, nurse, and other health care team members must communicate with each other as patient goals and outcomes are developed and interventions selected.
   d. Implementing: Verbal and nonverbal communication allows nurses to enhance basic caregiving measures and to teach, counsel, and support patients and their families.
   e. Evaluating: Nurses often rely on the verbal and nonverbal clues they receive from their patients to determine whether patient objectives or goals have been achieved.
   f. Documenting: Documentation data promotes continuity of care given by nurses and other health care team members.

6. Sample answers:
   a. Providing privacy: Providing privacy during nurse–patient interactions conveys caring and respect and preserves the patient's dignity.
   b. Maintaining confidentiality: The patient should know their right to privacy is respected. This conveys professionalism by the nurse, who shares what is necessary for care of the patient.
   c. Developing therapeutic communication skills: Nurses use therapeutic communication skills as part of a helping relationship. The nurse demonstrates truthfulness and open-mindedness, communicates needed knowledge and the care plan clearly and concisely, is flexible and concise, avoids words that may be interpreted

differently, and takes advantage of patient cues to communicate.

   d. Using silence as a tool: Silence can be appropriate. It allows time for the patient to initiate or continue speaking. Nurses should be aware of the different possible meanings of silence (the patient is comfortable with the nurse, the patient is demonstrating stoicism or exploring inner thoughts, the patient may be fearful, etc.).

7. A patient is recovering the day after a mastectomy. She is married with two school-aged children. When the nurse enters the patient's room, she finds the patient <u>with tears in her eyes and a worried expression on her face</u>. When asked how she is feeling, the patient replies "fine," although her <u>face is rigid, and her mouth is drawn in a firm line</u>. She is <u>moving her foot back and forth under the covers</u>. On further investigation, the nurse finds that the patient is worried about her children and her ability to be a healthy, functioning wife and mother again. After prompting, the patient says, "I don't know if my husband will still love me like this." She <u>sighs and falls silent,</u> reflecting upon her recovery. The nurse repositions the patient and <u>puts her hand over the patient's hand</u>. She <u>establishes eye contact</u> and suggests that things have a way of working out over time.

8. Sample answers:
   a. Orientation phase: By 8/6/25, the patient will call the nurse by her name. By 8/6/25, the patient will describe his freedoms/responsibilities within the institute.
   b. Working phase: By 8/10/25, the patient will list various classes/activities available to patients. By 8/10/25, the patient will express any anxieties he may have in his new environment to the nurse.
   c. Termination phase: By 8/25/25, the patient will meet the new nurse in charge of his care by the current, who will continue the relationship until their departure. By 8/27/25, the patient will report feeling good about his past care and look forward to his new relationship.

9. Sample answers:
   a. Warmth and friendliness: greets a patient with a pleasant smile
   b. Openness and respect: provides an honest explanation of a procedure
   c. Empathy: listens to a woman's lament over her miscarriage while helping her bathe
   d. Competence: quickly and smoothly inserts an indwelling catheter
   e. Consideration of patient variables: finds another nurse who speaks Spanish for her Latino patient

10. Sample answers:
   a. Failure to perceive the patient as a human being: The nurse should focus on the whole person, not simply the illness or dysfunction.
   b. Failure to listen: Nurses should be open to opportunities for communication by keeping an open mind and focusing on the patient's needs instead of their own needs.
   c. Use of inappropriate comments or questions: The nurse should avoid certain types of comments and questions (clichés, questions that probe for information, leading questions, comments that give advice, judgmental comments) that tend to impede communication.
   d. Changing the subject: The nurse should avoid changing the subject; the patient may be ready to discuss something and may be frustrated if put off by a change in topic.
   e. Giving false assurance: The nurse should not try to convince the patient that things are going to turn out well when knowing the chances are not good. False assurance may give patients the impression the nurse is not interested in their problems.

11. Sample answers:
   a. Bullying: Anger and aggressive behavior between nurses, or nurse-to-nurse hostility, has been labeled horizontal violence or bullying, lateral violence, and professional incivility. Bullying affects patient safety because the toxic environment produces negative impacts teamwork. Deterioration in the quality of care and a greater potential for an error occurs. It creates a toxic work environment and generates considerable emotional and physical consequences on those being bullied.
   b. Organizational response: Organizations should publish and enforce a policy related to incivility. Tactics against bullying include education for the staff, holding staff accountable, zero tolerance policies toward disruptive behaviors, protection for those who report the behaviors, training leaders to role model professional standards of behavior, surveillance and reporting systems put in place to identify unprofessional behaviors, and emphasis placed on the importance of documenting bullying behaviors.

APPLYING YOUR KNOWLEDGE

CRITICAL THINKING QUESTIONS

1. Answers will vary with student experience.
2. Answers will vary with student experience.
3. Answers will vary with student experience.
4. Answers will vary with student experience.

REFLECTIVE PRACTICE: CULTIVATING QSEN COMPETENCIES

Sample Answers

1. Patient-centered care: What communication skills will the nurse use to complete an assessment of Irwina?
   The nurse should orient the patient to their presence before initiating conversation, face her, and speak directly to her. Communicate important

information in a quiet environment with little distraction; keep the conversation simple and concrete, using gestures/pantomime if needed to augment what is stated. The nurse must be patient and give Irwina time to respond. Obtain an interpreter if the language barrier interferes with communication and gathering assessment data. Attempts should be made to contact family, if available.

2. Patient-centered care/safety: What would be a successful outcome for this patient?
Irwina provides information to the nurse for the assessment and agrees to her daughter's participation in the interview.

3. Patient-centered care/safety: What intellectual, technical, interpersonal, and/or ethical/legal competencies are most likely to bring about the desired outcome?
Intellectual: ability to incorporate knowledge of the goals and phases of helping relationships as a component of the patient's care plan
Interpersonal: strong people skills including the ability to communicate and interact effectively with patients who have hearing or cognitive deficits
Ethical/legal: ability to advocate for Irwina who may be unable to do so herself, due to language and hearing problems

4. Teamwork and collaboration: What resources might be helpful for Irwina?
Interpretation services, consultation with an audiologist, assessment of confusion with a neurology or psychiatry consult, family members

---

PRACTICING FOR NCLEX
MULTIPLE-CHOICE QUESTIONS

1. d	**2.** d	**3.** a	**4.** b	**5.** a
6. c	**7.** c	**8.** d	**9.** b	**10.** c
11. a				

ALTERNATE-FORMAT QUESTIONS
Multiple-Response Questions

1. a, b
2. a, b, c, d, f
3. b, d f
4. a, c, d, f
5. a, b, c, f
6. a, c, f
7. b, c, d
8. b, c, d, e

Sequencing Questions

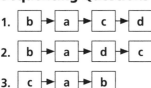

1. b → a → c → d
2. b → a → d → c
3. c → a → b

CHAPTER 9

ASSESSING YOUR UNDERSTANDING
FILL IN THE BLANKS

1. promoting
2. helping
3. cognitive
4. affective
5. patient
6. Motivation
7. evidence-based
8. coach
9. counselor
10. empower

MATCHING EXERCISES
Matching Exercise 1

1. b	**2.** c	**3.** a	**4.** e	**5.** d

Matching Exercise 2

1. d	**2.** b	**3.** a	**4.** d	**5.** b
6. d				

Matching Exercise 3

1. c	**2.** b	**3.** d	**4.** a	**5.** a
6. d				

Matching Exercise 4

1. d	**2.** b	**3.** a	**4.** c

SHORT ANSWER

1. Sample answers:
   a. Promoting health: Nurses teach/counsel patients concerning health practices that lead to a higher level of wellness.
   b. Preventing illness: Nurses can teach patients health practices that help prevent specific illnesses or dangerous situations. Examples include promoting immunizations, diet, exercise, or medication safety.
   c. Restoring health: Nurses can teach patients self-care practices that will facilitate recovery such as encouraging mobility.
   d. Facilitating coping: Nurses can assist patients and their families to come to terms with the patient's illness and necessary lifestyle modifications.
2. Sample answers:
   a. The nurse in the helping relationship demonstrates sensitivity and concern by creating a nonthreatening learning environment with time for questions.
   b. Honest and open communication can provide the adult learner with a realistic preview of what will be involved and allow them to retain some control over what is taught.
   c. Present new information clearly and in amounts that patients can comprehend to prevent them from becoming discouraged or overwhelmed.

3. Sample answers:
   a. Demonstration: Take the patient through the exercises and have them demonstrate them in return.
   b. Print material: Give a brochure that explicitly describes and diagrams the exercises you wish them to learn.
   c. Discussion: Have a conversation with the patient about the exercises and their desire and ability to perform them.

4. Sample answers:
   a. Content must be prioritized such that essential or survival information is thoroughly taught first, and less important content is saved for another time.
   b. Teamwork and cooperation allow nurses to meet deadlines for teaching. If teaching is needed beyond hospitalization, the nurse can schedule additional learning opportunities through home care nurses, outpatient programs, or referrals to community-based programs.

5. Sample answers:
   a. Formal: Planned teaching that is provided to fulfill learner objectives (e.g., viewing a film on diabetes)
   b. Informal: Unplanned teaching that represents the majority of nurse–patient interactions (e.g., a nurse showing a mother the proper way to hold an infant, walking the patient through blood glucose testing, while performing the procedure)

6. Sample answers:
   a. Cognitive domain: Oral questioning, quizzes
   b. Affective domain: Patient's verbal response indicating a attitudes, values, and feelings
   c. Psychomotor domain: Return demonstration of a procedure or skill

7. Sample answers:
   a. Short-term counseling: Situational crisis (e.g., a nurse counsels a housebound patient after a fire destroys her bedroom)
   b. Long-term counseling: Developmental crisis (e.g., a nurse counsels an adolescent about the dangers of drugs and alcohol)
   c. Motivational counseling: Discussion of feelings and incentives with the patient (e.g., a nurse counseling a woman in a shelter about dignity and autonomy when she states she is leaving her abusive spouse)

8. Sample answers:
   a. Identifying the new knowledge, attitudes, or skills that are necessary for patients and family members to manage their health care
   b. Assessing learning readiness
   c. Assessing the patient's ability to learn
   d. Identifying patient strengths and personal resources the nurse can tap

9. Answers will vary with student experiences.

10. Sample answers:
    a. Ensuring health care instructions are understandable and designed to support patient goals

    b. Including patient and family as partners in the teaching–learning process
    c. Using interactive teaching strategies
    d. Remembering that teaching and learning processes rely on strong interpersonal relationships with patients and their families

11. Sample answers, student may list 3 of the following.
    a. Ignoring the restrictions of the patient's environment
    b. Failing to accept that patients have the right to change their minds
    c. Using medical jargon
    d. Failing to negotiate goals
    e. Duplicating teaching that other team members have done

APPLYING YOUR KNOWLEDGE
CRITICAL THINKING QUESTIONS

1. a. First, the nurse assesses readiness to learn and learning needs. The nurse could open the discussion by asking if the patient if they are open to hearing about the effects of obesity on arthritis pain. The nurse can explain this relationship and, if met with positive response from the patient, continue with various teaching strategies.
   b. Sample Response: Lecture/discussion, the nurse could explain the role of simple carbohydrates and fats on weight, how many calories must be burned to lose 1 lb, and the need for exercise to burn more calories. Demonstration/role-playing, the nurse could provide a sample menu and jointly construct meal menus meeting to the goal, or role-play dining out and requesting no fats be added to the prepared meal.
   c. Answers will vary based on nurse and patient.

2. Responses will vary with student experience.

3. Responses will vary with student experience.

REFLECTIVE PRACTICE: CULTIVATING QSEN COMPETENCIES
Sample Answers

1. Patient-centered care/safety: What should be the focus of patient teaching for this couple? Patient teaching should focus on health maintenance and promotion for the mother and fetus. The nurse begins by assessing the cultural practices and knowledge they may bring to the session. Teaching topics might include proper nutrition including the benefits of folic acid supplements and prenatal vitamins, substances to avoid when pregnant (tobacco, alcohol, cat litter, x-rays, etc.), methods of childbirth, and parenting skills. The nurse should encourage the couple's choice of childbirth planning and provide as much information as possible on home births.

2. Patient-centered care/safety: What would be a successful outcome for Marco and Claudia? By next visit, the couple lists the benefits of home childbirth versus other methods and signs up for a class on comfort measures during delivery and

newborn care. In collaboration with the birth attendant, Marco and Claudia will have considered a backup plan for potential complications arising during home birth.

3. Patient-centered care: What intellectual, technical, interpersonal, and/or ethical/legal competencies are most likely to bring about the desired outcome? Intellectual: knowledge of how to design an appropriate teaching program for childbirth and parenting, including cultural practices and preferences Interpersonal: ability to establish trusting relationships with patients to foster teaching and learning; being a cheerleader for the couple as they learn about childbirth and newborn care. Ethical/legal: strong sense of accountability for the health and well-being of patients that translates into a commitment to getting patients the information they need

4. Teamwork and collaboration/informatics: What resources might be helpful for this couple? Prenatal classes or videos; printed and AV materials on pregnancy, childbirth, and parenting; evidence-based information on birth attendant/midwife, home delivery, and birth plan. Document the mother's vital signs, weight and fetal heart rate, the new family's expectations, and all teaching in the electronic health record

PRACTICING FOR NCLEX
MULTIPLE-CHOICE QUESTIONS

1. a   2. b   3. d   4. a   5. c
6. b   7. d   8. d   9. d   10. a

ALTERNATE-FORMAT QUESTIONS
Multiple-Response Questions

1. a, b, e, f
2. b, c, e
3. c, d, f
4. a, e, f
5. a, c, d, e
6. b, c, d
7. b, c, d
8. a, b, c, d

Prioritization Questions

1. At the first patient encounter
2. c

CHAPTER 10

ASSESSING YOUR UNDERSTANDING
FILL IN THE BLANKS

1. Leadership
2. explicit (legitimate), implied
3. emotional
4. autocratic
5. democratic/participative
6. servant leadership
7. Quantum
8. transactional
9. Transformational
10. Magnet
11. just culture
12. management
13. shared governance
14. preceptor

MATCHING EXERCISE

1. e   2. g   3. a   4. b   5. d
6. g

SHORT ANSWER

1. The experienced mentor has common interests, and acts as a role model who can advise and support the protégé, ease the new nurse into their responsibilities, and provide information and network links. Mentors suggest options for the protégé's growth, identify helpful resources, answer questions, and provide honest feedback. The mentor does not receive a financial reward.

2. List the steps you would employ to change visiting hours from a few hours daily to open visitation, 24 hours a day. How would you handle people who resist the change? Answers will vary with student experience, Unfreezing, introduce the need for families to be with the loved ones, research that shows patients are less anxious and fare better. Moving: Refreezing: open visiting hours become the norm. Identify a problem, inform about the change, begin the change process, evaluate the process. Educate those who resist but continue the process.

3. a. Threat to self: Loss of self-esteem and the belief that more work will be required and that social relationships will be disrupted. Explain the proposed change to everyone affected in simple, concise language so they know how they will be affected by it.
   b. Lack of understanding: The people who will be affected by the change should be involved in the change process. When they understand the reason for and benefits of the change, they are more likely to accept it.
   c. Limited tolerance for change: Some people do not like to function in a state of flux or disequilibrium. Expedite the change so there is only a short period of confusion and explain this tactic to the employees involved.
   d. Disagreements about the benefits of the change: Resistance may occur when the information available to the change agent is different from that received by people resisting the change. If the information available to the resisters is more accurate and relevant than the information available to the change agent, then resistance may be beneficial.
   e. Fear of increased responsibility: People often worry about having more complex responsibilities placed on them, particularly if they are

unprepared for them. Since communication is the key to understanding, opportunities should be provided for open communication and feedback. Incentives may be helpful in obtaining a commitment to change.

4. **a.** Avoiding: There is awareness of the conflict situation, but the parties involved decide to either ignore the conflict, or avoid, or postpone its resolution. The conflict has not been resolved and may resurface later in an exaggerated form.

   b. Collaborating: This is a joint effort to resolve the conflict with a win–win solution. All parties set aside previously determined goals, determine a priority common goal, and accept mutual responsibility for achieving this goal. This focus on problem solving is based on mutual respect, honest communication, and shared decision making.

   c. Competing: This approach results in a win for one party at the expense of the other group. This win–lose confrontation can leave the loser frustrated, with a desire to "get even" in the future. This strategy may be used when one party has more knowledge regarding the situation, or when resistance is appropriate because of ethical concerns or unsafe patient care practices.

   d. Compromising: For this technique to be effective, both parties must be willing to relinquish something of equal value. If that does not occur, either or both parties may feel that they have lost the conflict and given up more than the other group.

   e. Cooperating/accommodating: One party makes a conscious decision to let the other group win and may collect an "IOU" for use in the future. This party's original loss may result in a more positive outcome in the future.

   f. Smoothing: Smoothing is an effort to compliment the other party and focus on agreement rather than disagreement, thus reducing the emotion in the conflict. The original conflict is rarely resolved with this technique.

5. Leaders have five major sources of power in their power grid. Define the type of power listed below and state the typical reason they fail or succeed.

   a. Coercive power is the "stick" of leadership where staff are sanctioned for failing to comply with the leader's desires. Coercive power relies on fear but rarely inspires nurses to work with a leader for the long term.

   b. Legitimate power emanates from a position or title. It can be short-lived if the leader is ineffective because to be influential, leaders must have followers.

   c. Reward power is based on a leader's ability to give something of value in return for performance. Nurse leaders have reward and recognition power that needs to be used in a meaningful, sustainable, and practical way.

   d. Expert power is built on the individual's specialized knowledge and access to information. Many nurse leaders struggle with giving up their expert power as clinicians when moving into a leadership role.

   e. Referent or relationship power is built on a leader's personal brand. Leaders with referent power are respected and have what is sometimes called "social capital" because people chose to follow them.

APPLYING YOUR KNOWLEDGE
CRITICAL THINKING QUESTIONS

1. Sample answers:
   a. As a leader, how would you handle this situation? You might call a quick huddle to explain the situation and ask for cooperation, state you heard the comment about quitting, and tell the nurses you will advocate for better staffing ratios with the nurse manager and DON. Determine if they would like to assign "buddies" to help each other with breaks or turning; you could assist them where there are gaps in care.

   b. What type of leadership style would you feel most comfortable using? Democratic to listen and autocratic in that changes to staffing will not occur that shift.

   c. What do you anticipate the outcome will be or should be? The nurses will feel heard, supported, and come together to provide safe patient care.

2. Answers will vary with student experience.
3. Answers will vary with student experience.
4. Sample answers:
   a. Communication: Answer questions honestly, respecting the patient's dignity and autonomy.

   b. Problem-solving: Ask the patient what they would like to see happen.

   c. Management: Collaborate with interprofessional team to provide sufficient rest, visitation, and other activities the patient deems important. Attempt to assign the same team of nurses/AP for consistency.

   d. Self-evaluation: Ask yourself if there were other ways to meet the patient and family needs.

REFLECTIVE PRACTICE: CULTIVATING QSEN COMPETENCIES
Sample Answers

1. Patient-centered care/teamwork and collaboration: How might the nurse empower Rehema with the knowledge and ability to be a leader of her peers? The nurse could help Rehema identify her strengths, evaluate how she accomplishes work, clarify her values, and determine how she can contribute to the community by being a leader in her school. The nurse can also empower Rehema by directing her to resources to be knowledgeable about STIs and feel confident in her role as a leader.

2. Patient-centered care/teamwork and collaboration: What would be a successful outcome for Rehema? By next visit, Rehema describes the incidence of STIs and lists interventions to prevent spreading these diseases.

By next visit, Rehema states that she feels confident in her ability to lead a discussion with fellow students on STIs.

3. Patient-centered care/teamwork and collaboration: What intellectual, technical, interpersonal, and/or ethical/legal competencies are most likely to bring about the desired outcome?

Intellectual: Ability to identify leadership skills appropriately and apply personal leadership skills to a variety of patient situations; knowledge of the incidence and prevention of STIs

Interpersonal: Strong people skills; ability to communicate with and instill confidence in patients

Ethical/legal: Ability to advocate for fellow students and their partners, providing them with accurate and sound information

4. Patient-centered care/teamwork and collaboration/safety: What resources might be helpful for Rehema?

Information on STIs, collaboration with the health center, ability to uphold student's dignity and autonomy while focusing on their safety, information on leadership styles and how to propose and overcome resistance to change

---

PRACTICING FOR NCLEX
MULTIPLE-CHOICE QUESTIONS

1. a   **2.** b   **3.** c   **4.** c   **5.** a
6. d

ALTERNATE-FORMAT QUESTIONS
Multiple-Response Questions

1. c, e, f
2. a, c, f
3. b, c, d
4. b, d, f
5. c, d, f

Sequencing Question

1. 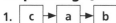 c → a → b

CHAPTER 11

ASSESSING YOUR UNDERSTANDING
FILL IN THE BLANKS

1. outpatient
2. Ambulatory
3. Respite
4. Hospice
5. voluntary
6. therapist
7. primary

8. supply
9. uninsured
10. errors
11. High-reliability
12. Primary
13. consumers

MATCHING EXERCISES
Matching Exercise 1

1. f   **2.** d   **3.** a   **4.** b   **5.** e
6. c

Matching Exercise 2

1. f   **2.** e   **3.** c   **4.** d   **5.** b
6. a

SHORT ANSWER

1. a. DRGs encourage early discharge from the hospital and have created a new acutely ill population who need skilled care at home.
  b. There are increasing numbers of older adults living longer in the community (aging in place) with multiple chronic illnesses.
  c. With more sophisticated monitoring and technology, people can be kept alive and comfortable in their own homes.
  d. Health care consumers demand that services be humane and provisions be made for a dignified death at home.
2. a. Primary care offices: Make health assessments, assist health care providers, administer vaccines, and provide health education.
  b. Ambulatory care centers and clinics: A nurse practitioner may run these centers, which usually provide walk-in services and are open at times other than traditional office hours.
  c. Mental health centers: Nurses who work in mental health/crisis intervention centers must have strong communication and counseling skills, must be thoroughly familiar with community resources specific to the needs of patients being served and the ethical and legal impact of interventions.
  d. Rehabilitation centers: These centers use a health care team composed of health care providers, nurses, physical therapists, occupational therapists, and counselors.
  e. Long-term care centers: Help patients maintain function and independence with concern for the living environment, as well as for the health care provided. Provide direct care, supervise others, serve as administrators, and teach.
3. a. Surgical procedures
  b. Diagnostic tests
  c. Medications
  d. Physical therapy
  e. Counseling
  f. Health education
4. DRGs: Diagnosis-related groups; this plan pays the hospital a predetermined, fixed amount defined by the medical diagnosis or specific procedure rather

than by the actual cost of hospitalization and care. DRGs were implemented by the federal government in an effort to control rising health care costs. If the cost of hospitalization is greater than that assigned, the hospital must absorb the additional cost. However, if the cost is less than that assigned, the hospital makes a profit.

5. When patients come in contact with many different health care providers (e.g., registered nurses, licensed practical nurses, nursing assistants, nurse specialists, physical therapists, dietitians, and students) and are frequently seen by other specialists called in on consultation or to do surgery, the patient may become confused about care and treatment. This fragmentation of care may result in the loss of continuity of care, resulting in conflicting plans of care, too much or too little medication, and higher health care costs.

APPLYING YOUR KNOWLEDGE
CRITICAL THINKING QUESTIONS

1. The nurse assesses which resources are lacking (e.g., windshield survey, community meeting), gains partnership from the community, investigates available resources, plans, and implements for change.
2. Answers will vary with student experience.
3. Answers will vary with student experience.
4. Sample answer: PT provides exercises and recommendations for mobility and ambulation, OT provides ability to maintain ADLs such as cooking, housekeeping; both promote safety. The PA assists and works under the physician; the physician retains the ultimate responsibility for diagnosis and treatment. The social worker uses specialized knowledge related to insurance reimbursement, obtains needed equipment, and can provide counseling; the chaplain provides spiritual guidance and may also provide counseling. The nurse, as a member of the interprofessional team, will interact with all disciplines, and this knowledge will enable the nurse to contact the appropriate team member.
5. Answers will vary with student experience.

REFLECTIVE PRACTICE: CULTIVATING QSEN COMPETENCIES
Sample Answers

1. Patient-centered care: What nursing interventions might the nurse employ to assist Margaret with her caregiver duties?
The nurse can provide Margaret with information about how to access respite care and make referrals for her. However, since Medicaid and most insurance providers do not cover the costs of respite care, the nurse should also check community services that may provide respite care for free. Margaret's husband may qualify for hospice care, and the nurse can arrange for this service.
2. Patient-centered care/safety: What would be a successful outcome for this patient and his wife?

Margaret verbalizes her ability to provide care and maintain the patient's safety. She agrees to respite care and hospice care programs, stating she will accept any services available to her.
3. Patient-centered care: What intellectual, technical, interpersonal, and/or ethical/legal competencies are most likely to bring about the desired outcome?
Intellectual: knowledge of the various types of health care services and settings available to meet the needs of families caring for dying patients
Technical: ability to provide technical assistance to meet the needs of families of patients on hospice
Interpersonal: ability to work with different available resources to ensure everyone's access to safe, quality health care
Ethical/legal: knowledge of ethical and legal principles related to patients with terminal illnesses
4. Patient-centered care/teamwork and collaboration: What resources might be helpful for Margaret?
Home physical therapy and a lift, respite care, hospice services, community services

PRACTICING FOR NCLEX
MULTIPLE-CHOICE QUESTIONS

1. c   2. b   3. d   4. d   5. c
6. c   7. d   8. d   9. b   10. b
11. b

ALTERNATE-FORMAT QUESTIONS
Multiple-Response Questions

1. a, b, e
2. c, d, f
3. a, c, d, e
4. a, b, c, d
5. a, b, d
6. b, e, f

CHAPTER 12

ASSESSING YOUR UNDERSTANDING
FILL IN THE BLANKS

1. community-based
2. religion, race, age, occupation
3. *Healthy People*
4. huddles
5. AMA (or, against medical advice)
6. admission
7. pre-entry
8. Ambulatory
9. Coordination, care
10. **C**oncerned, **U**ncomfortable, **S**afety
11. navigator
12. wristband

CORRECT THE FALSE STATEMENTS

1. F, nurse
2. F, decreasing

3. T
4. T
5. F, copy
6. F, health care provider's order

SHORT ANSWER

1. Sample answers:
  a. Assist the patient or seek permission, check with relatives, neighbors, or fellow members of their house of worship, or club members who could help; if necessary, employ interprofessional collaboration by checking with social worker who will have knowledge of community services.
  b. Describe the procedure to the patient, including sensations the patient may experience or medications such as sedation or anesthesia that are typically given, so they will know what to expect.
  c. Ask the patient about any insurance, Medicare, or Medicaid; check with the social worker to determine whether procedures are covered and what amount the patient will be responsible for. Refer to the appropriate agencies if necessary.

2. This process verifies that all medications have been correctly ordered (or discontinued when warranted) upon admission, with each transfer, and upon discharge, to ensure accuracy as the patient moves through the health care system.

3. **a.** Discharge planning: Exchanges information among the patient, caregivers, and those responsible for home care while the patient is in the institution and after the patient returns home
  b. Interprofessional collaboration: Meets the patient's and family's physical, psychological, sociocultural, and spiritual needs in all settings and at all levels of health
  c. Involving patient and family in planning: Ensures that patient and family needs are consistently met as the patient moves from one level of care to another

4. **a.** Assess the patient's need for nursing care related to admission.
  b. Include consideration of biophysical, psychosocial, environmental, self-care, educational, and discharge planning factors in each patient's assessment.
  c. Involve the patient and family in care as appropriate.
  d. Nursing staff members should collaborate, as appropriate, with health care providers and members of other clinical disciplines to make decisions regarding the patient's need for nursing care.
  e. Assess the need for continuing care in preparation for discharge, and document referrals for such care in the patient's medical record.

5. **a.** Transfer within the hospital setting: Patient's belongings and/or furniture are moved; patient's records are moved or made available electronically; medications must be correctly labeled for the new room; and other departments must be notified as appropriate. Other hospital departments must be notified of the transfer. If transfer is to a new floor, the nurse at the original area gives a verbal report about the patient to the nurse at the new area. The report should include the patient's name, age, providers, admitting diagnosis, surgical procedure (if applicable), current condition and manifestations, allergies, medications and treatments, laboratory data, and any special equipment that will be needed to provide care. Patient goals and nursing care priorities are identified, and the existence of advance directives is noted. Accurate, concise, and complete verbal communication is essential.
  b. Transfer to a long-term facility: All the patient's belongings are carefully packed and sent to the facility; prescriptions and appointment cards for return visits to the health care provider's office may be sent; patient is discharged from hospital setting, but a copy of the chart may be sent to a long-term care facility along with a detailed assessment and care plan.
  c. Discharge from a health care setting: Check patient discharge order, instructions, equipment and supplies, and financial arrangements. Assist the patient to dress and pack belongings; check for written order for future services; transport patient to car and assist as necessary; make necessary recordings on records and complete discharge summary.

6. The patient is informed of any possible risks of leaving. A form must be signed that releases the provider and health care institution from any legal responsibility for the patient's health status; the patient must be informed of risks before signing the form; the signature of the patient must be witnessed; and the form becomes part of the patient's record.

7. Position the bed in its highest position; arrange the furniture in the room to allow easy access to the bed. Open the bed by folding back the top bed linens. Assemble necessary equipment and supplies. Assemble special equipment and supplies (e.g., oxygen therapy equipment) and make sure it is working properly. Adjust the physical environment of the room. The nurse can delegate these tasks to the AP.

8. Sample answers:
  a. Knowledgeable and skilled: A nurse knows the proper procedure for administering IV fluids and competently administers them.
  b. Independent in making decisions: A home health care nurse encounters a situation in which caregiver burden is suspected and schedules respite care for the caregiver.
  c. Accountable: A home health care nurse learns how to perform advanced procedures when caring for acutely ill patients in the home.

9. ISBARQ stands for:
   I: Introduction: The nurses involved in the hand-off identify themselves, their roles, and their jobs.
   S: Situation: The nurse performing the handoff describes the chief complaint, diagnosis, treatment plan, and patient wants and needs.
   B: Background: The nurse performing the hand-off lists the vital signs, mental and code status, medications, and lab results.
   A: Assessment: The nurse performing the handoff gives the current patient provider's assessment of the patient.
   R: Recommendation: The nurse performing the handoff identifies pending lab results and what needs to occur over the next few hours and any other recommendations for care that are appropriate.
   Q: Question and answer: The nurses provide time for questions and answers regarding the patient situation.
   SBAR communication includes only Situation, Background, Assessment, and Recommendation; ISBARQ adds Introduction and Question and answer.

APPLYING YOUR KNOWLEDGE
CRITICAL THINKING QUESTIONS

1. Sample answer:
   The nurse ensures someone is remaining with the patient for 24 hours after anesthesia. The nurse teaches the patient and their support person about new medications including antibiotics and pain medication. Instructions on how to manage the dressing and when to contact the health care provider or return to the hospital are given. The nurse navigator may arrange home PT and follow up with home care to assess the wound and vital signs.

2. Sample answer:
   Determine what the older adult prefers. Investigate needed care. Determine who will safely transfer them into and out of bed, so they do not develop complications of bedrest. Assess who will be home to supervise their care (family or home care aid), meals, toileting, etc. Finally, which environment will be safest?

REFLECTIVE PRACTICE: CULTIVATING QSEN COMPETENCIES
Sample Answers

1. Patient-centered care/safety: How might the admitting nurse respond to the patient, given the intellectual disability, admission, and condition?
   The nurse should speak reassuringly, explaining the admission process and assessing the patient's respiratory system. The nurse should also describe the care that will be provided in simple terms. The patient should have a fall risk assessment and oxygenation checked frequently, to maintain his safety.

2. Patient-centered care/safety: What would be a successful outcome for this patient?
   The nurse ensures the patient is physically safe and tries all means of communication. Respiratory distress, adventitious breath sounds, and/or pulse oximetry readings normalize.

3. Patient-centered care: What intellectual, interpersonal, and/or ethical/legal competencies are most likely to bring about the desired outcome?
   Intellectual: knowledge of intellectual disability and the settings available to meet the needs of a patient with profound intellectual disability
   Interpersonal: ability to establish trusting professional relationships with patients, family/caregivers, and health care professionals in different practice settings to ensure continuity of care
   Ethical/legal: knowledge of the nurse's legal and ethical obligations as patients are transferred between home and different practice settings

4. Teamwork and collaboration/informatics: What resources might be helpful for the nurse working with this patient?
   Information on communicating with patients with intellectual disability, communicating with health care professionals who have worked with Jeff. Documenting the above along with effective communication techniques in the electronic health record.

PRACTICING FOR NCLEX
MULTIPLE-CHOICE QUESTIONS

1. c	**2.** a	**3.** d	**4.** c	**5.** d
6. c				

ALTERNATE-FORMAT QUESTIONS
Multiple-Response Questions

1. a, c, e, f
2. b, c, f
3. c, e
4. b, e, f
5. a, c, f

Sequencing Question

1.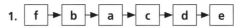

f → b → a → c → d → e

CHAPTER 13

ASSESSING YOUR UNDERSTANDING
FILL IN THE BLANKS

1. patient-centered
2. implementing
3. Quality and Safety Education for Nurses (QSEN)
4. thoughtful
5. evaluation
6. knowledge
7. diagnosing (and analyzing)
8. judgment

9. noticing, diagnosing, intervening, evaluating
10. map
11. Reflective

MATCHING EXERCISES

Matching Exercise 1

1. a	**2.** d	**3.** e	**4.** b	**5.** c
6. a	**7.** e	**8.** b	**9.** c	**10.** e
11. d	**12.** a			

Matching Exercise 2

1. a	**2.** b	**3.** d	**4.** a	**5.** c
6. b				

SHORT ANSWER

1. **a.** Experienced clinicians
   b. Texts and journals
   c. Institutional policies and procedures and professional groups and writings
2. Patient:
   a. Scientifically based, holistic, individualized care
   b. Opportunity to work collaboratively with nurses
   c. Continuity of care
   Nursing:
   a. Achievement of a clear and efficient plan of action by which the entire nursing team can achieve results for patients through collaboration and communication
   b. Satisfaction that the nurse is making an important difference in the lives of patients
   c. Opportunity to grow professionally when evaluating the effectiveness of interventions and variables that contribute positively or negatively to the patient's goal achievement
3. **a.** Determining the need for nursing care: The nursing process provides a framework that enables the nurse to systematically collect patient data and clearly identify patient strengths and problems.
   b. Planning and implementing the care: The nursing process helps the nurse and patient develop a holistic plan of individualized care that specifies mutually agreed upon goals and the nursing actions most likely to assist the patient to meet those goals and execute the care plan.
   c. Evaluating the results of the nursing care: The nursing process provides for evaluation of the care plan in terms of patient goal achievement.
4. **a.** Defining the nursing process: The nursing process is a systematic method that directs the nurse, with the patient's participation, to accomplish the following: (1) assess the patient to determine the need for nursing care, (2) determine nursing diagnoses for actual and potential health problems, (3) identify expected outcomes and plan care, (4) implement the care, and (5) evaluate the results.
   b. Primary goals of the nursing process: The goals of the nursing process are to help the nurse manage each patient's care scientifically, holistically, and creatively to promote wellness, prevent disease or illness, restore health, and facilitate coping with altered functioning.
   c. Skills necessary for successful use of the nursing process: The skills necessary to use the nursing process successfully include intellectual, technical, interpersonal, and ethical/legal skills, as well as the willingness to use these skills creatively when working with patients.
5. Sample answers:
   a. Systematic: Each nursing task is a part of an ordered sequence of activities, and each activity depends on the accuracy of the activity that precedes it and influences the actions that follow it.
   b. Dynamic: There is great interaction and overlapping among the five steps; no one step in the process is a one-time phenomenon; each step is fluid and flows into the next step.
   c. Interpersonal: The human being is always at the heart of nursing. The nursing process ensures that nurses are patient centered rather than task centered.
   d. Outcome oriented: The nursing process offers a means for nurses and patients to work together to identify specific goals related to wellness promotion, disease and illness prevention, health restoration, and coping with altered functioning that are most important to the patient and match them with appropriate nursing actions.
   e. Universally applicable in nursing situations: Once nurses have a working knowledge of the nursing process, they can apply it to well or ill patients, young or old patients, in any type of practice setting.
6. **a.** Purpose of thinking: This helps to discipline thinking by keeping all thoughts directed to the goal.
   b. Adequacy of knowledge: It is important to judge whether the knowledge available to you is accurate, complete, and relevant. If you reason with false information or lack important data, it is impossible to draw a sound conclusion.
   c. Potential problems: As you become more skilled in critical thinking, you will learn to "flag" or remedy pitfalls to sound reasoning.
   d. Helpful resources: Wise professionals are quick to recognize their limits and seek help in remedying their deficiencies.
   e. Critique of judgment/decision: Ultimately, you must identify alternative judgments or decisions, weigh their merits, and reach a conclusion.
7. Sample answers:
   a. Practice a necessary skill until you feel confident in its execution before performing it on a patient.
   b. Take time to familiarize yourself with new equipment before using it in a clinical procedure.
   c. Identify nurses who are technical experts and ask them to share their secrets.
   d. Never be ashamed to seek assistance if you feel unsure of how to perform a procedure or manage equipment.

8. Answers will vary with student experience.
9. Answers will vary with student experience.
10. Sample answers:
   a. "I'm Nurse Brown and I'll be your nurse this week. What would you like to accomplish with this time, and how can I help you get through this period?"
   b. "What family members do you expect to see while you are here? Would you trust them to make decisions about your care if you were unable to do so yourself?"
   c. "What are your goals, hopes, and dreams in life? How do you hope to accomplish them? How will your hospitalization affect these goals?"
   d. "Tell me about your life at home/school/work. Is there anyone or anything in particular that you will miss during your recuperation?"
11. a. Do I know the legal boundaries of my practice?
    b. Do I own my personal strengths and weaknesses and seek assistance as needed?
    c. Am I knowledgeable about, and respectful of, patient rights?
    d. Does my documentation provide a legally defensible account of my practice?
12. a. Open-mindedness: A nurse is open to learning new ideas from a patient.
    b. Profound sense of the value of the person: A nurse goes to bat for a homeless woman who needs medical care.
    c. Self-awareness and knowledge of own beliefs and values: A nurse examines her own beliefs to see how they affect her practice.
    d. Sense of personal responsibility for actions: A nurse is committed to using expertise to provide health care to those who need it.
    e. Caring about well-being of patients and acting accordingly: A nurse is committed to learning new techniques to be the best nurse possible for patients.
    f. Leadership skills: A nurse uses leadership skills to persuade nurses to join professional nursing organizations.
    g. Bravery to question the "system": A nurse questions the staffing choices of a superior after working several shifts short-staffed.

APPLYING YOUR KNOWLEDGE
CRITICAL THINKING QUESTIONS

1. Answers will vary.
2. Begin by assessing that a problem exists, who it affects and if you have the skills to intervene. As a nurse-to-be, you may bring these problems and the data you've collected to campus leaders, if beyond your scope of learning. Nurses have an obligation to participate to their level of practice, act as role models, and answer questions using accurate and up-to-date information.
3. Answers will vary.

REFLECTIVE PRACTICE: CULTIVATING QSEN COMPETENCIES
Sample Answers

1. Patient-centered care/safety: How might the nurse use blended nursing skills to respond to this patient situation?
   The nurse should assess the reasons Charlotte is not attending the planned teaching session. The nurse considers possible reasons including fear, fatigue, lack of knowledge of possible consequences if the wound is not kept clean (i.e., infection), and being overwhelmed with family and work responsibilities. The nurse should use blended skills to advocate for this family and seek out possible resources (such as help from relatives or the community) to help ensure safe care.
2. Patient-centered care/safety: What would be a successful outcome for this patient and her family?
   Charlotte states the importance of proper wound care, demonstrates changing the dressings on her daughter's wound and the consequences (infection, poor wound healing) of omitting this from care.
3. Patient-centered care: What intellectual, technical, interpersonal, and/or ethical/legal competencies are most likely to bring about the desired outcome?
   Intellectual: knowledge of the science of nursing care related to wound care
   Technical: ability to competently change dressings on a wound and teach this skill to the caretaker
   Interpersonal: ability to counsel Charlotte who is finding it difficult to respond to the challenge of caring for her daughter at home
   Ethical/legal: commitment to patient safety and quality care, including the need to report problem situations immediately
4. Teamwork and collaboration/informatics: What resources might be helpful for Charlotte?
   Counseling services, community services, help from relatives or friends, home care/wound care nurse, printed materials on wound care. Document each time you made an appointment to teach Charlotte and all missed appointments, the appearance of the wound and dressings applied.

PRACTICING FOR NCLEX
MULTIPLE-CHOICE QUESTIONS

1. c	2. d	3. b	4. c	5. c
6. d	7. b	8. c	9. b	10. c
11. c	12. d			

ALTERNATE-FORMAT QUESTIONS
Multiple-Response Questions

1. a, b, c
2. c, e, f
3. a, c, d, e
4. b, e, f
5. b, d, e
6. a, b, c, d, e, f

Sequencing Questions

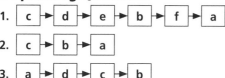

1. c → d → e → b → f → a
2. c → b → a
3. a → d → c → b

CHAPTER 14

ASSESSING YOUR UNDERSTANDING
FILL IN THE BLANKS

1. Critical
2. deductive
3. inductive
4. reasoning
5. judgment
6. Situation(al)
7. noticing
8. NCLEX
9. process
10. cumulative
11. Competency
12. knowledge
13. beginner
14. they
15. ABC

MATCHING EXERCISES

1. d   2. e   3. b   4. f   5. a
6. c

SHORT ANSWER

1. Answers will vary.
2. Answers will vary.
3. Answers will vary.
4. Assessing and noticing are closely aligned; analysis and diagnosis is aligned with interpreting; intervening and responding are also similar. Evaluating or reflect on the patient outcome allows us to return to assessing/noticing. Reflecting in Tanner's model also involves evaluating the nurses' response and becoming aware of areas of practice to strengthen or change in similar situations.
5. Be attentive to accurate assessments and nursing language through practice on varied patients, by reading the electronic health record and asking questions. Ask the primary nurse how they knew what to do, what cues they noticed and how they determined what recommendations they made/will make to the health care provider and, what prompted the nurse to follow up. Be attentive to the roles of all team members as they visit your patient and write in the health record. Start integrating NCLEX-style practice questions into your study plan early in the nursing program to increase comfort with the types of questions that will appear on the licensure exam.

APPLYING YOUR KNOWLEDGE
CRITICAL THINKING QUESTIONS

1. Underline cues you notice in the following scenario.

   You receive a report on a patient admitted with a <u>change in mental status and syncope</u>. The patient has a <u>history of diabetes</u>, and their <u>blood glucose was low upon arrival</u>.

2. "Could you tell me what brought you here today? How are you feeling now? Were you aware your blood glucose level was low? Are you able to check your blood glucose at home with a glucometer? I'd like to review the signs and symptoms of hypoglycemia and its treatment if that's OK with you."

REFLECTIVE PRACTICE: CULTIVATING QSEN COMPETENCIES
Sample Answers

1. Ashley can focus on learning as much as possible about each concept presented in school. As the one responsible for her learning, she can use textbooks, current evidence, and notes to go beyond memorization and ask herself how this is used for patients and how the material can be translated into congruence with the nursing process.
2. The student learns to provide patient-centered care by talking with patients, determining their preferences, values, and knowledge of their health problems. When the student meets the patient, the student has prepared for any procedures, medications, teaching, and documentation needed. The student also observes the patient's nonverbal cues and congruence with what is said and what the patient does.
3. The student attends to all health care professionals that enter the room, seeking an understanding of their roles. Further, the student observes their primary nurse to learn why they reach out to other team members and what the nurse hopes the outcome of these interactions will be. The student can request to follow their patients to other departments to observe the activities and goals to care for each.
4. When participating in care, the student can determine the reason certain care is given and seek to determine if this focuses on safety and current evidence and research. The student can begin a lifelong habit of reading current journal articles.
5. Ashley can use the electronic health record to review previous documentation as part of the data collection and assessment before meeting the patient. She can read other team members consultations and recommendations, learning to recognize patterns for care and written communication. The student can review the EMAR to begin to correlate pharmacologic therapy to the patient condition. Additionally, the student becomes acquainted with electronic sources for evidence based literature and applies this information to practice.

PRACTICING FOR NCLEX

MULTIPLE-CHOICE QUESTIONS

1. b	**2.** c	**3.** b	**4.** c	**5.** b
6. a	**7.** c	**8.** d	**9.** a	**10.** b

ALTERNATE-FORMAT QUESTIONS

Multiple-Response Questions

1. b, c, d, f
2. a, b, c,
3. a, b, c, d, e

Prioritization Question

1. b

CHAPTER 15

ASSESSING YOUR UNDERSTANDING

FILL IN THE BLANKS

1. patient, support, record
2. initial
3. validation
4. PCAM (or, Patient Centered Assessment Method)
5. focused
6. emergency
7. minimum

MATCHING EXERCISES

Matching Exercise 1

1. c	**2.** e	**3.** d	**4.** b	**5.** a
6. f				

Matching Exercise 2

1. O	**2.** S	**3.** O	**4.** S	**5.** S
6. O				

SHORT ANSWER

1. **a.** Make a judgment about a person's health status.
   b. Make a judgment about a patient's ability to manage his or her own health care.
   c. Make a judgment about a patient's need for nursing.
   d. Refer the patient to a health care provider or other health care professional.
   e. Plan and deliver thoughtful, person-centered, holistic nursing care that draws on the patient's strengths and promotes optimum functioning, independence, and well-being.
2. Sample answers:
   a. A nursing student auscultates a blood pressure of 74/50, and asks the instructor to check her assessment because the earlier blood pressure was 122/78
   b. When the patient states one thing, but behavior indicates a different response (denying smoking when the bathroom smells like cigarette smoke)
3. Sample answers:
   a. How have you been feeling recently?
   b. Can you tell me about any health problems you've experienced?
4. **a.** Purposeful: The nurse identifies the purpose of the nursing assessment (comprehensive, focused, emergency, time-lapsed) and then gathers the appropriate data.
   b. Prioritized: The nurse gets the most important information first.
   c. Complete: The nurse identifies all patient data to understand a patient's health problem and develop a care plan to maximize health promotion.
   d. Systematic: The nurse gathers the information in an organized manner.
   e. Accurate: The nurse continually verifies what is heard with what is observed and uses other senses to validate all questionable data.
   f. Relevant: The nurse determines what type of data and how much data to collect for each patient.
   g. Recorded in a standard manner: The nurse records the data according to facility policy so that all caregivers can easily access the data.
5. Sample answers:
   a. Change since previously seen
   b. Cluster of symptoms related to potential complications of their medical problem
   c. Any patient needs
6. **a.** New onset of extreme dyspnea (answers will vary).
   b. S: This is Susan, I'm calling about Mr. Jones who has extreme dyspnea and anxiety.
   c. B: Patient was admitted with an exacerbation of asthma yesterday and does not have nebulizer treatments ordered.
   d. A: VS are T 99.2, P 122, RR 32, BP 156/88, Pulse oximetry reading 90%.
   e. R: Could you please order mini-nebulizer treatments now?
7. **a.** Patient's health orientation: Patients must identify potential and actual health risks and explore habits, behaviors, beliefs, attitudes, and values that influence levels of health.
   b. Patient's developmental stage: Nursing assessments are modified according to the patient's developmental stage.
   c. Patient's culture: When assessing patients from different cultural backgrounds (e.g., racial, ethnic, religious, socioeconomic), nurses must remember all the influences of cultural factors. Consideration of the patient's culture begins with how the nurse approaches the patient and whether the nurse makes direct eye contact or shakes the person's hand.
   d. Patient's need for nursing: Whether the nurse will interact with the patient for a short or long period and the nature of nursing care needs influence the type of data the nurse collects.

APPLYING YOUR KNOWLEDGE

CRITICAL THINKING QUESTIONS

1. Sample questions: "Could you tell me what brought you to the ED today?" "Do you recall feeling dizzy? Your blood sugar on admission was quite low; did you eat today?" "What medications do you take for your diabetes? For other conditions? Any OTC or herbal supplements?" "I see you

have diabetes and a foot ulcer; do you have any other medical history?"
2. Answers will vary.

REFLECTIVE PRACTICE: CULTIVATING QSEN COMPETENCIES
Sample Answers
1. Patient-centered care/safety: How might the nurse facilitate Susan's ability to cope with disability? The nurse should assess the patient's body image and self-esteem needs. Working collaboratively with other members of the health care team, the nurse could then prepare a nursing care plan that specifically addresses these needs.
2. Patient-centered care/safety: What would be a successful outcome for this patient?
By discharge, Susan will verbalize the need to remain physically active, discuss measures for safety with activities, and consider joining a support group if she needs support.
3. Patient-centered care/evidence-based practice: What intellectual, interpersonal, and/or ethical/legal competencies are most likely to bring about the desired outcome?
Intellectual: knowledge of the signs and symptoms of MS, supportive services for patients with MS, information on most current evidence on management and medications for MS
Interpersonal: demonstration of caring and strong communication skills to assist patients with coping with life-changing diagnoses
Ethical/legal: referral to National MS Society for information on disease, support groups or counseling for patient or patient and spouse, strong advocacy skills and a willingness to use them for patients needing assistance or equipment for home
4. Teamwork and collaboration: What resources might be helpful for Susan?
Family counseling, printed materials on MS, support groups

PRACTICING FOR NCLEX
MULTIPLE-CHOICE QUESTIONS
| 1. d | 2. d | 3. c | 4. a | 5. c |
| 6. b | 7. d | 8. d | 9. d | 10. d |

ALTERNATE-FORMAT QUESTIONS
Multiple-Response Questions
1. c, d, f
2. b, c, f
3. c, d, f
4. a, b, e, f
5. a, c, d

Prioritization Questions
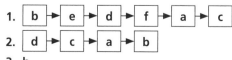
1. b → e → d → f → a → c
2. d → c → a → b
3. b

CHAPTER 16

ASSESSING YOUR UNDERSTANDING
FILL IN THE BLANKS
1. diagnoses
2. analyzes
3. problem
4. prevent (or reduce, resolve)
5. etiology (underlying cause), signs, symptoms
6. collaborative
7. cues
8. standard (or norm)
9. cluster
10. syndrome

MATCHING EXERCISES
| 1. c | 2. a | 3. b | 4. d | 5. a |
| 6. c | 7. d | | | |

CORRECT THE FALSE STATEMENTS
1. F, nursing diagnoses
2. F, standard or norm
3. T
4. F, cluster of significant data
5. F, etiology
6. T
7. T
8. T
9. F, analyzes
10. F, risk

SHORT ANSWER
1. a. Uses legally inadvisable language
   b. √
   c. Identifies responses not necessarily unhealthy
   d. Says the same thing as problem
   e. Identifies problems/etiologies that cannot be altered
   f. √
   g. √
   h. Reverses clauses
   i. Writes diagnosis in terms of needs
   j. Includes a medical diagnosis
2. Sample answers:
   a. Were you able to pass any urine today? Is your urine stream weak or strong?
   b. Can you tell me why you take each of these medications? Do you know which doctors prescribed each of them?
   c. You seem overwhelmed by the changes in your life? Are you feeling powerless to deal with your health problem?
   d. Were you able to get some sleep last night? What do you usually do to help you sleep? Did the noise on the unit keep you awake?
3. Sample answers:
   a. Blood pressure: the nurse determines the presence of hypotension or shock versus hypertension as risk factor for multiple health problems
   b. Growth and development: the nurse assesses patients of all ages to compare their chronological

age to their developmental age to detect problems or plan care

c. Diagnostic laboratory study: deviations from standard/normal values or therapeutic values are used to monitor safe medication use, detect risk factors for diseases

4. a. Are my data accurate and complete?

b. Have I correctly distinguished normal from abnormal findings and decided if abnormal data may be signs and symptoms of a specific health problem?

c. Have I made and validated deductions or opinions that follow logically from patient cues?

d. Has the patient or the patient's surrogates (if able to do so) validated that these are important problems?

e. Have I given the patient or the patient's surrogate an opportunity to identify problems that I have missed?

f. Is each diagnosis supported by evidence? Might these cues signify a different problem or diagnosis?

g. Have I tried to identify what is causing the actual or potential problem and what strengths/resources the patient might use to avoid or resolve the problem?

h. Have I followed facility guidelines to correctly document diagnostic statements in a way that clearly communicates patient problems to other health care professionals?

i. Is this a problem that falls within nursing's independent domain, or does it signify a medical diagnosis or collaborative problem?

5. The two-part health problem provides an underlying cause to direct care, but it lacks the signs and symptoms to support how the nurse concluded that the correct problem was identified like the three-part statement has.

6. Sample answers

a. The home care nurse is visiting Mr. Klinetob, age 86, whose <u>wife of 52 years died 6 months ago</u>. He has degenerative joint disease and has talked for years about having "just a touch of arthritis," which never kept him from being up and about. His family reports <u>he sits in his room and has no desire to engage in self-care activities</u>. He tells the nurse <u>he is "too stiff" in the morning to bathe, and "I just don't seem to have the energy."</u> The nurse notices that <u>his hair is matted and uncombed, his face has traces of previous meals, and he has a strong body odor.</u>
Health problem: Grief (or depression)
Etiology: Death of spouse
Signs and symptoms: Loss of energy, sits in room, does not engage in self-care activities, matted and uncombed hair, food particles on face, and strong body odor

b. Ms. Adams sustained a right-sided stroke that resulted in <u>left hemiparesis</u> (paralysis on the left side of the body) and <u>left-sided "neglect."</u> She <u>ignores the left side of her body</u> and actually denies its existence, <u>stating it belongs to the patient in the next bed.</u> <u>This patient was previously quite active:</u> <u>she walked for 45 to 60 minutes four or five times a week and was an avid swimmer.</u>
Health problem: Unilateral neglect
Etiology: Decreased cerebral perfusion
Signs and symptoms: Left hemiparesis (paralysis), ignores the left side of her body stating it belongs to someone else

APPLYING YOUR KNOWLEDGE
CRITICAL THINKING QUESTION

1. Sample answers:
   Health problem: Impaired gas exchange
   Etiology: Possible infection/inflammation
   Signs and symptoms: Pulse oximetry reading <95%, dyspnea, tachypnea, pallor, reports fear of COVID-19 infection

REFLECTIVE PRACTICE: CULTIVATING QSEN COMPETENCIES
Sample Answers

1. Patient-centered care: What health problem could the nurse consider appropriate for Martin? How might the nurse advocate for Martin to ensure that he gets tested for colon cancer?
   Health problem: Anxiety related to constipation, possible bowel alterations, fear of colon cancer. The nurse suggests guaiac testing of the stool by the health care provider. Also the nurse suggests speaking to the primary care provider to discuss scheduling a colonsocpy and to request a consult with a gastroenterologist.

2. Patient-centered care/safety: What would be a successful outcome for this patient?
   Martin states the warning signs of colon cancer and agrees to schedule a colonoscopy. He discusses appropriate self-management for constipation.

3. Patient-centered care/evidence-based practice: What intellectual, interpersonal, and/or ethical/legal competencies are most likely to bring about the desired outcome?
   Intellectual: knowledge of gastrointestinal elimination, including hemorrhoids and risk factors for colon cancer
   Interpersonal: work collaboratively with other members of the health care team to meet the needs of patients
   Ethical/legal: ability to serve as a trusted and effective patient advocate to counsel patients with bowel alterations

4. Teamwork and collaboration: What resources might be helpful for Martin?
   The nurse reports the findings to the health care provider, works collaboratively with them to resolve the problem. The nurse suggests consultations with other health care professionals (gastroenterologist, dietician) and provides educational materials on colon cancer, diet plans to prevent constipation.

5. Informatics: In what way will the nurse use the electronic health record to document Martin's care?
   The nurse documents the patient's concern about bloody stool, results of the guaiac test, teaching,

and the suggestion to the patient to follow up with a colonoscopy.

PRACTICING FOR NCLEX

MULTIPLE-CHOICE QUESTIONS

1. c   **2.** a   **3.** d   **4.** c   **5.** c
6. b   **7.** a

ALTERNATE-FORMAT QUESTIONS

Multiple-Response Questions

1. b, c, e, f
2. a, b, c, d
3. a, b, d
4. b, c, d, f

Prioritization Questions

1.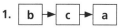

2. a
3. b

CHAPTER 17

ASSESSING YOUR UNDERSTANDING

FILL IN THE BLANKS

1. outcome
2. informal
3. initial, ongoing, discharge
4. patient
5. evaluative (evaluation)
6. evidence-based
7. nurse-initiated
8. (health care) provider–initiated
9. algorithm
10. practice

MATCHING EXERCISE 1

1. f   **2.** c   **3.** d   **4.** b   **5.** e
6. a

MATCHING EXERCISE 2

1. b   **2.** a   **3.** c   **4.** a   **5.** b

MATCHING EXERCISE 3

1. c   **2.** b   **3.** d   **4.** e   **5.** c
6. a

SHORT ANSWER

1. a. Teach patient and parent(s) the proper technique for using an inhaler with spacer; teach indications for use of inhaler.
   b. Walk with patient the length of the hallway at least three times daily, encouraging her to arise slowly and dangle prior to getting out of bed.
   c. Assess patient's weight loss goal; teach patient about "MyPlate," which suggests eating mostly whole grains and vegetables, with lean meats.
2. Pain
3. a. Setting priorities: Before developing or modifying the care plan, the prioritized list of nursing diagnoses should be reviewed to determine whether they are correctly ranked as high priority, medium priority, or low priority.
   b. Writing goals/outcomes that determine the evaluative strategy: For each problem statement in the care plan, at least one goal must be written that, if achieved, demonstrates a direct resolution of the problem statement.
   c. Selecting appropriate evidence-based nursing interventions: Nursing interventions should be consistent with standards of care; realistic; compatible with patient's values, beliefs, and psychosocial background; valued by patient and family; and compatible with other planned therapies.
   d. Communicating the nursing care plan: Nursing orders are in writing and thus communicate to the entire nursing staff and health care team the specific nursing care to be implemented for the patient.
4. A succinct rationale statement demonstrates that the student is deliberately choosing the nursing intervention because of its high probability to effect the desired change. You should always be prepared to explain why you are doing intervention "a" as opposed to intervention "b" or "c." You should know how likely it is that the proposed intervention will achieve the desired outcomes and what the associated risks are.
5. a. Evaluate effectiveness of pain medication for patient every 2 hours.
   b. Assess patient for available friends and family who are supportive of the patient.
   c. Assess patient's room for variety of colors, textures, visual stimulation.
   d. Teach patient to perform daily strengthening exercises and ambulate with the walker.
6. a. Nursing care related to basic human needs: The nursing care plan should concisely communicate to caregivers data about the patient's usual health habits and patterns obtained during the nursing history that are needed to direct daily care (e.g., requires assistance setting up food tray).
   b. Nursing care related to nursing diagnoses: The plan should contain goals/outcomes and nursing interventions for every nursing diagnosis, as well as a place to note patient responses to the care plan; for instance, if the nursing diagnosis is impaired skin integrity related to mobility deficit, a goal should be written to turn patient frequently and assess for skin breakdown.
   c. Nursing care related to the medical and interdisciplinary plan of care: The care plan should record current medical orders for diagnostic studies and specified related nursing care; for instance, if a diagnostic test is scheduled for the morning, appropriate fasting measures should be included in the care plan.
7. a. Have changes in the patient's health status influenced the priority of nursing diagnoses?
   b. Have changes in the way the patient is responding to health and illness or the care

plan affected those nursing diagnoses that can be realistically addressed?

   c. Are there relationships among diagnoses that require that one be worked on before another can be resolved?

   d. Can several patient problems be dealt with together?

8. **a.** Mrs. Myers will state the impact of sugars/simple carbohydrates on blood sugar by beginning 2/16/25.

   b. After viewing video on smoking, Mrs. Gray identifies three dangers of smoking.

   c. √

   d. √

   e. By next visit, patient will state three benefits of psychotherapy.

   f. √

9. Sample answers:

   a. By 11/12/25, patient will consume 2,500 mL of liquid daily; skin turgor will be brisk.

   b. By next visit, patient will discuss her fears with her partner and report a willingness to resume sexual activity.

   c. By 6/4/25, patient will report a decrease in the number of stress incontinent episodes (less than one per day) following performance of pelvic floor exercises.

   d. After receiving medication education, patient reports improved pain control to tolerable level of 3/10 or less.

10. **a.** Set priorities consistent with standards and facility policies, identifying and recording expected patient outcomes, selecting evidence-based nursing interventions, and recording the care plan.

   b. When providing patient-centered care, the goal is to keep the patient and the patient's interests and preferences central in every aspect of planning.

   c. Keep the "big picture" in focus. What are the discharge goals for this patient, and how should this direct each shift's interventions?

   d. Trust clinical experience and judgment but be willing to ask for help when the situation demands more than your qualifications and experience can provide; value collaborative practice.

   e. Respect your clinical intuition, but before establishing priorities, identifying outcomes, and selecting nursing interventions, be sure that research supports your plan.

   f. Recognize personal biases and keep an open mind.

11. **a.** What problems need immediate attention, and what could happen if I wait to attend to them?

   b. Which problems are my responsibility, and which do I need to refer to someone else?

   c. Which problems can be dealt with by using standard plans (e.g., critical paths, standards of care)?

   d. Which problems are not covered by protocols or standard plans but must be addressed to ensure a safe hospital stay and timely discharge?

12. **a.** S: safe

   b. M: measurable

   c. A: attainable

   d. R: realistic

   e. T: time-bound

APPLYING YOUR KNOWLEDGE
CRITICAL THINKING QUESTIONS

1. Sample answers:

   a. Mother states that child will require further testing and chemotherapy; mother will state consequences of chemotherapy on bone marrow and need to protect child from infection; parents will protect child from infection, report symptoms of anemia, thrombocytopenia, and leukopenia.

   b. Patient will state reason for initiation of airborne isolation; patient will consume a balanced diet with sufficient protein (based on patient's usual weight); upon discharge, patient will state the need to continue long-term antitubercular medications.

   c. Patient demonstrates normal mentation and skin turgor after rehydration with normal saline 200 mL/h; blood glucose returns to normal within 24 to 48 hours; upon discharge, patient demonstrates proper use of glucometer.

2. Outcome determination is a critical skill for successfully intervening with patients. If the outcomes specified in the care plan are not valued by the patient or do not contribute to the prevention, resolution, or reduction of the patient's problems or the achievement of the patient's health expectations, the care plan may be ineffective. Similarly, if social determinants of health create barriers that prevent the patient from realizing the outcomes, these need to be explored.

REFLECTIVE PRACTICE: CULTIVATING QSEN COMPETENCIES
Sample Answers

1. Patient-centered care/evidence-based practice: How might the nurse respond to Glenda's questions regarding dietary supplements?
The nurse can teach Glenda about consuming a heart healthy lower-salt diet with healthy fats diet with fruits, vegetables, and complex carbohydrates, such as the DASH or Mediterranean diet. The nurse can encourage her to begin an exercise program, such as walking each day or joining a gym. The nurse could also refer the patient to a dietitian to explain the types of diets and diet supplements that are available, including diets that are healthy and foods to avoid with high blood pressure.

2. Patient-centered care/evidence-based practice: What would be a successful outcome for this patient?
Glenda lists three high-sodium foods, heathy versus "bad" fats and the benefits she looks forward to by following a heart healthy diet and exercising.

3. Patient-centered care/evidence-based practice: What intellectual, technical, interpersonal, and

ethical/legal competencies are most likely to bring about the desired outcome?

Intellectual: knowledge of evidence-based recommendations for needed information to develop a care plan that meets the needs of a patient desiring to improve their overall health and fitness

Technical: ability to use the Internet to research evidence-based literature to obtain knowledge to develop a care plan for the patient

Interpersonal: ability to empathize with patients, sharing their struggles and celebrating their achievement of valued goals

Ethical/legal: ability to serve as a trusted and effective patient advocate who supplies evidence-based recommendations

4. Teamwork and collaboration: What resources might be helpful for Glenda?

Printed materials on healthy diets, exercise plans, referrals to nutritionist or other professionals (such as fitness trainers, gym)

PRACTICING FOR NCLEX

MULTIPLE-CHOICE QUESTIONS

1. d   **2.** a   **3.** c   **4.** b   **5.** c
6. b

ALTERNATE-FORMAT QUESTIONS

Multiple-Response Questions

1. a, c, d, f
2. a, c
3. b, d
4. a, d, f
5. a, d, e, f
6. c, d, f
7. a, b, c, d
8. b, c, e

Prioritization Questions

1.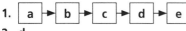
2. d

CHAPTER 18

ASSESSING YOUR UNDERSTANDING

FILL IN THE BLANKS

1. Protocols
2. Standing
3. Community (or public health)
4. indirect
5. Collaborative
6. adverse
7. outcome
8. bundle
9. informatics

MATCHING EXERCISES

1. a   **2.** b   **3.** a   **4.** c   **5.** b
6. c

CORRECT THE FALSE STATEMENTS

1. F, nurse
2. T
3. F, Protocols
4. F, nurse
5. T
6. T
7. T
8. F, insufficient (or not sufficient)
9. F, reassess the strategy
10. T

SHORT ANSWER

1. Sample answers:
   a. Teach patients and families about the interprofessional plan of care and clarify/interpret findings within the nurses' scope of practice.
   b. Prepare patients to participate maximally in the care plan before and after discharge.
   c. Serve as a liaison among the members of the health care team.
2. Sample answers:
   a. Nurse variable: nurse with overwhelming outside concerns
   b. Patient variable: patient who gives up
   c. Health care variable: understaffing causing overworked nurses
3. Sample answers:
   a. Nurses teach and motivate patients, families, and communities to participate actively in seeking health, preventing disease and illness, recovering health, and learning to cope with altered functioning to promote effective self-care.
   b. The nursing actions planned to promote patient goal/outcome achievement and the resolution of health problems should be carefully executed. It is important that the nurse use time wisely to maximize each patient encounter to help the patient achieve his or her goals/outcomes.
4. Sample answer:
   The nurse assesses activities Mr. Franks participated in prior to admission and determine if another resident has similar interests or his interests can be accommodated by the activities team. The nurse uses creativity to engage Mr. Franks and have him show interest in himself and others. If this plan is ineffective, Mr. Franks may need a psychological or psychiatric evaluation to assess for depression or difficulty with adjustment to his new environment.
5. Sample answer:
   Along with receiving care for pregnancy, this patient should receive education on planning economical, nutritious meals. Collaboration with the social worker can assist the patient in locating community or government services that could provide some relief in this area.
6. Sample answers:
   a. Administering a prescribed medication to a patient
   b. Lobbying for a new recreational facility in a long-term care facility

---

   c. Participating in a vaccination campaign at a local mall

7. a. The right task

   b. The right circumstance

   c. To the right person

   d. With the right directions and communication

   e. With the right supervision and education

APPLYING YOUR KNOWLEDGE

CRITICAL THINKING QUESTIONS

1. a. Answers will vary.

   b. Answers will vary.

2. Answers will vary.

REFLECTIVE PRACTICE: CULTIVATING QSEN COMPETENCIES

Sample Answers

1. Patient-centered care: What might be the nurse's response when advocating for Antoinette and her family?
The nurse's first responsibility is to her patient. In this case, the nurse assesses the patient's dietary intake and family life that may contribute to her failure to thrive. The nurse determines if there is an educational need, poverty, or impaired coping regarding a child with developmental delay. A referral to social services may needed to help the family with childcare and resources. The nurse should also investigate any community services available to help this family.

2. Patient-centered care: What would be a successful outcome for this patient?
By next visit, Antoinette is in the normal height and weight for her age and is reaching more appropriate developmental milestones. Antoinette's grandmother states that she will receive help from community services.

3. Patient-centered care: What intellectual, technical, interpersonal, and ethical/legal competencies are most likely to bring about the desired outcome?
Intellectual: knowledge of growth and development, information necessary to implement the nursing interventions that effectively meet the nursing needs of a toddler with physical and developmental delays
Technical: ability to competently adapt procedures and equipment to meet the needs of patients across the life span
Interpersonal: ability to work collaboratively with members of the health care team to implement the interdisciplinary care plan
Ethical/legal: ability to participate as a trusted and effective patient advocate

4. Teamwork and collaboration: What resources might be helpful for this family?
Social services, community services, counseling services, support group for parents of children with disability, nutritional counseling

PRACTICING FOR NCLEX

MULTIPLE-CHOICE QUESTIONS

1. b   **2.** c   **3.** d   **4.** c   **5.** b

6. d   **7.** a   **8.** d

ALTERNATE-FORMAT QUESTIONS

Multiple-Response Questions

1. a, b

2. a, e, f

Prioritization Question

1. b.

CHAPTER 19

ASSESSING YOUR UNDERSTANDING

FILL IN THE BLANKS

1. terminate, modify, continue

2. patient

3. outcome

4. criteria

5. psychomotor, physiologic

6. judgment

7. Standards

8. Clinical

9. quality

10. retrospective

MATCHING EXERCISES

Matching Exercise 1

1. e   **2.** c   **3.** a   **4.** d   **5.** b

Matching Exercise 2

1. a   **2.** b   **3.** b   **4.** a   **5.** a

6. b

SHORT ANSWER

1. Sample answers:

   a. Cognitive: Ask the patient to repeat the information or to apply the new knowledge to their everyday situations, such as stating foods high in sodium.

   b. Psychomotor: Ask the patient to demonstrate the new skill, such as a dressing change.

   c. Affective: Observe the patient's behavior and conversation for signs that the outcomes are achieved. The patient's statement will indicate a change in values or attitudes, such as valuing their health.

2. a. Identifying evaluative criteria: Evaluative criteria are the patient goals/outcomes developed during the planning step and must be clearly identified to determine whether they can be met by the patient.

   b. Determining whether these criteria and standards are met: Because evaluative criteria reflect desired changes or outcomes in patient behavior, and because nursing actions are directed toward these outcomes, they become the core of evaluation to determine whether the plan has been effective.

   c. Terminating, continuing, or modifying the plan: Reviewing each step of the nursing process helps to determine whether goals have been met and whether the plan should be terminated, continued, or modified.

3. Sample answers:
   a. Patient: Is the patient motivated to learn new health behaviors?
   b. Nurse: Do the nurses come to work well rested and ready to help their patients?
   c. Health care system: Is a healthy nurse-to-patient ratio important to the institution?

4. The nurse reevaluates each preceding step of the nursing process for accuracy and may need to monitor patient outcomes more frequently:
   a. If needed, collect new assessment date.
   b. Add or revise diagnoses as needed.
   c. Modify or rewrite patient goals and outcomes.
   d. Revise the nursing orders.

5. Assess the patient's usual and current sleep–rest pattern, anxiety (especially after visitors leave), medications taken; collaborate with the interprofessional team, including the pharmacist and health care providers. Consider PT to promote additional activity during the day, which may promote sleep. Review evidence-based literature for additional ideas.

6. a. Structure: An audit focused on the environment in which care is provided. Evaluation is based on physical facilities and equipment, organizational characteristics, policies and procedures, fiscal resources, and personnel resources.
   b. Process: An audit that focuses on the nature and sequence of activities carried out by the nurse implementing the nursing process. Evaluation is based on acceptable levels of performance of nursing actions related to patient assessment, diagnosis, planning, implementation, and evaluation.
   c. Outcome: Outcome evaluations focus on measurable and demonstrable changes in the health status of the patient or the results of nursing care.

7. a. Delete or modify the nursing diagnosis: After evaluating the data, the nurse may decide the nursing diagnosis is inadequate and delete or change the diagnosis.
   b. Make the goal statement more realistic: The nurse should determine the effectiveness of the goal and adjust the goal to meet the patient's needs.
   c. Adjust the time criteria in the goal statement: If the time period was too short to accomplish the goal, it may need to be extended.

   d. Change nursing interventions: Reevaluate the nursing interventions and change the ones that were ineffective; tailor the interventions to the patient's needs.

8. *Quality by inspection* focuses on finding deficient workers and removing them. Nurses and others working in a setting using this approach may be afraid to admit a mistake or error and wrongly attempt to hide a problem which may result in serious harm to patients. *Quality as opportunity,* on the other hand, focuses on finding opportunities for improvement and fosters an environment that thrives on teamwork, with people sharing the skills and lessons they have learned. This helps create a just culture.
The rest of the answer will vary.

9. a. Nurses measure patient outcome achievement.
   b. Nurses measure how effectively nurses help targeted groups of patients to achieve their specific goals.
   c. Nurses (peer review) or managers measure the competence of individual nurses.
   d. Nurses measure the degree to which external factors, such as different types of health care services, specialized equipment or procedures, or socioeconomic factors, influence health and wellness.

10. The HCAHPS is the Centers for Medicare and Medicaid Services' publicly reported patient satisfaction program. The program provides consumers with information about a hospital's performance in key areas of communication, pain control, timeliness of care, discharge instructions, hospital cleanliness, and treatment with courtesy and respect. The survey was designed to produce data that allow objective and meaningful comparisons of hospitals on topics important to consumers. Public reporting creates new incentives for hospitals to improve quality of care and enhance public accountability through transparency. Are you helping or hurting your hospital? How would patients answer these questions about your interactions: how often did nurses treat you with courtesy and respect, listen carefully to you, and explain things in a way you could understand? During this hospital stay, after you pressed the call button, how often did you get help as soon as you wanted it?

APPLYING YOUR KNOWLEDGE
CRITICAL THINKING QUESTIONS

1. Sample answers:
   a. Broken rules: refusing to use equipment, preferring to adhere to the "way we've always done it." Manager or charge nurse reminds nurse(s) of current evidence and escalates disciplinary process for not following policy or procedure.

b. Mistakes: investigates causes of error, determining whether nurse needs education, there is a process or equipment problem, works with interdepartmental staff to resolve.

c. Lack of support: nurses report short staffing to manager, charge nurse, and DON; they may bring up unionizing.

d. Incompetence: breaks aseptic technique, fails to recognize signs of impending shock in a postoperative patient; determines if nurse is not motivated to learn or needs education. Sets date for follow-up evaluation.

e. Poor teamwork: Manager determines if nurse is not motivated to work as a team or needs education. Holds team meeting, sets date for follow-up evaluation with named individuals.

f. Disrespect: brings incident to nurses' attention; depending on level of incivility and with whom, various levels of discipline may result.

g. Micromanagement: the charge nurse constantly questions nurses' decisions or if they have followed-up on diagnostic tests. Nurse speaks to manager to question if they feel they are not timely in their care; matter may be resolved.

2. Answers will vary.

REFLECTIVE PRACTICE: CULTIVATING QSEN COMPETENCIES

Sample Answers

1. Patient-centered care/safety: What should be the focus of an evaluation of Ms. Otsuki's nursing care plan conducted by the home health care nurse? The nurse should evaluate Ms. Otsuki's understanding of generic and trade names of her medications, especially Lasix and furosemide. The nurse assesses for additional problems with understanding, compliance with the medication regimen, and for polypharmacy in an older adult related to confusion. The nurse asks the patient to consider using a compartmental pillbox, filled weekly by herself and her daughter, as a safety check. A secondary concern is to determine if the patient is capable of managing her health care and medications with only a daily visit from her daughter.

2. Patient-centered care/safety: What would be a successful outcome for this patient? By next visit, Ms. Otsuki states the purposes, dosages, and frequency of administration of the drugs she is taking. She has obtained and filled a weekly pillbox with her daughter. By next visit, the patient verbalizes that she feels comfortable with the medication administration and is receiving help with home management from her daughter and/or the visiting nurse who provides medication teaching and follow-up.

3. Patient-centered care/evidence-based practice: What intellectual, technical, interpersonal, and ethical/legal competencies are most likely to bring about the desired outcome?

Intellectual: Knowledge about pharmacology and polypharmacy, especially in the older adult. Ability to incorporate knowledge of assessment, diagnosing, planning, and implementing nursing care for the underlying disorder and medications
Technical: ability to use a documentation system competently to record the patient's progress toward outcome achievement
Interpersonal: ability to identify and respond to the changing needs of a patient experiencing different alterations in health status
Ethical/legal: commitment to evaluating patient achievement of outcomes in a timely fashion and to addressing whatever is interfering with outcome achievement within the scope of nursing practice

4. Teamwork and collaboration: What resources might be helpful for Ms. Otsuki?
Social services, home nurse care visit, community services, printed materials on the drugs she is taking, compartmentalized pillboxes

PRACTICING FOR NCLEX
MULTIPLE-CHOICE QUESTIONS
1. a **2.** c **3.** b **4.** d **5.** b
6. d **7.** d **8.** d **9.** c **10.** b

ALTERNATE-FORMAT QUESTIONS
Multiple-Response Questions
1. a, e
2. a, b, c
3. c, e, f
4. a, b, d

Prioritization Question
1. a

CHAPTER 20

ASSESSING YOUR UNDERSTANDING
FILL IN THE BLANKS
1. electronic
2. variance (or occurrence)
3. minimum
4. OASIS
5. instrument
6. change-of-shift (or hand-off)
7. incident (or variance or occurrence)
8. conference
9. communication
10. medication
11. graphic
12. background, assessment
13. referral

MATCHING EXERCISES
1. f **2.** c **3.** b **4.** e **5.** d
6. a

SHORT ANSWER

1. **a.** Nursing care data related to patient assessments
    b. Nursing diagnoses or patient needs
    c. Nursing interventions
    d. Patient outcomes

2. **a.** Change-of-shift/hand-off reports: Given by a primary nurse to the nurse replacing them, or by the charge nurse to the nurse who assumes responsibility for continuing care of the patient. Can be written, oral, or audiotaped.
    b. Telephone orders: The nurse transcribes the order on an order sheet, and it must be co-signed by the health care provider within a set time. Similarly, the nurse enters the order into the electronic health record. Used for emergencies, the facilities' policies must be followed regarding telephone orders including a witness when required, and a read-back to the provider.
    c. Transfer and discharge reports: Nurses report a summary of a patient's condition, treatment, and care when transferring or discharging patients.
    d. Reports to family members and significant others: Nurses must keep the patient's family and significant others updated about the patient's condition and progress toward goal achievement.
    e. Incident reports: A tool used by health care agencies to document the occurrence of anything out of the ordinary that results in or has the potential to result in harm to a patient, employee, or visitor.
    f. Conferring about care: To consult with a colleague or interprofessional team member to exchange ideas or to seek information, advice, or instructions.
    g. Consultations and referrals: When nurses detect problems they cannot resolve because the problems lie outside the scope of independent nursing practice, they consult with, or make referrals to other professionals.
    h. Nursing and interdisciplinary team care conference: Nurses and other health care professionals frequently confer in groups to plan and coordinate patient care.
    i. Nursing care rounds: A group of nurses visit selected patients, often at the patient's bedside to gather information, evaluate nursing care, and provide the patient with an opportunity to discuss their care.

3. **a.** Communication: The patient record helps health care professionals from different disciplines who interact with the same patient at different times to communicate with one another.
    b. Care planning: Each professional working with the patient has access to the patient's baseline and updated data and can see how they are responding to the treatment plan from day to day. Modifications of the plan are based on these data.
    c. Quality process and performance improvement: Charts may be reviewed to evaluate the quality of nursing care and the competence of the nurses providing that care.
    d. Research: The record may be studied by researchers to determine the most effective way to recognize or treat specific health problems. The aim is to promote evidence-based practice in nursing and quality health care.
    e. Decision analysis: Information from records review often provides the data needed by strategic planners to identify needs and the means and strategies most likely to address these needs.
    f. Education: Health care professionals and students reading a patient's chart can learn a great deal about the clinical manifestations of health problems, effective treatment modalities, and factors that affect patient goal achievement.
    g. Credentialing, regulation, and legislation: Documentation allows reviewers to monitor health care providers' and the health care facility's compliance with standards governing the profession and provision of care.
    h. Legal documentation: Patient records are legal documents that may be entered into court proceedings as evidence and play an important role in implicating or absolving health providers charged with improper care.
    i. Reimbursement: Patient records are used to demonstrate to payers that patients received the intensity and quality of care for which reimbursement is being sought.
    j. Historical document: Because the notations in patient records are dated, they provide a chronologic account of services provided. Obtaining patient's old medical records can provide context for current problems.

4. **a.** Nurses should identify themselves and the patient and state their relationship to the patient.
    b. Nurses should report concisely and accurately the change in the patient's condition and what has already been done in response to this change.
    c. Nurses should report the patient's current vital signs and clinical manifestations.
    d. Nurses should have the patient record at hand so that knowledgeable responses can be made to the health care provider's inquiries.
    e. Nurses should record concisely the time and date of the call, what was said to the health care provider, and the health care provider's response and read back any changes to the orders.

5.

Documentation Method	Description/Advantages/Disadvantages
SOURCE-ORIENTED RECORD	**Description:** Each health care group keeps data on its own separate form. Notations are entered chronologically, with most recent entry being nearest the front of the record. **Advantages:** Each discipline can easily find and chart pertinent data. **Disadvantages:** Data are fragmented, making it difficult to track problems chronologically with input from different groups of professionals.
PROBLEM-ORIENTED MEDICAL RECORDS	**Description:** Organized around a patient's problems; contributes collaboratively to care plan. SOAP is used to organize data entries in the progress notes. **Advantages:** Entire health care team works together in identifying a master list of patient problems and contributes collaboratively to care plan. **Disadvantages:** Some nurses believe that the SOAP method focuses too narrowly on problems and advocate a return to the traditional narrative format.
PIE—PROBLEM, INTERVENTION, EVALUATION	**Description:** Unique in that it does not develop a care plan; the care plan is incorporated into the progress notes in which problems are identified by a number. A complete assessment is performed and documented at the beginning of each shift. **Advantages:** It promotes continuity of care and saves time since there is no separate care plan. **Disadvantages:** Nurses need to read all the nursing notes to determine problems and planned interventions before initiating care.
FOCUS CHARTING	**Description:** Its purpose is to bring the focus of care back to the patient and the patient's concerns. A focus column is used that incorporates many aspects of a patient and patient care. The focus may be a patient strength, problem, or need. **Advantages:** Holistic emphasis on the patient and patient's priorities; ease of charting. **Disadvantages:** Some nurses report that DAR categories (Data, Action, Response) are artificial and not helpful when documenting care.
CHARTING BY EXCEPTION	**Description:** Shorthand documentation method that makes use of well-defined standards of practice; only significant findings or "exceptions" to these standards are documented in the narrative notes. **Advantages:** Decreased charting time, greater emphasis on significant data, easy retrieval of significant data, timely bedside charting, standardized assessment, greater communication, better tracking of important responses, and lower costs. **Disadvantages:** None noted.
CASE MANAGEMENT MODEL	**Description:** Interdisciplinary documentation tools clearly identify those outcomes that select groups of patients are expected to achieve on each day of care. Collaborative pathway is part of a computerized system that integrates the collaborative pathway and documentation flowsheets designed to match each day's expected outcomes. **Advantages:** Reduced charting time by 40% and increased staff satisfaction with the amount of paperwork from 0% to 85%. **Disadvantages:** Works best for "typical" patients with few individualized needs.
OCCURRENCE OR VARIANCE CHARTING	**Description:** Variances from the plan are documented; for example, when a patient fails to meet an expected outcome, or a planned intervention is not implemented in the case management model. **Advantages:** Decreased charting time; only variances are charted. **Disadvantages:** Loss of individualized care.
ELECTRONIC HEALTH RECORDS	**Description:** Comprehensive computer systems have revolutionized nursing documentation in the patient record. **Advantages:** The nurse can call up the admission assessment tool and key in the patient data, develop the care plan using computerized care plans, add new data to the patient data base, receive a work list showing treatments, procedures, and medications, and document care immediately. **Disadvantages:** Policies should specify what type of patient information can be retrieved, by whom, and for what purpose (privacy).

6. Sample answer:
Draw a single line through the error, write "mistaken entry"; add correct information; date and initial the entry. If you record information in the wrong chart, write "mistaken entry—wrong chart" and sign off. Follow similar guidelines in electronic records.

APPLYING YOUR KNOWLEDGE
CRITICAL THINKING QUESTIONS

1. Provide responses with empathy for the difficult decision the daughter made to place her mother in long-term care and the physical pain her mother endured after fracturing her hip. Educate the daughter on best practices and accreditation standards related to physical and chemical restraints, explaining the various safety mechanisms including bed alarms and keeping the bed very low to the floor. Additionally, many facilities use a certain color socks or gown to indicate the patient is a fall risk. If the patient is very restless or agitated, a family care conference can discuss pharmacologic intervention.
2. The nurse summarizes the patient's history and progress since admission, describes the patient's current mobility, independence, and emotional response to the amputation.
3. Answers will vary.

REFLECTIVE PRACTICE: CULTIVATING QSEN COMPETENCIES
Sample Answers

1. Patient-centered care/safety: What should be the focus of discharge teaching for Phillippe and his wife?
The nurse should provide a report of Phillippe's condition and care that concisely summarizes all the patient data that his wife will need to provide immediate care. Safety issues, such as not driving for 24 hours after sedation, reporting bleeding, and resuming their previous diet as indicated are included. Any medications and follow-up appointments should be discussed and written in the discharge summary.
2. Patient-centered care/safety: What would be a successful outcome for this patient?
The patient and his wife state that they will make a follow-up appointment that day. They indicate that they will call the health care provider for bleeding and that Phillippe can eat when he returns home.
3. Patient-centered care/evidence-based practice: What intellectual, interpersonal, and ethical/legal competencies are most likely to bring about the desired outcome?
Intellectual: assessment of aspirin or anticoagulants before the procedure (a contraindication to proceed), knowledge of colonoscopy as a diagnostic measure, and need for follow-up; most current

evidence regarding removing polyps and frequency of reexamination.
Interpersonal: ability to demonstrate that what matters is communicating the care plan so that coordination of care is achieved
Ethical/legal: ability to incorporate ethical and legal principles that guide decision making related to a patient needing discharge teaching
4. Teamwork and collaboration/informatics: What resources might be helpful for this patient? Discharge teaching including medication, diet, activity, and follow-up appointments. In many hospitals, the patient can make an appointment through the electronic patient portal.

PRACTICING FOR NCLEX
MULTIPLE-CHOICE QUESTIONS

1. d	**2.** d	**3.** c	**4.** b	**5.** b
6. c	**7.** a	**8.** c	**9.** c	

ALTERNATE-FORMAT QUESTIONS
Multiple-Response Questions

1. a, d, f
2. a, b, e, f
3. c, d, e, f
4. a, c, f
5. b, e, f
6. a, b, c, d, e

Ordered Response

1.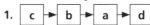

Prioritization Question

1. b

CHAPTER 21

ASSESSING YOUR UNDERSTANDING
FILL IN THE BLANKS

1. clinical information system
2. electronic health record
3. informatics
4. superuser
5. usability
6. portal
7. data visualization
8. Big
9. environmental
10. unit

MATCHING EXERCISES
Matching Exercise 1

1. a	**2.** e	**3.** f	**4.** d	**5.** b
6. c				

Matching Exercise 2

1. e	**2.** a	**3.** c	**4.** b	**5.** d
6. f				

SHORT ANSWER

1. **a.** Improve quality, safety, efficiency, and reduce health disparities
   b. Engage patients and family
   c. Improve care coordination and population and public health
   d. Maintain privacy and security of patient health information
2. **a.** Better clinical outcomes
   b. Improved population health outcomes
   c. Increased transparency and efficiency
   d. Empowered people
   e. More robust research data on health systems
3. **a.** Data: Discrete entities that are described without interpretation
   b. Information: Data that have been interpreted, organized, or structured
   c. Knowledge: Information that is synthesized so that relationships are identified
   d. Wisdom: Appropriate use of knowledge to manage and solve human problems
4. Sample answers:
   a. Analyze and plan: The nurse questions the advantages and disadvantages of switching to an electric health record system and how it will affect the current nursing workflow. The nurse analyzes the data and strategizes with colleagues to help implement the change.
   b. Design: The nurse helps to design a new work area that incorporates the use of new, upgraded computers and mobile computers to create and access electronic health records.
   c. Test: The nurse collaborates with coworkers to create a testing plan that includes the use of testing scripts to ensure all components of the system are working as designed.
   d. Train: The head nurse schedules an in-service to train all employees involved in the use of EHRs. The nurse incorporates the five steps of ADDIE (analysis, design, development, implementation, and evaluation), in the training development process.
   e. Implement: The nurse ensures all testing and training has been completed, end users have been educated, and support resources are ready for any questions that arise prior to "flipping the switch." Nurse superusers are available to assist if help is needed.
   f. Maintain: The nurse oversees the new technology and keeps the system up and running through the allocation of resources and attention to detail.
   g. Evaluate: The nurse takes steps to evaluate the effectiveness of the EHR and how it has improved the practice.
5. **a.** Usability: The extent to which a product can be used by specified users to achieve specified goals with effectiveness, efficiency, and satisfaction in a specified context of use. Making clinical systems easy to use, intuitive, and supportive of nurses' workflow is what usability is all about. Comprehensive tools for usability evaluation can be found through a number of sources both internal and external to the health care IT industry.
   b. Optimization: Strategies to improve processes, maximize effective use, reduce errors, reduce costs, eliminate workflow inefficiencies, improve clinical decision support, and improve end-user skills and satisfaction with the system. Nurses in all settings can participate in organization-wide committees that discuss and make recommendations for improvements to the system.
   c. Standard terminologies: Nursing terminologies identify, define, and code care delivery concepts in an organized structure to represent nursing knowledge. Without the ability to aggregate and analyze data entered into the EHR, it is a challenge to represent nursing's contribution to patient outcomes and to the organization's bottom line.
   d. Interoperability: The ability of a system to exchange electronic health information with and use electronic health information from other systems without special effort on the part of the user. This means that all people, their families, and health care providers should be able to send, receive, find, and use electronic health information in a manner that is appropriate, secure, timely, and reliable to support the health and wellness of people through informed, shared decision making. With the right information available at the right time, people and caregivers can be active partners and participants in their health and care.
   e. Security and privacy: Nurses are responsible to minimize the risk of harm to patients and providers through both system effectiveness and individual performance. Ensuring secure and appropriate access to clinical systems starts with good management of passwords.
6. **a.** Better health outcomes
   b. Chronic condition management
   c. Timely access to care
   d. Patient retention
   e. Patient-centered medical home recognition
7. **a.** Telehealth: continuing medical education, provider training
   b. Telecare: exercise tracking tool, medication reminder systems
   c. Telemedicine: conducting diagnostic tests, accessing specialists not from the patient's geographical area

APPLYING YOUR KNOWLEDGE
CRITICAL THINKING QUESTIONS

1. Answers will vary.
2. Sample answer:
   If a colleague posted a sticky note on a workplace computer, removing it and returning it to them is prudent. Remind them that anyone who has access

to their entries in the electronic health record or other areas of the information system, can chart with their identity and they would have difficulty proving the documentation, if false or not consistent with standards, was entered by another party.

3. Sample answer:
Data can be obtained from medical devices such as physiologic/ hemodynamic monitors; radiology, laboratory, and pathology systems; ventilators; wearable devices; blood glucose monitors, financial databases; genomics information; open sources; patient portals; real-time location systems; smart pumps; social media. Examples of data retrieval that impact care/safety: Nurses frequently bypass alerts and guardrails on IV pumps, leading to errors. The questions of whether the process is too burdensome, there are too many screens or education is necessary can be explored. Risk and intervention: remote blood glucose monitoring allows the nurse to intervene where potentially dangerous patterns of high or low blood glucose exist.

REFLECTIVE PRACTICE: CULTIVATING QSEN COMPETENCIES

1. Patient-centered care/safety: What should be the focus of an evaluation of Frank's nursing care plan. How can informatics be of help in this case?
The nurse can use historical electronic health records to determine the causes of the four recent admissions and include them in the care plan. Frank may require a home care nurse to assess his oxygenation, a home health aide to assist with ADLs, hygiene, and meals. If he wears or needs home oxygen, oxygen safety and long tubing (a trip hazard) to reach the bathroom and kitchen is needed. Frank would be identified as high risk for readmission based on population health analytic tools, directing appropriate referrals.

2. Patient-centered care/safety: What would be a successful outcome for this patient?
After receiving home health care visits, Frank states that he is taking his medicine daily, the aide has prepared meals for him to warm, he is eating more regularly, and his energy and activity level has increased. He is hoping to continue to gain energy so he can go outside when the home health aide is present.

3. Patient-centered care/evidence-based practice: What intellectual, technical, and interpersonal competencies are most likely to bring about the desired outcome?
Intellectual: knowledge of the effects of COPD on the body, best practices to relieve breathlessness and manage other symptoms of COPD
Technical: ability to use informatics technology to identify Frank as a high-risk patient
Interpersonal: ability to work with Frank in a trusting relationship to help him receive the care and services he needs

4. Teamwork and collaboration/informatics: What resources might be helpful for Frank?

Home health care nursing services to assess and plan care, home health aide for ADLs, social services, respiratory therapist visits, home PT for reconditioning.

PRACTICING FOR NCLEX
MULTIPLE-CHOICE QUESTIONS

| 1. d | 2. c | 3. b | 4. b | 5. a |
| 6. a | 7. c | 8. a | 9. a | 10. b |

Multiple-Response Questions

1. a, b, e
2. b, e
3. b, c, d, e

Sequencing Questions

1.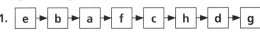

2.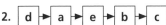

CHAPTER 22

ASSESSING YOUR UNDERSTANDING
FILL IN THE BLANKS

1. proximodistal
2. genital
3. 1, faith
4. adult
5. Pharmacogenetics
6. assimilation
7. operational
8. self, roles
9. chromosomes
10. thrive

MATCHING EXERCISES
Matching Exercise 1

| 1. b | 2. g | 3. e | 4. h | 5. g |
| 6. a |

Matching Exercise 2

| 1. c | 2. f | 3. a | 4. d | 5. b |
| 6. e |

CORRECT THE FALSE STATEMENTS

1. T
2. F, regular and predictable
3. F, different
4. T
5. F, id
6. T
7. T
8. F, preconventional level, stage 1, punishment and obedience orientation
9. F, 29 and 34
10. T
11. T
12. T

SHORT ANSWER

1.

Theorist and Theory	Basic Concepts of Theory	Stages of Development
EXAMPLE **Sigmund Freud** Psychoanalytic theory	Stressed the impact of instinctual drives on determining behavior: unconscious mind, the id, the ego, the superego, stages of development based on sexual motivation.	Oral stage Anal stage Phallic stage Latent stage Genital stage
Erik Erikson Psychosocial theory	Based on Freud, expanded to include cultural and social influences in addition to biologic processes: 1. Stages of development 2. Developmental goals or tasks 3. Psychosocial crises 4. Process of coping	Trust vs. mistrust Autonomy vs. shame/doubt Initiative vs. guilt Industry vs. inferiority Identity vs. role confusion Intimacy vs. isolation Generativity vs. stagnation Ego integrity vs. despair
Robert J. Havighurst Developmental tasks	Living and growing are based on learning; person must continually learn to adjust to changing social conditions, developmental tasks.	Infancy and early childhood Middle childhood Adolescence Young adulthood Middle adulthood Later maturity
Roger Gould Psychosocial development	Gould studied men and women between the ages of 16 and 60 years, labeling the central theme for the adult years as "transformation," with specific beliefs and developmental phases.	Ages 18 to 22 Ages 22 to 28 Ages 29 to 34 Ages 35 to 43 Ages 43 to 50 Ages 50 to 60
Daniel Levinson Moral development	Levinson and associates (1978) based their theory on the organizing concept of "individual life structure." The theory centered on the belief that the pattern of life at any point in time is formed by the interaction of three components: the self (values, motives), the social and cultural aspects of one's life (family, career, religion, ethnic background), and the set of roles in which one participates (husband, father, friend, student).	Early adult transition Entering the adult world Settling down Midlife transition The pay-off years
Jean Piaget Cognitive development	Learning occurs as result of internal organization of an event, which forms a mental schema and serves as a base for further schemata as one grows and develops.	Sensorimotor stage Preoperational stage Concrete operational stage Formal operational stage
James Fowler Faith development	Theory of spiritual identity of humans; faith is reason one finds life worth living; six stages of faith.	Intuitive–projective faith Mythical–literal faith Synthetic–conventional faith Individuative–reflective faith Conjunctive faith Universalizing faith

2. **a.** Preconventional level: Follows intuitive thought and is based on external control as child learns to conform to rules imposed by authority figures. Example: Child learns that he will be sent to his room if he writes on the walls.
   b. Conventional level: This level is obtained when a person becomes concerned with identifying with significant others such as parents and shows conformity to their expectations. Example: A college student gets all As in college so their parents will think highly of them.
   c. Postconventional level: This level is associated with moral judgment that is rational and internalized into one's standards or values. Example: A bank teller resists the urge to steal money from a customer's account because it is against the law.
3. Sample answer: Kohlberg's theory focuses on cultural effects on perceptions of justice or interpersonal relationships and Gilligan's the male morality of justice. However, Gilligan also speaks to women's moral development–based ethic of care.
4. Sample answers:
   a. Freud: The 6-year-old is between the phallic and latency stage and will be experiencing increased interest in biologic sex differences and conflict and resolution of that conflict with parent of same sex.
   b. Erikson: The 6-year-old is becoming achievement oriented, and the acceptance of parents and peers is paramount.
   c. Havighurst: The 6-year-old is ready to learn the developmental tasks of developing physical skills, wholesome attitudes toward self, getting along with peers, sexual roles, conscience, morality, personal independence, etc. An illness could stall these processes.
   d. Piaget: The 6-year-old is in the preoperational stage, including increased language skills and play activities allowing child to better understand life events and relationships.
   e. Kohlberg: Moral development is influenced by cultural effects on perceptions of justice in interpersonal relationships. Moral development begins in early childhood and could be affected by a traumatic illness.
   f. Gilligan: Females develop a morality of response and care, level 1 being selfishness: a woman may tend to isolate herself to avoid getting hurt.
   g. Fowler: The 6-year-old is in stage 1—intuitive–projective faith. Children imitate the religious gestures and behaviors of others, primarily their parents, without a thorough understanding of them.
5. **a.** Superego
   b. Identity versus role confusion
   c. Formal operations stage
   d. Synthetic–conventional faith

6. Sample answer: The family plays a vital role in wellness promotion and illness prevention. Family values and cultural heritage influence interpretation of illness. A health problem of any family member can affect the remainder of the unit. Many health practices are shared by the family. Sometimes, the family may be the cause of illness.

APPLYING YOUR KNOWLEDGE
CRITICAL THINKING QUESTIONS
1. Answers will vary by theory.
   Toddler: Toddlerhood spans trust versus mistrust and autonomy versus shame and doubt where uncertainty; development of hope. This child explores the limits of abilities so that safety and fall prevention is a priority. They develop a will and will begin to anticipate events such as painful procedures. The child will need to know that the surgeon will make her "better," there will be a bandage on her chest, she will get medicine if she has an "ouchie," her mommy and daddy can stay with her, and she will have to do exercises for breathing. Painful procedures would not be performed in her bed, rather in a treatment room, when possible.
   School-aged child: Erikson's concrete operational stage: Develops logical thinking; incorporates others' perspectives; uses abstract thinking and deductive reasoning; tests beliefs to establish values. Will be curious about equipment and procedures, can ask questions about the importance (and danger) of the heart and surgery. Will likely follow directions not to pull out tubes, drains, monitor wires. May want to see religious leader or pray with family before the procedure. This child spans the formal operational stage where they adopt life-guiding values or religious practices.
   Adolescent: Is able to understand much of what an adult would about the surgery and postoperative recovery. *Identity versus role confusion where thy will explore personal identity and a sense of self; development of fidelity. They span intimacy versus isolation (young adulthood):* Development of happy relationships and a sense of commitment, safety, and caring; development of love. Will likely miss their friends or want them to visit, resume activities quickly and see friends. A telephone or tablet to keep in touch, when able will be helpful.
2. Answers will vary with student experience.

REFLECTIVE PRACTICE: CULTIVATING QSEN COMPETENCIES
Sample Answers
1. Patient-centered care/safety: What developmental considerations may affect care planning for Joseph? The developmental tasks of later adulthood include adjusting to decreasing physical strength and health, adjusting to retirement and reduced

income, and establishing physical living arrangements. The nurse assesses the patient's self-esteem needs related to his feelings of dependency on health care providers and his family. The nurse bases the care plan on interventions to foster feelings of personal dignity and worth, such as offering choices of times for ADLs, meals, procedures. The nurse validates his role as head of household and his ability to care for himself and others, offering education about recovery from hip fracture and how he can still care for others in nonphysical ways until he recovers. The nurse emphasizes proper use of assistive devices such as a walker, to help restore his independence.

2. Patient-centered care/safety: What would be a successful outcome for this patient?
Joseph states that he is willing to participate in his care plan and work toward accepting the assistance of others when necessary. He is free from falls, injury, uses assistive devices correctly.

3. Patient-centered care/evidence-based practice: What intellectual, technical, interpersonal, and/or ethical/legal competencies are most likely to bring about the desired outcome?
Intellectual: ability to apply knowledge of developmental theories to nursing care planning, follow standardized care plan/clinical pathway for hip fracture as a framework for care and quality, anticipates need for pain management. Also suggests nutritional intake to promote wound healing.
Technical: ability to provide dressing changes, pain management, discharge teaching as needed
Interpersonal: ability to use therapeutic communication to meet the patient's emotional and spiritual needs; validates the patient's dignity and worth especially at this time of decreased mobility
Ethical/legal: ability to advocate for Joseph's unmet developmental needs

4. Teamwork and collaboration: What resources might be helpful for Joseph and his family?
Home health care services, home physical therapy post discharge, raised toilet seat and assistive devices per surgeon and PT, community services.

PRACTICING FOR NCLEX
MULTIPLE-CHOICE QUESTIONS

1. a	**2.** b	**3.** a	**4.** c	**5.** b
6. c	**7.** c	**8.** d	**9.** a	**10.** c
11. b				

ALTERNATE-FORMAT QUESTIONS
Multiple-Response Questions

1. b, d, e
2. a, c, d
3. b, d, e
4. a, c, f

Sequencing Questions

1. c → e → b → a → d
2. c → b → e → a → d → f

Prioritization Question

1. a

CHAPTER 23

ASSESSING YOUR UNDERSTANDING
FILL IN THE BLANKS

1. endoderm
2. embryonic
3. Apgar
4. bonding
5. failure, thrive
6. Developmental
7. toddlers
8. type 2 diabetes
9. Adolescence

MATCHING EXERCISES
Matching Exercise 1

1. f	**2.** d	**3.** d	**4.** f	**5.** a
6. e	**7.** c			

SHORT ANSWER

1. **a.** P
   b. A
   c. I
   d. N
   e. N
   f. T
   g. T
   h. A
   i. S
   j. A
2. **a.** I
   b. S
   c. A
   d. S
   e. S
   f. A
   g. A
   h. T
   i. P
3. **a.** Pre-embryonic stage: Lasts about 3 weeks; zygote implants in the uterine wall and has three distinct cell layers: ectoderm, endoderm, and mesoderm.
   b. Embryonic stage: fourth to eighth week; rapid growth and differentiation of the germ cell layers, all basic organs established, bones ossify, and human features are recognizable.

c. Fetal stage: 9 weeks to birth; continued growth and development of all body organs and systems take place.

4. a. Gross motor behavior and skills
b. Fine motor behavior and skills
c. Language acquisition
d. Personal and social interaction

5. Sample answers:
a. "Easy": Infant sleeps, eats, and eliminates easily; smiles spontaneously; cries in response to significant needs.
b. "Slow to warm": Infant is more passive and distant than the "easy" infant.
c. "Difficult": Infant has volatile and labile responses, often is a restless sleeper, is highly sensitive to noises, and eats poorly.

6. a. Colic is inconsolable crying or fussing in an infant that lasts more than 3 hours, occurs more than 3 days per week, and lasts for more than 3 weeks, although the more-than-3-weeks pattern is not always considered in the determination of colic. Colic durations tend to be high across the first 6 weeks of life (17% to 25%) and then decrease between 6 and 12 weeks of life (11%), then down to 0.6% at 10 to 12 weeks. The nurse should educate the parents about colic and teach them measures to help relieve the symptoms.
b. Failure to thrive is a condition of inadequate growth in height and weight resulting from the infant's inability to obtain or use calories needed for growth. Collection of serial height, weight, and head circumference measurements on a reference scale such as a growth chart are helpful in determining this clinical finding. Underlying physical causes should be ruled out first; if the cause is psychosocial, specialized health interventions are warranted.
c. Sudden infant death syndrome (SIDS) refers to the sudden death of an infant under the age of 1 year when consideration of the infant's history, a postmortem examination, and investigation of the scene where the death occurred fails to reveal a cause of death. Sudden unexpected infant death syndrome (SUID) is an all-encompassing term used for sudden, unexplained infant deaths where the cause of death cannot readily be identified prior to an investigation. The rate of infant deaths attributed to SIDS has declined significantly since the early 1990s when the Safe to Sleep campaign promoted placing infants on their back to sleep rather than in the prone position.
d. Child maltreatment and adverse childhood experiences are any recent act or failure to act on the part of a parent or caretaker which result in death, serious physical or emotional harm, sexual abuse or exploitation; or an act or failure to act which presents an imminent risk of serious harm. Health care professionals must recognize and report abuse of children and provide interventions for high-risk families.
e. Accidents—such as motor vehicle crashes, poisonings, burns, drowning, choking and aspirations, and falls—are the major cause of death in toddlers. While choking is a hazard for infants, the toddler's mobility and increasing independence heightens this risk. Parents need education to prevent and intervene when a child is choking.

7. Sample answers:
a. Toddler: A toddler begins to understand object permanence, following simple commands and anticipating events. The perception of body image begins, and the toddler uses short sentences. The nurse should be aware that the toddler may experience separation anxiety; parents should be included in the preparation; language should be clear and simple.
b. Preschooler: A preschooler may have fear of pain and body mutilation, as well as separation anxiety that must be recognized by the nurse. The child needs much reassurance and parental support. A preprocedure visit should be scheduled if possible; allowing the child to practice on a doll may be helpful.
c. School-aged child: Body image, self-concept, and sexuality are interrelated. The school-aged child has well-developed language skills and ability to store information in long-term memory. The procedure should be explained clearly and thoroughly to child and caregivers.
d. Adolescent and young adult: The adolescent tries out different roles, personal choices, and beliefs in the stage called identity versus role confusion. Self-concept is being stabilized, with the peer group acting as the influential body. The nurse should be aware of the adolescent's need to understand the procedure and its benefits/risks.

8. Sample answers:
a. Infant: The most important role of the nurse is the prevention of illness and promotion of wellness through teaching family members. Teaching may range from scheduling immunizations to counseling parents who have a baby born with AIDS.
b. Toddler: The role of the nurse is in wellness promotion, helping caregivers find the means of helping toddlers through encouraging independence while setting firm limits. Safety measures for parents of active toddlers should be taught.
c. Preschooler: Promoting wellness continues for the preschooler, with emphasis on teaching accident prevention and safety, infection

control, dental hygiene, and play habits and encouraging self-esteem.

d. School-aged child: Areas of concern for school-aged children are traffic, bicycle, and water safety. Substance abuse teaching should be included, and communicable conditions should be discussed. Nurses should work with parents and teachers to recognize mental health disorders and to encourage physical fitness and positive self-identity.

e. Adolescent and young adult: Nurses should educate adolescents and family members about substance abuse, motor vehicle accidents, nutrition, and sex. Nurses and parents should be aware of the adolescent's need to belong to a peer group, be like everyone else, and try on different roles.

9. a. Prepubescence: Secondary sex characteristics begin to develop, but the reproductive organs do not yet function.

b. Pubescence: Secondary sex characteristics continue to develop, and ova and sperm begin to be produced by the reproductive organs.

c. Postpubescence: Reproductive functioning and secondary sex characteristics reach adult maturity.

10. a. Meningococcal conjugate
b. Hepatitis B
c. TDAP

APPLYING YOUR KNOWLEDGE
REFLECTIVE PRACTICE: CULTIVATING QSEN COMPETENCIES
Sample Answers

1. Patient-centered care/evidence-based practice: What should be the focus of the nursing care plan developed for Darlene?
The immediate focus should be the health habits of the mother and their effect on the fetus. The nursing care plan should include education regarding the detrimental effects of smoking and drinking alcohol on the fetus, the necessity to control nausea, and eat a protein-rich diet. She could benefit from a referral to counseling and/or social services, including shelter.

2. Patient-centered care/evidence-based practice: What would be a successful outcome for this patient?
By the end of the visit, the patient states that she values her health and the health of her unborn baby enough to stop smoking and drinking alcohol. She voices the importance of adequate protein

in her diet and taking a prenatal vitamin. By the next visit, she reports that her nausea is under control, and she is able to eat two to three healthier meals a day. She agrees to meet with the social worker.

3. Patient-centered care/evidence-based practice: What intellectual, technical, interpersonal, and ethical/legal competencies are most likely to bring about the desired outcome?
Intellectual: knowledge of the developmental needs of the fetus and the effects of maternal age and behaviors, sufficient vitamins, especially folic acid to prevent neural tube defects, well-balanced diet with sufficient protein, smoking and alcohol consumption on the fetus
Technical: ability to assess maternal vital signs and fetal heart tones, provide the technical nursing assistance necessary to assess and meet the needs of a pregnant person and her fetus
Interpersonal: ability to demonstrate nonjudgmental attitude when interacting in potentially emotionally charged situations, such as a teen experiencing a high-risk pregnancy and bouts of homelessness.
Ethical/legal: knowledge of the nurse's legal and ethical obligations in cases of maternal–fetal conflict

4. Teamwork and collaboration: What resources might be helpful for this patient?
Counseling services for Darlene's emotional support and to weigh the pros and cons of keeping the baby, social services, community services, support groups, printed materials on healthy pregnancy behaviors

PRACTICING FOR NCLEX
MULTIPLE-CHOICE QUESTIONS

| 1. c | 2. b | 3. a | 4. b | 5. c |
| 6. b | 7. c | 8. d | 9. c | 10. c |

ALTERNATE-FORMAT QUESTIONS
Multiple-Response Questions

1. a, d, e, f
2. b, c, e
3. b, d, e
4. b, e
5. a, c, e, f
6. a, b, f

Chart/Exhibit Questions

1. 7
2. 3
3. 10

CHAPTER 24

ASSESSING YOUR UNDERSTANDING

FILL IN THE BLANKS

1. cross-linkage
2. middle
3. sandwich
4. 60, 74; 75, 84; 85
5. ageism
6. wear, tear
7. review, reminiscence
8. Alzheimer's
9. Gerontology
10. Sleep, eating (feeding), incontinence, falls, breakdown

CORRECT THE FALSE STATEMENTS

1. T
2. F, 90s
3. F, hyperplasia (benign)
4. T
5. F, less
6. F, elasticity
7. F, 85
8. T
9. T
10. F, Dementia

SHORT ANSWER

1. **a.** Middle adulthood:
   Physiologic development: The early years are marked by maximum physical development and functioning. As time passes, gradual internal and external changes occur.
   Psychosocial development: Usually a time of increased personal freedom, economic stability, social relationships, increased responsibility, and awareness of one's own mortality.
   Cognitive, moral, and spiritual development: Intellectual abilities change from those of the young adult. There is increased motivation to learn. Problem-solving abilities remain, although response time may be slightly longer.
   b. Older adulthood:
   Physiologic development: The process of aging becomes more rapid. All organ systems undergo some degree of decline, and the body becomes less efficient.
   Psychosocial development: Most continue their activities from middle adulthood and adapt intuitively to gradual limitations of aging.
   Cognitive, moral, and spiritual development: Cognition does not change appreciably with aging; an older adult continues to learn and solve problems, and intelligence and personality remain consistent.
2. Sample answers:
   a. Physical examination every year

   b. Pelvic examination with Pap test every 5 years for females
   c. Eye examination with test for glaucoma every 1 to 2 years
   d. Maintenance of current immunizations
   e. Cancer screening
3. **a.** Genetic theory: Explains that lifespan depends to a great extent on genetic factors.
   b. Immunity theory: Focuses on the functions of the immune system, which declines steadily after young adulthood.
   c. Free radical theory: The free radical theory is based on oxidative stress. Free radicals, formed during cellular metabolism, are molecules with unpaired, high-energy electrons that seek to combine with another molecule. This electron pairing disrupts cell membranes and affects DNA and protein synthesis. Over time, irreversible damage results from the accumulated effects of this damage. Antioxidants are thought to protect against this type of free radical damage.
   d. Disengagement theory: Maintains that an older adult withdraws from societal interactions because it is mutually desired and satisfying for both the person and society.
   e. Activity theory: Successful aging involves the ability to maintain high levels of activity and functioning.
4. Alzheimer's disease (AD) is characterized by the formation of amyloid plaques and tangles of tau proteins, which have an impact on brain structure and function. It is progressive and ultimately fatal. In mild or early AD, forgetfulness and impaired judgment may be evident. Over several years, the person progresses to moderate or middle AD, and becomes increasingly confused, forgetting family and becoming disoriented in familiar surroundings. When the ability to perform simple activities of daily living is lost, the older adult enters the severe or late stage of AD. Safety is important; the person requires constant supervision and care, often in a long-term care facility.
5. **a.** Integumentary: Wrinkling and sagging skin with decreased elasticity; dryness and scaling are common.
   b. Musculoskeletal: Muscle mass and strength decrease.
   c. Neurologic: Temperature regulation and pain perception become less efficient.
   d. Cardiopulmonary: The body is less able to increase heart rate and cardiac output with activity.
   e. Gastrointestinal: Malnutrition and anemia become more common.
   f. Genitourinary: Blood flow to the kidneys decreases with diminished cardiac output.

APPLYING YOUR KNOWLEDGE
CRITICAL THINKING QUESTIONS

1. Problem-solving abilities remain consistent although response time may be slightly longer. Provide sufficient time for answers to questions, respecting that there are more memories to process and a desire to think a problem through before responding. Provide ample time to complete an activity, or help the older adult modify an activity. For example, suggest an older adult with arthritis to use an electric can opener rather than a manual one, or a person with heart disease may need 3 hours to garden, resting several times, rather than the 1 hour gardening used to require. Older adults experience role changes, decreased earning capacity, and loss of social and intimate relationships, which are stressful. The nurse can encourage socialization through senior centers, groups, religious services. Accept that sexual activity does not stop in old age and encourage its expression. Encourage new hobbies, increased involvement in community, church, or family affairs, volunteer work or new career, if desired to avoid social isolation and depression.

2. Assess for previous falls, fear of falling and conduct a fall risk assessment. Teach the older adult to replace dim light with brighter bulbs, remove trip hazards such as scatter rugs and avoid small pets. Consider affixing a bell to a small pet's collar as a warning they are approaching. Ensure the older adult has well-fitting shoes and slippers. Exercises such as walking can help maintain strength. Assess for proper use of assistive devices.

3. Answers will vary.

REFLECTIVE PRACTICE: CULTIVATING QSEN COMPETENCIES
Sample Answers

1. Patient-centered care/safety: How might the nurse use blended nursing skills to provide holistic, developmentally sensitive care for this patient? The nurse begins by assessing the patient's strengths, quantifying alcohol consumption, determining how he has been managing his diabetes and that he has a glucometer, and screens for depression. The nurse can point out that skills from the patient's previous roles can be used in new roles or in a new context. For example, a manager or administrator may continue to use their leadership talents in community or volunteer organizations. The nurse encourages the patient to remain physically active as part of helping with mood, diabetes management, and socialization, even if he simply walks out of doors. The nurse encourages the pa-

tient to build on old interests, asking what he used to like to do, and encouraging him to find similar activities here. The nurse can gently remind the patient that the calories in alcohol can negatively impact his diabetes. Also, the nurse can encourage the patient to find a spiritual community, if open to that.

2. Patient-centered care/safety: What would be a successful outcome for this patient? By next visit, the patient will report that he began walking in the neighborhood and met a few neighbors, attended a BBQ, and is drinking less. He states that he is amazed that his blood glucose levels are better.

3. Patient-centered care/safety: What intellectual, technical, interpersonal, and ethical/legal competencies are most likely to bring about the desired outcome? Intellectual: knowledge of the theories of aging as they relate to the changes faced by the aging adult. Able to synthesize knowledge of diabetes, nutrition/alcohol intake, exercise, and outcomes of diabetes for patient education. Technical: ability to adapt necessary skills and techniques to address the changes associated with the aging adult. Ensure patient uses a glucometer. Interpersonal: ability to establish trusting professional relationships with adult patients of different ages, respecting their developmental needs Ethical/legal: ability to practice in an ethically and legally defensible manner, maintaining the rights of the aging adult

4. Teamwork and collaboration: What resources might be helpful for this patient? Ensure he has a primary health care provider. Community services, social networks, physical fitness facility/programs, nutrition classes

PRACTICING FOR NCLEX
MULTIPLE-CHOICE QUESTIONS

1. c	2. a	3. d	4. b	5. c
6. a	7. d	8. b	9. b	10. c
11. c				

ALTERNATE-FORMAT QUESTIONS
Multiple-Response Questions

1. c, e, f
2. a, c, d
3. c, d, e
4. a, c, f

Prioritization Question

1. d

CHAPTER 25

ASSESSING YOUR UNDERSTANDING

FILL IN THE BLANKS

1. Quality, Safety, Nurses
2. Centers, Control, Prevention
3. aerobic, anaerobic
4. positive, negative
5. flora
6. reservoirs
7. portal, entry
8. antibody, antigen
9. health care–associated infection
10. iatrogenic
11. fungi
12. medical, surgical

MATCHING EXERCISES

Matching Exercise 1

1. e	2. a	3. d	4. c	5. b
6. f				

Matching Exercise 2

1. b	2. a	3. e	4. c	5. d
6. f				

CORRECT THE FALSE STATEMENTS

1. T
2. T
3. F, Hand hygiene
4. F, Transient bacteria
5. T
6. T
7. T
8. F, surgical asepsis
9. T

SHORT ANSWER

1. a. Number of organisms
   b. Virulence of the organism
   c. Competence of a person's immune system
   d. Length and intimacy (extent, duration) of the contact between a person and the microorganism
2. Sample answers:
   a. Other humans: Tuberculosis
   b. Animals: Rabies
   c. Soil: Tetanus
3. a. Gastrointestinal tract
   b. Genitourinary tract
   c. Blood and tissue
4. Sample answers:
   a. Direct contact: transmission of disease through touching, kissing, or sexual contact
   b. Indirect contact: personal contact with contaminated food, water, etc.
   c. Vectors: mosquitoes, ticks, and lice transmit organisms from one host to another
   d. Fomite: an inanimate object, such as equipment or countertops

   e. Airborne: spread of droplet nuclei through coughing, sneezing, or talking
5. a. Inflammatory response: A protective mechanism that eliminates the invading pathogen and allows tissue repair to occur.
   b. Immune response: Reactions by the body to an invading foreign protein such as bacteria or, in some cases, the body's own proteins. The body responds to an antigen by producing an antibody.
6. a. Intact skin and mucous membranes protect the body against microbial invasion.
   b. The normal pH levels of gastric secretions and of the genitourinary tract help to ward off microbial invasion.
   c. The body's white blood cells influence resistance to certain pathogens.
   d. Age, sex, race, and hereditary factors influence susceptibility.
7. a. Assessing: Early detection and surveillance techniques. The nurse should inquire about immunization status and previous or recurring infections, observe nonverbal cues, and obtain the history of the current disease. The nurse should assess vital signs, and laboratory studies (WBC and culture results).
   b. Diagnosing/problem identification: The direction or focus of nursing care depends on health problems that accurately reflect the patient's condition such as hyperthermia, hypotension, or inflammation.
   c. Planning: Effective nursing interventions to control or prevent infection. Nurses review assessment data and consider the cycle of events that results in infection control to formulate patient or community goals. The nurse plans to administer antimicrobial medications, checking for medication allergy prior to administering.
   d. Implementing: The nurse uses principles of aseptic technique to halt the spread of microorganisms and minimize the threat of infection, administers antimicrobials, and provides teaching to prevent spread of infection. During a public health crisis, the nurse, with public health officials, provides education and immunization to individuals and communities.
   e. Evaluating: The nurse determines if the patient has remained safe and free from infection or if an existing infection has been controlled or eliminated. Outcome measures can include decreasing WBC, fever, and transmission of disease in the community. The nurse practices antimicrobial stewardship.
8. Sample answers:
   a. Patient's home: Wash hands before preparing food and before eating; wash fresh fruits and vegetables prior to consuming. Use individual personal care items such as washcloths, towels, and toothbrushes.

b. Public facilities: Wash hands after using any public bathroom; use individually wrapped drinking straws.

c. Community: Use sterilized combs and brushes in beauty and barber shops; examine food handlers for evidence of disease. Individuals to wear a mask in public spaces if immunosuppressed.

d. Health care facility: Use standard aseptic techniques to prevent further spread of a present organism and prevent nosocomial infections. Do not admit visitors with infections. Offer influenza, pneumococcal, and other relevant vaccines.

9. a. Constant surveillance by infection control committees and nurse epidemiologists

b. Written infection prevention practices for all facility personnel

c. Use evidence-based practices that promote optimal physical condition in patients

10. a. Nature of organisms present: Some organisms are easily destroyed, whereas others can withstand certain commonly used sterilization and disinfection methods.

b. Number of organisms present: The more organisms present on an item, the longer it takes to destroy them.

c. Type of equipment: Equipment with narrow lumens, crevices, or joints requires special care. Certain items may be damaged by sterilization methods.

d. Intended use of equipment: The need for medical or surgical asepsis influences the methods used in the preparation and cleaning of equipment.

e. Available means for sterilization and disinfection: The choice of chemical or physical means of sterilization and disinfection takes into consideration the availability and practicality of the means.

f. Time: Time is a key factor. Failure to observe recommended time periods for disinfection and sterilization significantly increases the risk for infection and is considered negligent.

11. a. Hospital: The infection control nurse is responsible for educating patients and staff about effective infection control techniques and for collecting statistics about infections. This nurse monitors compliance with staff PPD, influenza vaccine, among others.

b. Home care setting: The infection control nurse's duties include surveillance for facility-associated infections, as well as education, consultation, performance of epidemiologic investigations and quality improvement activities, and policy and procedure development.

12. Effective nursing interventions can control or prevent infection. The nurse maintains medical asepsis; assesses vital signs and other signs of infection; and provides prescribed dressings, topical and systemic antimicrobials. The nurse reviews patient data, considers the cycle of events that result in the development of an infection, and incorporates infection control as a patient goal.

13. Use standard precautions for the care of all patients in the ER. For a patient with known or suspected TB, airborne precautions are initiated promptly. When entering the room, per CDC guidelines, a high-efficiency particulate air (HEPA) filter respirator or N95 respirator certified by NIOSH must be worn.

APPLYING YOUR KNOWLEDGE
CRITICAL THINKING QUESTIONS

1. Sample answer:
General symptoms of infections or sepsis typically include fever, malaise, and site-specific signs and symptoms such as cough or pus in a wound. If not responsive to treatment, severe infections and sepsis, which can set up an inflammatory response in the body, can lead to death.

2. Answers will vary.

3. Answers will vary. In your discussion, consider the concepts of altruism, beneficence, and the consequences of turning away patients due to personal objections.

REFLECTIVE PRACTICE: CULTIVATING QSEN COMPETENCIES
Sample Answers

1. Patient-centered care/safety: How might the nurse respond to Giselle in a holistic manner that respects her human dignity, while at the same time maintaining a safe environment for her?
The nurse validates the patient's worth as a person, and emphasizes the need for safety, a face mask if suggested by the health care provider and meticulous hand washing. The nurse asks what the patient believes will best protect her during Sunday school classes, if the health care provider agrees she may attend. The nurse suggests Giselle teach her students about taking medicine to help her "get better" (or other age-appropriate words) and the need to have them help protect her including handwashing or using alcohol-based hand sanitizer. The nurse listens respectfully, spending time in conversations with her about her life experiences, and allowing her to express negative feelings. Giselle can encourage love and belonging by having students draw pictures or write her letters of support in lieu of hugs. The nurse can help Giselle to recognize her strengths and explore other options to fulfill her love and belonging as well as self-esteem needs.

2. Patient-centered care/safety: What would be a successful outcome for Giselle?
Giselle will remain free from infection; she will state three actions she can take to prevent infection.

3. Patient-centered care/evidence-based practice: What intellectual, technical, interpersonal, and ethical/legal competencies are most likely to bring about the desired outcome?
   Intellectual: the patient must possess knowledge of the effects on their immune system and interventions to minimize them
   Technical: ability to apply appropriate infection control precautions, medications used for leukopenia, and monitoring techniques for infection assessment
   Interpersonal: ability to communicate care and compassion to patients requiring infection control precautions
   Ethical/legal: demonstration of a commitment to safety and quality; strong advocacy abilities
4. Teamwork and collaboration: What resources might be helpful for this patient?
   American Cancer Association, Cancer Support group, referral to counseling services, home health care visits

PRACTICING FOR NCLEX
MULTIPLE-CHOICE QUESTIONS

| 1. b | 2. d | 3. c | 4. a | 5. a |
| 6. c | 7. a | 8. b | 9. d | |

ALTERNATE-FORMAT QUESTIONS
Multiple-Response Questions

1. a, c, e
2. a, c, d
3. b, d, e
4. a, b, c, f
5. b, d, e
6. a, d, f
7. a, b, c, e

Sequencing Questions

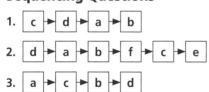

1. c → d → a → b
2. d → a → b → f → c → e
3. a → c → b → d

CHAPTER 26

ASSESSING YOUR UNDERSTANDING
FILL IN THE BLANKS

1. physiologic, temperature, pulse (heart rate), respiration, blood pressure. Pulse oximetry, pain
2. 9 cm, 18 cm
3. +1/4 (weak, on a scale of 0–4)
4. 100°F
5. 102.2
6. 37.5
7. Hypertension (high blood pressure)
8. falls/injury
9. Korotkoff
10. Doppler

DEVELOPING YOUR KNOWLEDGE BASE
IDENTIFICATION

1. a. Temporal
   b. Carotid
   c. Brachial
   d. Radial
   e. Femoral
   f. Popliteal
   g. Posterior tibial
   h. Dorsalis pedis

MATCHING EXERCISES
Matching Exercise 1

| 1. b | 2. e | 3. c | 4. f | 5. a |
| 6. d | | | | |

Matching Exercise 2

| 1. e | 2. b | 3. c | 4. a | 5. d |
| 6. f | | | | |

Matching Exercise 3

| 1. d | 2. e | 3. a | 4. c | 5. f |
| 6. g | | | | |

SHORT ANSWER

1. a. Circadian rhythms: Predictable fluctuations in measurements of body temperature and blood pressure throughout 24 hours occur in a circadian rhythm. The blood pressure is usually lowest on arising in the morning. Blood pressure has been noted to rise as much as 5 to 10 mm Hg by late afternoon, and gradually falls again during sleep.
   b. Age: Body temperatures of infants and children respond more rapidly to hot and cold temperatures than adults. The older adult loses some thermoregulatory control and is at risk for harm from extremes in temperature.
   c. Biologic sex: Body temperature tends to fluctuate more in women than in men, probably from normal, cyclic fluctuations in the release of their sex hormones.
   d. Stress: The body responds to both physical and emotional stress by increasing the production of epinephrine. As a result, the metabolic rate increases, raising body temperature.
   e. Environmental temperature: Exposure to extreme cold without adequate protective clothing can result in heat loss severe enough to cause hypothermia. Exposure to extreme heat may result in hyperthermia or heat stroke.

2. See table below.

Type of Thermometer	Brief Description	Uses/Contraindication	Normal Reading
A. ELECTRONIC AND DIGITAL	Two nonbreakable probes, disposable probe covers	Measure oral, rectal, or axillary body temperature over a period of 1 to 60 seconds, depending on the site and product used	Site dependent
B. TYMPANIC MEMBRANE	Infrared sensors detect heat given off by tympanic membrane	Not used for infants up to age 3 months due to possible tympanic membrane damage	36.8–37.8°C (98.2–100°F)
C. DISPOSABLE SINGLE-USE	Nonbreakable temperature sensitive tape or patch applied to forehead or abdomen; registers temperature within seconds	Used to screen temperature of toddler or young child	Color changes at different temperature ranges
D. TEMPORAL ARTERY	Forehead or abdomen; changes color at different temperatures	Newborns	37.1–38.1°C (98.7–100.5°F)
E. AUTOMATED MONITORING DEVICE	Measure body temperature, pulse, and blood pressure automatically	Used in various health care settings to measure body temperature, pulse, respirations, and blood pressure simultaneously	Site dependent

3. a. The middle three fingers may be used to palpate all peripheral pulse sites.
   b. A stethoscope may be used to auscultate the apical pulse.
   c. Doppler ultrasound may be used to assess pulses that are difficult to palpate or auscultate.
4. a. Pumping action of the heart: When the amount of blood pumped into the arteries increases, the pressure of blood against arterial walls also increases.
   b. Blood volume: When blood volume is low, blood pressure is also low because there is less fluid to exert pressure on the arterial wall.
   c. Viscosity of blood: The more viscous the blood, the higher the blood pressure.
   d. Elasticity of vessel walls: The elasticity of the walls, in addition to the resistance of the

arterioles, helps to maintain normal blood pressure.
5. a. A decrease in peripheral tissue perfusion: lower blood pressure, sluggish capillary refill, weak pulses, difficulty obtaining pulse oximetry readings
   b. Loss of fluid volume: weak peripheral pulses, lower BP, orthostatic hypotension, tachycardia
   c. Bounding pulses, tachycardia, elevated BP, resulting edema/swelling makes it difficult to palpate peripheral pulses
   d. Reduced cardiac output: weaker pulses, lower blood pressure, low saturation of oxygen
   e. Anxiety: stress response increased pulse, BP
6. 124
7. See table below.

Age	Temperature °C °F	Pulse beats/min	Respirations breaths/min	Blood Pressure mm Hg
Newborns	36.2–37.7 97.2–99.9	95–170	30–60	60–70/40
Infants	35.6–37.6 96–99.7	85–170	30–50	85/37
Toddler	35.6–37.2 96–99	70–150	20–40	88/42
Child	35.6–37.2 96–99	65–130	15–25	95/57
Adolescent	35.8–37.5 96.4–99.5	60–115	12–20	102/60
Adult	35.8–37.5 96.4–99.5	60–100	12–20	<120/80

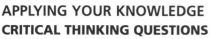

APPLYING YOUR KNOWLEDGE
CRITICAL THINKING QUESTIONS

1. Answers will vary. Nurses need to use various devices based on facility/unit availability and preferences, best practices, and for infection control purposes. Any uncertainty related to accuracy of an assessment should be validated by the primary nurse, instructor, or other health care provider.
2. Remind the resident that the BP will be falsely elevated impacting treatment; further this action is not consistent with safe, quality practice.

REFLECTIVE PRACTICE: CULTIVATING QSEN COMPETENCIES
Sample Answers

1. Patient-centered care/evidence-based practice: What might be causing Noah's reaction to the nurse's attempt to assess a tympanic temperature? Noah may be reacting out of fear of strange people and situations. His behavior is also consistent with the pain of otitis. Taking a tympanic temperature is contraindicated with ear infection because the movement of the tragus may cause severe discomfort.
2. What would be a successful outcome for Noah? Noah exhibits calmness upon examination and allows the nurse to perform necessary assessments. The patient receives needed treatment (antibiotics and fluids if indicated).
3. Patient-centered care: What intellectual, technical, and interpersonal competencies are most likely to bring about the desired outcome?
   Intellectual: knowledge of how to tailor vital signs technology to meet the developmental needs of a 2-year-old with probable otitis
   Technical: ability to correctly use the equipment necessary to assess and document vital signs
   Interpersonal: ability to establish a trusting relationship with children and their families
4. Teamwork and collaboration: What resources might be helpful for the nurse caring for Noah?
   Stuffed animal to demonstrate the procedures for taking vital signs, knowledge of distraction techniques to use when performing procedures on children

PRACTICING FOR NCLEX
MULTIPLE-CHOICE QUESTIONS

1. c	2. c	3. c	4. a	5. b
6. c	7. d	8. b	9. b	

ALTERNATE-FORMAT QUESTIONS
Multiple-Response Questions

1. a, b, c, e
2. a, e, f
3. b, c, e
4. c, d, f
5. b, c, f
6. a, b, c, d

Sequencing Question

1. d → e → b → a → c

CHAPTER 27

ASSESSING YOUR UNDERSTANDING
FILL IN THE BLANK

1. history, physical
2. therapeutic
3. Dignity
4. respiration
5. consent
6. quotes
7. bell, diaphragm
8. Snellen
9. symmetry
10. Pain

CORRECT THE FALSE STATEMENTS

1. T
2. F, tricuspid
3. F, mitral
4. T

IDENTIFICATION QUESTIONS: ANATOMY REVIEW

1. a. Liver
   b. Stomach
   c. Spleen
   d. Transverse colon
   e. Descending colon
   f. Small intestine
   g. Sigmoid colon
   h. Bladder
   i. Appendix
   j. Cecum
   k. Ascending colon
2. a. Malleus
   b. Incus
   c. Semicircular canals
   d. Facial nerve
   e. Cochlear and vestibular branch
   f. Cochlea
   g. Oval window
   h. Round window
   i. Eustachian tube
   j. Stapes and footplate
   k. Tympanic membrane

MATCHING EXERCISES
Matching Exercise 1

1. a	2. b	3. a	4. d	5. c
6. b	7. e	8. c	9. b	10. d

Matching Exercise 2

1. e	2. a	3. b	4. c	5. f
6. d				

Matching Exercise 3

1. c	2. e	3. d	4. f	5. b
6. a				

Matching Exercise 4

1. a	2. b	3. c	4. d

Complete the Chart

1.

Cranial Nerve	Name	Function	Method of Assessment
II	Optic	Visual acuity	Test visual acuity with Snellen eye chart and visual fields
II, III, VI	Optic Oculomotor Abducens	Pupil constriction/reaction to light, cardinal fields of gaze	Movement of eyes and lids, PERLA
V	Trochlear	Downward, inward eye movement	Patient moves eyes downward and inward, following finger or penlight
VII	Facial	Sensorimotor nerve that innervates the muscles of the face and functions to provide the taste sensation of the anterior two thirds of the tongue	Ask the patient to raise eyebrows, smile, show teeth, and puff out cheeks
VIII	Acoustic	Sense of hearing	Whisper word next to patient's ear
IX	Glossopharyngeal	Pharyngeal movement and swallowing	Motor nerve; ask patient to open the mouth and say "aaah"; observing the upward movement of the soft palate
XII	Hypoglossal	Movement of the tongue; strength of the tongue	Ask the patient to stick out tongue and push tongue against cheek

2.

Technique	Definition	Assessment/Observation
a. Inspection	Process of deliberate, purposeful observations performed in a systematic manner	Body size, color, shape, position, symmetry, norms, and deviations from norm
b. Palpation	Technique that uses sense of touch	Temperature, turgor, texture, moisture, vibrations, shape
c. Percussion	The act of striking an object against another object to produce a sound	Location, shape, size, and density of tissues
d. Auscultation	The act of listening to sound produced in the body, using stethoscope	Lung and bowel sounds; heart and vascular sounds

SHORT ANSWER

1. **a.** Establish a nurse–patient relationship.
   b. Gather data about the patient's general health status, integrating physiologic, psychological, cognitive, sociocultural, developmental, and spiritual dimensions.
   c. Identify patient strengths.
   d. Identify existing and potential health problems.
   e. Establish a base for the nursing process.
2. **a.** Ophthalmoscope
   b. Otoscope
   c. Nasal speculum
   d. Vaginal speculum
   e. Tuning fork
   f. Percussion hammer
3. **a.** Patient's age and/or developmental level
   b. Patient's cognitive and physical condition (mobility) and energy level
   c. Need for privacy
   d. Time constraints
4. **a.** Patient: Consider physiologic and psychological needs of the patient. Explain that a physical assessment will be performed by the nurse, that body structures will be examined, and that such assessments are painless. Have patient put on a gown and empty bladder.
   b. Environment: The time of the assessment should be mutually agreed on and should not interfere with meals or daily routines. The patient should be as free of pain as possible, and the room should be quiet, private, and offer warmth if patient needs to remove clothing.
5. **a.** Pitch—ranging from high to low
   b. Loudness—ranging from soft to loud
   c. Quality—for example, swishing or gurgling
   d. Duration—short, medium, or long

6. a. Edema: Use fingertip pressure to palpate a swollen (edematous) area; an indentation may remain after the pressure is released.

  b. Fluid loss: Pick up the skin in a fold; when fluid loss such as fluid volume deficit or dehydration exists, normal elasticity and fullness are decreased, and skin fold returns to normal slowly.

  c. Balance: Perform the Romberg's test by asking the patient to stand straight with feet together, both eyes closed and arms at the side. Wait 20 seconds and observe for swaying and ability to maintain balance. Be alert to prevent a patient fall or injury due to loss of balance.

7. a. Pupillary reaction: In a darkened room, ask patient to look straight ahead, bring the penlight from side of patient's face, and shine the light on one of the pupils. Observe pupil's reaction; normal finding is pupillary constriction. Repeat procedure in the same eye and observe the other eye—normally it too will constrict, producing a consensual response. Repeat the entire procedure with the other eye.

  b. Accommodation: Hold the forefinger about 10 to 15 cm in front of the bridge of the patient's nose. Ask the patient to first look at the forefinger, then at a distant object, then the forefinger again. Normally, the pupil constricts when the patient looks at the finger and dilates when he or she looks at a distant object.

  c. Convergence: Hold a finger about 6 to 8 inches from the bridge of the patient's nose and move finger toward eyes. Normally, the patient's eyes converge toward midline (assume cross-eyed appearance).

8. Sample answers:

  a. Orientation: What is today's date?

  b. Immediate memory: What did you eat for lunch today?

  c. Past memory: When is your wedding anniversary?

  d. Abstract reasoning: Explain the proverb "a stitch in time, saves nine."

  e. Language: Would you read this passage from this book?

9. a. Biographical data: "What is your birth date?"

  b. Reason for seeking health care: "Why are you visiting the clinic today?"

  c. Present health history: "When did you notice these symptoms?"

  d. Past health history: "When did you have your last mammogram?"

  e. Family history: "Do you have any close relatives who have diabetes?"

  f. Functional health: "Are you able to prepare your own meals?"

  g. Psychosocial and lifestyle factors: "How do you manage stress in your life?"

  h. Review of systems: "Are you experiencing any abdominal distress?"

APPLYING YOUR KNOWLEDGE
CRITICAL THINKING QUESTIONS

1. Sample answers:

  a. Patient who is comatose: introduce yourself and explain what you are doing, touch the patient gently

  b. Patient who is uncooperative: explain the need for the assessment, request they cooperate, if unable or if the patient is a child or has dementia, perform the assessment quickly

  c. Patient who does not understand your language: obtain an interpreter (phone or person), introduce yourself by stating your name and pointing to yourself, show the patient your equipment (i.e., stethoscope and pantomime; use a picture board)

  d. Young child: allow the child to sit on the parent's lap, distract them with a toy, become skilled and quick

2. a. Answers will vary.

  b. Answers will vary. Consider obtaining the patient's permission, if an emergency requiring accuracy exists.

REFLECTIVE PRACTICE: CULTIVATING QSEN COMPETENCIES
Sample Answers

1. Patient-centered care/safety: What type of health assessments would the nurse caring for Billy conduct? The nurse performs an emergency assessment to determine the effects of the bee sting and the allergic reaction that occurred. Determine if the child has an EpiPen and use it based on standing orders and the criteria. Once Billy is stabilized, the nurse should perform a focused assessment and contact the parents, answering any questions they might have. Provide positive feedback to Billy for alerting you about the bee sting promptly.

2. Patient-centered care/safety: What would be a successful outcome for Billy and his family?
Have at least two self-injecting epinephrine pens at the camp; ensure Billy can demonstrate the proper method for self-injecting epinephrine. Billy is free from wheezing, signs of hypoxemia or anaphylaxis/shock.
Billy states methods to avoid bee stings in the future and emergency interventions in the event a bee sting occurs.

3. Safety/evidence-based practice: What intellectual, interpersonal, and ethical/legal competencies are most likely to bring about the desired outcome?
Intellectual: knowledge of the typical assessment findings associated with an allergic/hypersensitivity reaction, criteria for administering epinephrine
Interpersonal: ability to communicate and interact effectively with patients and their families during times of stress
Ethical/legal: knowledge of special regulations and legislation detailing nursing responsibilities when providing first aid in camp situations

4. Teamwork and collaboration/safety: What resources might be helpful?
Printed or AV materials on allergic reactions to insect bites and how to prevent and treat them; posting a visual on how to use the EpiPen throughout the camp. Ensure all nurses and designated counselors can use the EpiPen as well.

PRACTICING FOR NCLEX
MULTIPLE-CHOICE QUESTIONS

1. b	**2.** d	**3.** a	**4.** c	**5.** d
6. b	**7.** d	**8.** a	**9.** a	**10.** b
11. a	**12.** c	**13.** a	**14.** b	**15.** a

ALTERNATE-FORMAT QUESTIONS
Multiple-Response Questions

1. c, d, e
2. b, d, e
3. a, b, e
4. c, d, e

Hot Spot Question

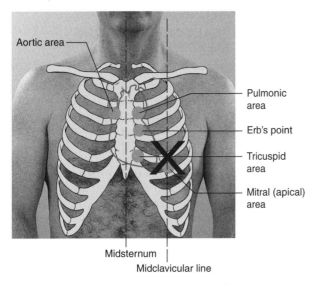

Prioritization Questions

1. c
2. b

Sequencing Question

1.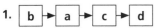
b → a → c → d

CHAPTER 28

ASSESSING YOUR UNDERSTANDING
FILL IN THE BLANKS

1. 13
2. choking
3. smoke
4. poison
5. adolescents
6. firearms
7. weapons
8. falls
9. same
10. event
11. root
12. restraint
13. Goals
14. injury
15. disaster
16. Bioterrorism

MATCHING EXERCISES
Matching Exercise 1

1. c	**2.** b	**3.** d	**4.** e	**5.** a
6. f				

Matching Exercise 2

1. a	**2.** b	**3.** e	**4.** d	**5.** c
6. c				

CORRECT THE FALSE STATEMENTS

1. T
2. T
3. T
4. F, home
5. F, children
6. T
7. T
8. F, falls
9. F, 14 and younger
10. T
11. F, increase
12. F, adult

SHORT ANSWER

1. Sample answers:
   a. Neonates and infants: mother who smokes, mother who drinks alcohol
   b. Toddler and preschooler: child abuse, expanded environment
   c. School-aged child: accidents, fire
   d. Adolescent: drug and alcohol consumption, motor vehicle crashes
   e. Adult: intimate partner violence, using alcohol to relieve stress
   f. Older adult: falls, elder abuse
2. Sample answers:
   a. Developmental considerations: A teenager who drinks and drives is at risk for accidents; an adult who is under stress at work is at risk for drug or alcohol abuse
   b. Lifestyle: A person who lives in a high-crime neighborhood is at risk for violence; a person who has a dangerous job is at risk for accidents
   c. Limitation in mobility: An older adult with an unsteady gait is at risk for falls; recent surgery or prolonged illness can temporarily affect mobility
   d. Limitation in sensory perception: Visual changes may cause a person to stumble, lose balance, and fall; a hearing deficit interferes

with normal communication and may result in a patient who is insensitive to alarms, horns, sirens, etc.

   e. Limitation in knowledge: A mother who does not know how to childproof her home puts her toddler at risk for accidents; an older adult person who does not know how to use their walker is at risk for falls

   f. Limitation in ability to communicate: Fatigue or stress, certain medications, aphasia, and language barriers are factors that can affect personal interchange and compromise the patient's ability to express urgent safety concerns

   g. Limitation in health status: A patient recovering from a stroke may have muscle impairment; many patients who fall also have a primary or secondary diagnosis of cardiovascular disease

   h. Limitation in psychosocial state: Depression may result in confusion and disorientation, accompanied by reduced awareness of environmental hazards; social isolation may be responsible for a reduced level of concentration

3. a. Nursing history: The nurse must be alert for any history of falls because a person with a history of falling is likely to fall again. Assistive devices should be noted. A history of drug or alcohol abuse should also be noted.

   b. Physical assessment: Nurses need to assess the patient's mobility status, ability to communicate, level of awareness or orientation, and sensory perception.

   c. Accident-prone behavior: Some people seem to be more likely than others to have accidents.

   d. Environment: The nurse must assess every setting in which the patient is at risk for injury, including the home, community, and health care facility.

4. Sample answers:
   a. Age older than 65 years
   b. Documented history of falls
   c. Slowed reaction time
   d. Disorientation or confusion

5. Sample answer: The nurse teaches the adults in the home about safety for toddlers and develops a plan focusing on childproofing the home. The plan includes the installation of cabinet locks; electrical outlet covers. Additionally included is locking medications, cleaners, removing or placing poisonous plants to higher levels, and keeping small or sharp objects out of reach.

6. Sample answers:
   a. Do your children's toys have small or loose parts?
   b. Have you ever left your infant in the bathtub to answer the phone?
   c. Do you have soft pillows or blankets in your infant's crib?

7. Sample answers:
   a. Screening programs for vision and hearing
   b. Fire prevention programs
   c. Drug and alcohol prevention programs

8. Sample answers:
   a. Impaired circulation
   b. Pressure injuries and diminished bone mass
   c. Fractures
   d. Altered nutrition and hydration
   e. Incontinence

10. **S:** 12 PM, patient wearing vest restraint
    B: Admitted with change in mental status and dehydration. Reports need to void frequently in spite of indwelling catheter and had continually gotten out of bed and walked to the bathroom until she fell yesterday at 8 PM and vest restraint applied.
    A: Patient's skin is intact at points of contact of the vest restraint, heels are lifted off the bed with pillows. Patient continues with confusion and frequently states she needs to use the bathroom to urinate.
    R: Remind patient she has an indwelling catheter, continue IV saline at 60 mL/h for dehydration.

11. The nurse completes the safety event report immediately after an accident and is responsible for recording the occurrence of the accident and its effect on the patient in the medical record. The circumstances of the accident and details concerning the patient's response, the examination, and treatment of the patient after the event are included in the report.

APPLYING YOUR KNOWLEDGE
CRITICAL THINKING QUESTIONS

1. Answers will vary.
2. Answers will vary.
3. The nurse explains about the IV and protects the IV with an arm board or mitts. The nurse can obtain an order to restrain the arm without the IV.

REFLECTIVE PRACTICE: CULTIVATING QSEN COMPETENCIES
Sample Answers

1. Patient-centered care/safety: What safety interventions might the nurse implement for this patient? Bessie should be advised to have clutter removed from the home and remove throw rugs and fire hazards. The nurse assesses for smoke detectors and suggests they are installed if absent. Bessie should be advised to wear shoes with rubber soles when walking in her home. The nurse assesses the patient is using the walker properly and if there is a need for additional PT. The patient may also benefit from a home alert system in case she falls and needs help.

2. Patient-centered care/safety: What would be a successful outcome for this patient? By the end of the visit, Bessie can state three safety issues in her home and formulates a plan to correct them. By the next visit, Bessie demonstrates walking freely through a clutter-free home with fire alarms installed.

3. Patient-centered care/safety: What intellectual interpersonal, and ethical/legal competencies are most likely to bring about the desired outcome?
Intellectual: knowledge of the safety and security needs of older adults and related nursing responsibilities and care
Interpersonal: ability to establish a therapeutic relationship with an older adult in order to communicate the need for safety interventions in the home
Ethical/legal: commitment to patient safety and quality care, including ability to report problem situations immediately

4. Teamwork and collaboration: What resources might be helpful for this patient?
Home health care services, home health aide for bathing and grooming, PT or home PT, housekeeping services, smoke detectors, home alert system

PRACTICING FOR NCLEX
MULTIPLE-CHOICE QUESTIONS

1. b	2. c	3. d	4. b	5. a
6. b	7. a	8. b	9. b	

ALTERNATE-FORMAT QUESTIONS
Multiple-Response Questions

1. b, c, e
2. a, b, e
3. a, b, d
4. a, c, f
5. a, b, c, e

Sequencing Question

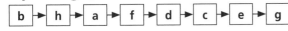

b → h → a → f → d → c → e → g

Prioritization Question

1. c

CHAPTER 29

ASSESSING YOUR UNDERSTANDING
FILL IN THE BLANKS

1. yang
2. holistic
3. Acupuncture
4. imagery
5. nutritional
6. aromatherapy
7. touch
8. platelets (or bleeding)
9. Allopathic
10. integrative

MATCHING EXERCISE

1. d	2. f	3. b	4. e	5. a
6. c				

SHORT ANSWER

1. a. Ayurveda: The aim of Ayurvedic medicine is to integrate and balance the body, mind, and spirit. Key concepts include universal interconnectedness among people, their health, and the universe as well as the body's constitution and life forces.
Nursing considerations: May include dietary needs, time set aside for self-care such as meditation, and desire to use or continue a herbal/supplement regimen.
   b. Yoga: A set of exercises that consist of various physical postures practiced to promote strength and flexibility, increase endurance, and promote relaxation.
Nursing considerations: Encourage patients to find a type of yoga that is compatible with their physical condition and goals. Some positions are contraindicated in patients with certain physical conditions.
   c. Qi gong: System of posture, exercise, breathing techniques, and visualization regulating *qi*.
Nursing considerations: Can be learned from videos/DVDs or in a class; encourage students to explore background of instructor.

2. a. Relaxation techniques: The goal is to increase the activity of the parasympathetic system (as opposed to sympathetic system) to influence the body–mind connection and reduce the effect of stress and stress-related illness. If tolerated, lavender aromatherapy may be used to further promote relaxation, enhancing pain relief measures.
   b. Meditation: Seeks to change one's physiology to a more relaxed state and alter one's perception to an increased openness/acceptance of reality.
   c. Imagery: Involves using all five senses to visualize an event or body process unfolding according to a plan.

3. a. Physically, a human being is an open energy system.
   b. Anatomically, a human being is bilaterally symmetric.
   c. Illness is an imbalance in a person's energy field.
   d. Human beings have natural abilities to transform and transcend their conditions of living.

4. Sample answer: Treatment would consist of first restoring the patient's power and then treating symptoms. Healing techniques may include native plants and herbs, animals, rituals, ceremonies, and purification techniques.

5. Sample answers:
   a. Nutritional therapy: Nutritional supplements, vitamins, minerals, herbs have been used to promote healing, decrease inflammation, and treat symptoms such as nausea. Caution the patient to seek guidance from the health care provider, as interactions with the treatment plan or contraindications may exist. The nurse assesses the patient's individual needs and preferences with respect to foods.
   b. Aromatherapy: It is believed that the fragrance of oils can evoke powerful memories and change people's perceptions and behaviors. Certain aromas may promote relaxation.

c. Music: It is believed that music is effective in reducing pain, decreasing anxiety, and promoting relaxation, thereby distracting persons from unpleasant sensations.

6. a. Biology-based practices: Using herbs and special diets
   b. Mind–body medicine: Using meditation or yoga
   c. Energy medicine: Using energy fields or magnetic fields
   d. Manipulative and body-based practices: Manipulating body parts

APPLYING YOUR KNOWLEDGE
CRITICAL THINKING QUESTION

1. Sample answers:
   a. The patient may benefit from nutrients or substances that ease diarrhea and nausea, stimulate appetite, and help maintain weight. Pain management with stretching, (gentle or chair) yoga, aromatherapy, or massage (touch) could be helpful. Music, meditation, and guided relaxation with music or nature sounds promote relaxation and augment pain management.
   b. Gentle touch, therapeutic touch, or relaxing massage may be beneficial in decreasing anxiety or agitation. Aromatherapy may stimulate remembering pleasant times.

REFLECTIVE PRACTICE: CULTIVATING QSEN COMPETENCIES
Sample Answers

1. Patient-centered care, safety, evidence-based practice: What type of CHA might the nurse suggest to promote relaxation for Sylvia?
   The nurse could teach mind–body techniques such as meditation, guided imagery, biofeedback, and relaxation to reduce stressful emotions and promote healing. The nurse educates the patient that herbal supplements are considered medications. She should check with the surgeon to ensure they will not promote bleeding or interfere with anesthesia surgery.

2. Evidence based practice, safety and informatics: What would be a successful outcome for Sylvia?
   On her next visit, Sylvia lists two CHA measures that promote relaxation and demonstrates the proper use of them. The nurse records this information in the electronic health record to ensure continuity of care. Using the electronic health record, the interprofessional team performs medication reconciliation that documents prescriptions, over-the-counter medications, and any herbals the patient takes.

3. Safety/evidence-based practice: What intellectual, technical, and interpersonal competencies are most likely to bring about the desired outcome?
   Intellectual: knowledge of available and appropriate complementary and alternative modalities; knowledge of those foods and herbals that may predispose bleeding on interactions with anesthetics or analgesics

Technical: ability to properly perform CHA and integrate these measures into patient care; medication reconciliation and communication using the electronic health record
Interpersonal: ability to work collaboratively with other members of the health care team to promote culturally competent care that includes the use of CHA

4. Teamwork and collaboration: What resources might be helpful for Sylvia?
   Community-based resources offering movement therapy, meditation, or stress reduction. Community resources and support for postsurgical recovery, based on the underlying problem and procedure performed.
   Other health care professionals using CHA, printed and AV materials on CHA, referral to special programs delivering CHA

PRACTICING FOR NCLEX
MULTIPLE-CHOICE QUESTIONS

1. a　2. c　3. b　4. c　5. a
6. d

ALTERNATE-FORMAT QUESTIONS
Multiple-Response Questions

1. a, b, e, f
2. a, b, c, f
3. a, b, c, d
4. c, d, e
5. b, d, f
6. a, c, d

Prioritization Question

1. c

CHAPTER 30

ASSESSING YOUR UNDERSTANDING
FILL IN THE BLANKS

1. suspension
2. generic
3. trade (manufacturer)
4. allergy
5. tolerance
6. Toxic
7. idiosyncratic
8. Teratogenic
9. surface
10. up, back
11. toxicity
12. filter
13. compatible
14. 100
15. reconstitution

FILL IN THE BLANKS

1. 1.5 mL
2. 0.5 tab (½ tab)
3. 3 tabs

4. 0.5 tab (½ tab)
5. 0.5 tab (½ tab)
6. 0.5 tab (½ tab)
7. 0.5 tab (½ tab)
8. 2 tabs
9. 0.5 mL
10. 1 capsule of 500 mg and 1 capsule of 250 mg. (3 capsules of 250 mg)

MATCHING EXERCISES

Matching Exercise 1

1. b.   2. a   3. e   4. c   5. d

Matching Exercise 2

1. f   2. d   3. a   4. c   5. e
6. b

Matching Exercise 3

1. f   2. b   3. d   4. c   5. a
6. e

SHORT ANSWER

1. a. Pharmaceutical: refers to the mechanism of action (MOA), physiologic effect (PE), and chemical structure (CS) of the drug
   b. Therapeutic: refers to the clinical indication for the drug or therapeutic action (e.g., analgesic, antibiotic, or antihypertensive)
2. a. Drug–receptor interactions: The drug interacts with one or more cellular structures to alter cell function.
   b. Drug–enzyme interactions: The drug combines with enzymes to promote the desired effect.
3. Sample answers:
   a. Developmental stage of patient: A child's dose of medication is smaller than an adult's dose.
   b. Weight: Drug doses for children should be calculated on weight (in kilograms) or body surface area. Doses for adults are based on a reference adult (e.g., a healthy adult age 18 to 65 years weighing 150 lb/68.18 kg).
   c. Genetic factors: Asian patients may require smaller doses of a drug because they metabolize it at a slower rate.
   d. Cultural factors: Herbal remedies may interfere with or counteract the action of the prescribed medication.
   e. Hepatic disease: Liver disease may affect drug action by slowing the metabolism of drugs.
   f. Time of administration: The presence of food in the stomach generally delays the absorption of oral medications.
4. Sample answers:
   a. The nurse knows that the patient is allergic to the drug.
   b. The nurse has difficulty reading the order.
   c. The nurse knows the drug will be harmful to the patient.
5. a. Stock supply system (computerized automated dispensing cabinets [ADCs]): A large cabinet containing stock medications for the unit is used. The nurse accesses the system with a username and password, calling up a medication list for a specific patient or a list of available medications. In many systems, only medications entered for a specific patient are available for withdrawal at any one time.
   b. Unit-dose dispensing system: The pharmacist simplifies medication preparation by packaging and labeling each dosage for a 24-hour period. Computerized ADCs are a technology based on stock supply of unit-dose medications (see above).
   c. Medication cart: A typical cart contains individual drawers. Labeled with the patient's name, into which the medications for each patient are placed. If computers are not standard in every patient room and an EHR is used, there may also be a computer attached to the cart that allows for ready access to the eMAR by the administering nurse. The nurse moves the cart from room to room when dispensing medications.
   d. Barcode-enabled medication administration (BCMA): When using a computerized barcoded administration system, each patient and each nurse wear identification with a unique barcode to identify the person. Each drug is packaged with a barcode that includes its unique National Drug Code number to identify the form and dosage. The nurse scans his or her own ID, the patient's ID, and each package of medication to be administered. The system confirms the nurse's dispensing authority and the patient's ID, matching the patient with his or her medication profile. If any of the information is incorrect or does not match, an alert message will appear on the screen notifying the nurse of the discrepancy. The system also records the medication administration and stores the information.
6. a. Three checks: The medication label should be read (1) when the nurse reaches for the unit-dose package or container; (2) after retrieval from the drawer and compared with the eMAR/MAR or compared with the eMAR/MAR immediately before pouring from a multidose container; and (3) before giving the unit-dose medication to the patient, or when replacing the multidose container in the drawer or shelf.
   b. Eleven rights: Ensure that the (1) right medication is given to the (2) right patient in the (3) right dosage (in the right form) through the (4) right route at the (5) right time for the (6) right reason based on the (7) right (appropriate) assessment data using the (8) right documentation and monitoring for the (9) right response by the patient. Additional rights have been suggested to include (10) the right to education, ensuring that patients receive accurate and thorough information about the medication, and (11) the right to refuse, acknowledging that patients can and do refuse to take a medication.

7. Sample answers:
  a. Crush the medication (if appropriate for the type of medication) and add it to food or a drink so that the patient can swallow it.
  b. Allow the patient to suck on a piece of ice to numb their taste buds.
  c. Give the medication with generous amounts of water.
8. Sample answers:
  a. Route of administration: A longer needle is needed for an intramuscular injection than for intradermal or subcutaneous injection.
  b. Viscosity of the solution: Some medications are more viscous than others and require a large-lumen needle to be injected.
  c. Volume to be administered: The larger the amount of medication to be injected, the greater the capacity of the syringe.
  d. Body size: An obese person requires a longer needle to reach muscle tissue than a thin person.
  e. Type of medication: There are special syringes for certain uses, such as insulin or tuberculin syringes.
9. a. Assess the patient's condition immediately when the error is noted. Observe for adverse effects.
  b. Notify the nurse manager and the primary care provider to discuss possible courses of action based on the patient's condition.
  c. Report the incident following institutional policy. These may include an incident report, a quality assurance report, a risk assessment/root cause analysis report, or a variance report. These forms—generally called *special event*, *event*, or *unusual occurrence reports*—require an objective, complete account of the medication error. Include the steps taken after the error was recognized. For legal reasons, describe the error fully and accurately.
  d. Medication errors are a common allegation in nursing liability cases. Do not document in the patient's record the fact that an incident report was filed. Your institution is bound by state and national mandates to report certain incidents. Some of this reporting is voluntary and some is required. For example, reporting *near-miss* medication errors, in which an error almost occurred, is voluntary in some instances, but *sentinel events*, in which serious patient harm or death results from the error, require reporting.
10. a. Ampules: An ampule is a glass flask that contains a single dose of medication for parenteral administration. Medication is removed from an ampule, using a filter needle, after its thin neck is broken.
  b. Vials: A vial is a glass bottle with a self-sealing stopper through which medication is removed. Generally, an amount of air equivalent to the volume needed is injected into the vial prior

to drawing up the medication. The nurse can remove several doses from the same container.
  c. Prefilled cartridges: These provide a single dose of medication. The nurse inserts the cartridge into a reusable holder and clears the cartridge of excess air.
11. Fill in the missing information to explain how the following prescriptions would be administered. Use a pharmacology reference for medication information.
  a. Atenolol (Tenormin), 50 mg, PO BID, hold for BP less than 110 systolic
  Upon entering the room, the nurse introduces themselves and performs hand (1) hygiene. The nurse recognizes the medication name atenolol as the (2) generic name, when the patient refers to it as Tenormin. Next, the nurse (3) identifies the patient using (4) active identification of their name or (identification number, medical record number) and (5) date of birth, comparing it to the eMAR. The nurse assesses the patient's (6) vital signs prior to administering medications to avoid adverse reactions.
  The nurse teaches the patient that this medication is given by the (7) oral route and will be given (8) two times daily. Prior to administering this antihypertensive medication, the nurse notes the blood pressure is 102/70. Based on this assessment, the nurse plans to (9) withhold/hold the medication and (10) notify the prescriber. Documentation in the MAR and electronic health record will include (11) notation that the medication was withheld, (12) the patient's blood pressure, (13) the physician that was notified, and (14) any changes in the prescription.
  b. Heparin 5,000 unit subcutaneously twice daily
  After hand hygiene and patient (1) identification, the nurse explains that the medication is being given to prevent blood clots and that the injection will be given in the (2) abdomen. The nurse then selects an appropriate syringe for the (3) volume or amount of medication (generally 1 or 3 mL). First, the nurse injects a volume of air equivalent to the volume of heparin needed, keeping the vial on a flat surface. The nurse then inverts the vial, withdrawing the medication, ensuring there are no air (4) bubbles that could interfere with accurate dosing. The nurse performs the (5) recheck of the dose of medication and vial against the MAR (second check), and, prior to putting the vial away, checks the dose, syringe, and vial again (third check). The nurse gathers a fold of skin on the patient's abdomen and injects the medication at a 90-degree angle (45 degrees if the patient is extremely slender). When withdrawing the needle, the nurse applies (6) pressure, without rubbing the injection site.

c. NPH insulin 45 units daily SQ in the AM
After hand hygiene, active patient identification, and the first check of the vial of insulin against the eMAR, the nurse withdraws insulin from the vial using a(n) (1) insulin syringe. Prior to administering the insulin injection, the nurse assesses the patient's (2) fingerstick blood glucose, whether they have (3) eaten or had beverages, and the (4) site routinely used at that time of day. The nurse continues (5) premeal glucose monitoring and observes for (6) symptoms of hypoglycemia.

d. Nitroglycerin ointment (Nitro-Bid) 1/2 inch or 7.5 mg to anterior chest wall q8 hours
The nurse applies clean (1) gloves; removes the old patch, folding it, medication side facing (2) inward; and wipes the area as needed. Using the supplied paper, the nurse measures out (3) 1/2 inch(es). The nurse writes the (4) date, (5) time, and their initials on a piece of tape long enough to cover the patch. The nurse places the patch on a new, non-(6) hairy area on the anterior chest wall and secures it with tape, then documents the removal and new site of application. The nurse assesses the patient's blood (7) pressure before and after administration and for chest (8) pain and dizziness.

e. Oxycodone 5 mg with acetaminophen 325 mg 1 tablet PO
q4 hours PRN for pain
When the patient reports pain, clarify the (1) location and (2) severity of the patient's pain. Verify allergies and when the last doses were administered to ensure the (3) 4-hour interval has elapsed, and the maximum daily dose of acetaminophen is not (4) exceeded. Administer one tablet orally if indicated. Evaluate the medication's (5) effectiveness after administration. Assess for (6) sedation and presence of (7) constipation.

12. Medication administration.

13. Sample answer: Therapeutic drug level indicates optimal range of medication in the blood for a positive outcome without toxic effects. This medication should be withheld, and the prescriber notified. The nurse documents the level and that the medication is withheld on the MAR or per policy. In addition, the nurse documents the therapeutic drug level and any instructions from the prescriber in the electronic health record.

14. Sample answer: A peak and trough level are designed to ensure the therapeutic range of medication, in other words, neither too high (toxic) nor too low(ineffective). The trough level is drawn just before the medication dose; the peak is drawn 1 hour after the dose is administered. The nurse communicates results of the levels in report and to the health care provider. The provider may adjust the dose based on the outcome of the blood levels.

15. The nurse must recount the medication, determine if anyone on the unit had bypassed the safety features of the dispensing cabinet, and make a variance report. The nurse manager and pharmacy are notified.

16. The nurse enters the room, performs hand hygiene, and identifies the patient per policy. Generally, the nurse scans their ID, the patient ID bracelet, and each medication, comparing this to the eMAR and the package/bottle per the three checks. Once the process is complete, all monitoring has been completed, the patient may take the medication. The nurse may double-check once again, before discarding packages, based on facility procedure.

APPLYING YOUR KNOWLEDGE
CRITICAL THINKING QUESTIONS
Sample Answers

1. a. The nurse is obligated to question the prescription. The nurse may read progress notes, consults, or

Method	Ciprofloxacin
Dosage range	250–750 mg
Possible route of administration	PO
Frequency/schedule	BID
Desired effects	Cure/treat infection
Possible adverse effects	GI upset, nausea, diarrhea
Signs and symptoms of toxic drug effects	CNS stimulation, dizziness
Special instructions	Avoid antacids, vitamins
Nursing/collaborative management of adverse effects	Report severe diarrhea to provider

other portions of the electronic health record, but, if the question persists, the nurse must discuss the rationale for the medication with the provider. While the nurse may consult other experts on the unit, it is ultimately the nurse's responsibility to understand the purpose of a medication for each patient.

b. The nurse should recheck the order and pertinent provider notes in the electronic health record to determine if a new medication has been prescribed. If the medication is correct, the nurse could verify with the pharmacy that the medication is correct for its physical description and that there is a generic and trade name. If there is no information indicating the medication is correct, the nurse withholds the medication and clarifies with the provider.

REFLECTIVE PRACTICE: CULTIVATING QSEN COMPETENCIES
Sample Answers

1. Safety/teamwork and collaboration: How might the nurse use blended nursing skills to respond to this potential medication error? What resources might be helpful in preventing future errors?
   To determine that the medication was labeled incorrectly, the nurse would use the five rights of medication administration: (1) Give the right medication (2) to the right patient (3) in the right dosage (4) through the right route (5) at the right time. The nurse could call the pharmacy and have new medication delivered with the right patient's name. Teach patients about their medications, especially the purpose, and to question anything they do not understand; attend to all aspects of medication labeling.

2. Patient-centered care/safety: What would be a successful outcome for this patient?
   The patient receives the prescribed medication with his name on the label. The nurse adhered to the safety systems and procedures put in place by the facility.

3. Safety/evidence-based practice: What intellectual, technical, and ethical/legal competencies are most likely to bring about the desired outcome?
   Intellectual: ability to identify prescribed dose and medication, knowledge of intravenous antibiotic therapy, understanding systems wide safety features designed to prevent errors
   Technical: ability to safely administer IV antibiotics to a patient
   Ethical/Legal: ability to provide patient safety via accurate patient identification to ensure medications are delivered in the right dosage to the right patient

4. Informatics/safety: When the nurse scans the barcode, the system states that the medication and dose is correct. What action is safest, given the situation?
   The nurse follows the policy and best practice guidelines to ensure safe medication and adheres to safety systems guidelines. Next steps include active iden-

tification of the patient using two identifiers (if not completed first) and visual inspection of the medication label, dose, and expiration date. Additionally, the nurse follows the rights of medication administration, critically analyzing if it is safe to administer each medication, and documents clearly.

PRACTICING FOR NCLEX
MULTIPLE-CHOICE QUESTIONS

1. b	**2.** a	**3.** c	**4.** d	**5.** b
6. a	**7.** b	**8.** d	**9.** b	**10.** a
11. b	**12.** d	**13.** c	**14.** c	**15.** a
16. a	**17.** d	**18.** b	**19.** d	**20.** b
21. b				

ALTERNATE-FORMAT QUESTIONS
Multiple-Response Questions

1. a, c, d, e
2. b, e, f
3. a, b, c
4. b, d, e
5. a, c, d
6. b, e, f
7. b, d, f
8. a, b, d
9. b, d, e

Theory to Practice

1. d

Prioritization Question

1. d

CHAPTER 31

ASSESSING YOUR UNDERSTANDING
FILL IN THE BLANKS

1. surgery
2. urgency
3. elective
4. risk
5. maintenance
6. conscious (moderate or procedural)
7. Informed
8. Advance
9. universal
10. PACU
11. skin
12. void/urinate
13. frequent
14. endotracheal

MATCHING EXERCISES
Matching Exercise 1

1. a	**2.** c	**3.** d	**4.** b	**5.** d
6. b				

Matching Exercise 2

1. a, b, f
2. d

3. e
4. b
5. a, f

SHORT ANSWER

1. a. Preoperative phase: begins with the decision that surgical intervention is necessary and lasts until the patient is transferred to the operating room table
   b. Intraoperative phase: extends from admission to the surgical department to transfer to postanesthesia care unit (PACU)
   c. Postoperative phase: lasts from admission to the PACU to the complete recovery from surgery and the first health care provider follow-up visit

2. a. Based on urgency: may be classified as elective surgery (preplanned; patient choice), urgent surgery (necessary for patient's health; not emergency), or emergency surgery (preserves patient's life, body part, or body function)
   b. Based on degree of risk: may be classified as minor: performed in health care provider's office, an outpatient clinic, or a same-day, outpatient surgery setting (also referred to as ambulatory surgery), or major: requires hospitalization, is prolonged and has higher degree of risk, involves major body organs
   c. Based on purpose: descriptors include diagnostic, ablative, palliative, reconstructive, transplant, and constructive

3. a. Induction: begins with administration of the anesthetic agent and continues until patient is ready for incision
   b. Maintenance: continues from point of incision until near completion of procedure
   c. Emergence: starts as patient begins to emerge from the anesthesia and usually ends when patient is ready to leave the operating room

4. a. Description of the procedure or treatment
   b. Underlying disease process and its natural course
   c. Name and qualifications of the person performing the procedure or treatment
   d. Explanation of the common risks involved, including potential for damage, disfigurement, or death
   e. Patient's right to refuse treatment and withdraw consent
   f. Explanation of expected (not guaranteed) outcome, recovery, and rehabilitation plan and course of medication if prescribed

5. a. Cardiovascular disease: increased potential for hemorrhage and hypovolemic shock, hypotension, venous stasis, thrombophlebitis, and overhydration with IV fluids
   b. Pulmonary disorders: increased possibility of respiratory depression from anesthesia, postoperative pneumonia, atelectasis, and alterations in acid–base balance
   c. Kidney and liver function disorders: influence the patient's response to anesthesia, affect fluid and electrolyte as well as acid–base balance, alter metabolism and excretion of drugs, and impair wound healing
   d. Endocrine disorders: endocrine diseases, especially diabetes mellitus, increase the risk for hypoglycemia or acidosis, slow wound healing, and increased risk for postoperative infection and cardiovascular complications

6. a. Fear of the unknown: Encourage the patient to identify and verbalize fears; identify and correct incorrect knowledge; identify patient strengths.
   b. Fear of pain and death: Teach patient about usual pain management strategies, including medication, positioning, and frequent nursing assessment. Support the patient's spiritual needs through acceptance, participation in prayer, or referral to clergy or chaplain.
   c. Fear of changes in body image and self-concept: Identify the need for support systems during initial interview; arrange a preoperative visit from a person who has had the same procedure and adapted successfully.

7. The nurse is responsible for ensuring that the tests are ordered and performed, and the results are recorded in the patient's health record before surgery. The nurse reports abnormal findings such as blood glucose, coagulation studies, renal function, or others.

8. a. Surgical events and sensations: Tell the patient and family when surgery is scheduled; how long it will last; what will be done before, during, and after surgery; and what sensations the patient will be experiencing during the perioperative period, including referred pain. Inform the patient and family about expected tubes and drains that could be present postoperatively.
   b. Pain management: The patient should be informed that pain reported by the patient is the determining factor of pain control, pain will be assessed frequently after major surgery. There are many routes and modalities for pain management from intravenous, patient-controlled analgesia, oral agents, pressure-controlled pumps with soaker drains, and more. If concerned, inform the patient there is little danger of addiction to pain medications, and nonpharmacologic methods of pain control (relaxation techniques, TENS) are available.

9. a. Hygiene and skin preparation: Clean the skin with antibacterial soap to remove bacteria (preoperative showers or baths are taken before the scheduled surgery using chlorhexidine gluconate [CHG] soap; children and adult inpatients may be cleansed preoperatively with microfiber cloths impregnated with CHG antimicrobial skin antiseptic, which eliminates skin microorganisms and leaves an antimicrobial film on their skin). Shampoo the hair and clean the fingernails to help to reduce the number of organisms present on the body. Leave hair at the surgical site in place if possible or remove/clip only the hair that will interfere with the procedure.

b. Elimination: Emptying the bowel of feces is no longer a routine procedure, but the nurse should use preoperative assessments to determine the need for an order for bowel elimination. If an indwelling catheter is not in place, the patient should void immediately before receiving preoperative medications.

c. Nutrition and fluids: Diet depends on the type of surgery; patients need to be well nourished and hydrated before surgery to counterbalance fluid, blood, and electrolyte loss during surgery. Light meals such as tea and toast may be consumed up to 6 hours before surgery; fatty meals should be consumed up to 8 hours before surgery.

d. Rest and sleep: The nurse can facilitate rest and sleep in the immediate preoperative period by meeting psychological needs, carrying out teaching, providing a quiet environment, and administering prescribed bedtime sedative medications.

10. a. Maintain intact skin surfaces
   b. Remain free of neuromuscular damage
   c. Have symmetric breathing patterns

11. Sample answer: The nurse in the PACU provides vigilant monitoring during emergence from anesthesia and the first hours after surgery beginning with monitoring vital signs and quality of respirations, managing pain, maintaining IVs and fluid and electrolyte balance, stabilizing physiologic parameters (such as heart and respiratory rate), and preparing for the next level of care.

12. Sample answer: The person who will be changing the patient's dressing at home should demonstrate proper techniques in wound care and dressing change. Teaching should include the following information: (1) where to buy dressing materials and medical supplies, (2) signs and symptoms of infection, (3) need to eat well-balanced meals and drink fluids within prescribed limits, (4) how to modify activities of daily living (as needed), (5) need to wear disposable gloves when changing the dressing and wash hands before and after putting gloves on, and (6) how to dispose of old dressings.

13. Sample answers:
   a. Developmental considerations: Infants and older adults are at a greater risk from surgery than are children and young or middle-aged adults.
   b. Medical history: Pathologic changes associated with past and current illnesses increase surgical risk.
   c. Medications: Use of anticoagulants and certain herbals before surgery may precipitate hemorrhage.
   d. Previous surgery: Previous heart or lung surgery may necessitate adaptations in the anesthesia used and in positioning during surgery.
   e. Lifestyle: Cultural and ethnic background of the patient may affect surgical risk. Substance abuse issues should be identified and considered in the perioperative plan (e.g., pain management).

   f. Nutrition: Diabetes, malnutrition, and obesity increase surgical risk.
   g. Activities of daily living: Exercise, rest, and sleep habits are important for preventing postoperative complications and facilitating recovery.
   h. Sociocultural needs: The patient's cultural background may require that nursing interventions be individualized to meet needs in such areas as language, food preferences, family interaction and participation, personal space, and health beliefs and practices.

14. a. Vital signs: Assess temperature, blood pressure, and pulse and respiratory rates. Note that tachycardia and hypotension may indicate hemorrhagic shock or increased fluid requirements. Note deviations from preoperative and PACU data as well as symptoms of complications.
   b. Color and temperature of skin: Assess for coolness, pallor, cyanosis, and diaphoresis.
   c. Level of consciousness: Assess for orientation to time, place, and person as well as reaction to stimuli and ability to move extremities.
   d. Intravenous fluids: Assess type and amount of solution, flow rate, security and patency of tubing, and infusion site.
   e. Surgical site: Assess dressing and dependent areas for drainage; anticipate drainage may be bloody initially. Assess drains and tubes and be sure they are intact, patent, and properly connected to drainage systems. Collaborate with the provider if drainage seems excessive.
   f. Tubes and drains: Assess indwelling urinary catheter and gastrointestinal suction, etc. for drainage, patency, and amount of output.
   g. Pain management: Assess the patient for pain, determine which analgesic has been given, and the time of administration, if pertinent. Assess for and manage nausea and vomiting.
   h. Position and safety: Place the patient in the ordered position; if the patient is not fully conscious, place them in the side-lying position. Elevate side rails and place the bed in the low position.
   i. Comfort: Cover the patient with a blanket, maintain warmth, and assess for hypothermia. Reorient the patient to the room as necessary, and allow family members to remain with the patient, per policy, after the initial assessment is completed.

15. Sample answers:
   a. Nausea and vomiting: Provide oral hygiene as needed, avoid strong-smelling foods, and administer antiemetics.
   b. Thirst: Offer ice chips; maintain oral hygiene.
   c. Hiccups: Rebreathe into a paper bag; eat a teaspoon of granulated sugar.
   d. Surgical pain: Evaluate outcome of pain management frequently; offer nonpharmacologic measures to supplement medications.

APPLYING YOUR KNOWLEDGE
CRITICAL THINKING QUESTION

1. Sample answers:

a. The nurse performs an assessment with a focus on the cardiopulmonary system, considering smoking and lung damage that could complicate anesthesia and postoperative recovery. Preoperatively, the nurse teaches coughing and deep breathing, discusses early mobility, and explains/demonstrates use of the incentive spirometer to prevent pneumonia. The nurse explains to expect waking up with tubes and drains, such as an endotracheal tube or chest drains that may be placed during surgery. The nurse also discusses risk factors for coronary artery disease and the need to modify diet and increase exercise to prevent its progression.

b. The nurse conducts a focused GI and psychosocial assessment. The nurse assesses the patient's concerns related to the cancer diagnosis, surgery, and outcome. If a colostomy is planned, the nurse discusses the patient's perception of this as well as teaches the patient about available resources to learn to manage the device. The nurse listens to the patient's concerns about having cancer at a young age and concerns about their family as well as discusses pain management, coughing and deep breathing, and maintaining mobility.

REFLECTIVE PRACTICE: CULTIVATING QSEN COMPETENCIES
Sample Answers

1. Patient-centered care: How might the nurse use blended nursing skills to implement the perioperative care plan in a manner that respects Molly's human dignity and addresses her fears and concerns about the surgical experience?

The nurse should assess the patient's psychological, sociocultural, and spiritual dimensions, explaining that it is normal to have preoperative anxiety as is a major psychological stressor. The nurse can provide information about the surgery, anticipated postoperative care, frequent vital signs and assessments, needed peri pads, pain management, and education. The nurse can use cues obtained in a health history, including the underlying disorder prompting the surgery, to plan nursing interventions and emotional support for a successful recovery.

2. Patient-centered care/evidence-based practice: What would be a successful outcome for this patient? Following the nursing history, the patient verbalizes her fears regarding the surgery and lists three coping methods to reduce stress. The patient is able to verbalize the expected care postoperatively, including pain management and requesting pain medication before pain is out of control, coughing and deep breathing, use of the incentive spirometer, turning, and mobility. The patient is free from

infection and postoperative complications and is discharged without incident.

3. Evidence-based practice/safety: What intellectual, interpersonal, and/or ethical/legal competencies are most likely to bring about the desired outcome? Intellectual: ability to identify the common psychological patient responses before and after surgery, including pain management. The nurse ensures preoperative antibiotics are administered to prevent infection, per surgical protocol.

Interpersonal: ability to individualize communication and patient education based on patient needs.

Ethical/legal skills: ability to participate in care as a trusted and effective advocate, including advocating for a patient who is fearful. Completes preoperative checklist, validates surgical site, ensures lab and diagnostic tests are completed and available in the electronic health record.

4. Teamwork and collaboration/evidence-based practice: What resources might be helpful for Molly? Referral to psychological services if anxiety continues; home health aide if weak or needs assistance with ADLs.

Printed or AV materials of hysterectomies, counseling, support groups.

PRACTICING FOR NCLEX
MULTIPLE-CHOICE QUESTIONS

1. b	**2.** a	**3.** b	**4.** d	**5.** b
6. c	**7.** c	**8.** b	**9.** a	**10.** c
11. b	**12.** d	**13.** a	**14.** c	**15.** c

ALTERNATE-FORMAT QUESTIONS
Multiple-Response Questions

1. d, e, f
2. b, e, f
3. a, c, d
4. a, b, d, e
5. b, c, d, e
6. b, c, f
7. a, b, c, e
8. c, e, f

Sequencing Questions

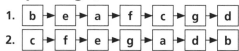

1. b → e → a → f → c → g → d
2. c → f → e → g → a → d → b

Prioritization Question

1. d

CHAPTER 32

ASSESSING YOUR UNDERSTANDING
FILL IN THE BLANKS

1. skin
2. gingivitis
3. diabetes

4. pediculosis
5. bariatric
6. Halitosis
7. rinsing
8. Lyme
9. powder
10. sebum

MATCHING EXERCISES

1. e   **2.** d   **3.** f   **4.** b   **5.** c
6. a

CORRECT THE FALSE STATEMENTS

1. F, ceruminous glands
2. T
3. F, noncircumcised
4. T
5. F, lowest
6. T
7. F, Oily
8. T
9. F, podiatrist
10. F, morning care (AM care)

SHORT ANSWER

1. a. Culture: Many people in North America place a high value on personal cleanliness, shower frequently, and use many products to mask odors. Culture may also dictate whether bathing is private or communal.
  b. Socioeconomic class: Financial resources often define the hygiene options available to people. The availability of running water and finances for soap, shampoo, etc., affects hygiene.
  c. Spiritual practices: Religion may dictate ceremonial washing and purification, which may be a prelude to prayer or eating or following death.
  d. Developmental level: Children learn different hygiene practices while growing up. Family practices may dictate morning or evening baths, frequency of shampooing, feelings about nudity, frequency of clothing changes, etc.
  e. Health state: Disease or injury may hinder a person's ability to perform hygiene measures or motivation to follow usual hygiene habits.
  f. Personal preference: People have personal preferences with regard to shower versus tub baths, bar soap versus liquid soap, etc.
2. a. Feeding
  b. Bathing and hygiene
  c. Dressing and grooming
  d. Toileting
3. First, the nurse assesses whether the parent has the financial means to buy the materials necessary for their infant's hygiene (shampoo, oil, powder, diaper rash ointment, etc.). If not, a social service recommendation may be indicated. If there is deficient knowledge regarding bathing an infant, the parent should be educated on the proper bathing techniques. If cradle cap is present on the scalp,

the nurse can teach removal with a soft brush and application of an emollient. The nurse can discuss the need for good hygiene for her baby, and a bath should be demonstrated with the parent providing a return demonstration.
4. a. Early morning care: The patient should be assisted with toileting and provided comfort measures designed to refresh the patient and prepare them for breakfast. The face and hands should be washed, and mouth care provided.
  b. Morning care (AM care): After breakfast, the nurse offers assistance with toileting, oral care, bathing, back massage, special skin care measures, hair care, cosmetics, dressing, and positioning. Bed linens are refreshed or changed.
  c. Afternoon care (PM care): The nurse should ensure the patient's comfort after lunch and offer assistance with toileting, handwashing, and oral care to nonambulatory patients.
  d. Hour-of-sleep care (HS care): The nurse again offers assistance with toileting, washing of face and hands, and oral care. A back massage helps the patient relax and fall asleep. Soiled bed linens or clothing should be changed, and the patient positioned comfortably.
  e. As-needed care (PRN care): The nurse offers individual hygiene measures as needed. Some patients require oral care every 2 hours. Patients who are diaphoretic may need their clothing or linens changed several times a shift.
5. Sample answers: Bathing cleanses the skin, acts as a conditioner, relaxes a restless person, promotes circulation, serves as musculoskeletal exercise, stimulates the rate and depth of respiration, promotes comfort, provides sensory input, improves self-esteem, and strengthens the nurse–patient relationship.
6. Sample answers: Provide the patient with articles for bathing and a basin of water that is at a comfortable temperature; place these items conveniently for the patient. Provide privacy; remove top bed linens and replace with a bath blanket. Place cosmetics in a convenient place with a mirror and light, and supply hot water and a razor for a patient who wishes to shave. Assist patients who cannot reach to bathe themselves completely.
7. Sample answers: A towel bath can be accomplished with little fatigue to the patient. The towel remains warm during the short procedure. Patients state that they feel clean and refreshed. The oil in the bathing solution eliminates dry, itchy skin.
8. a. Lips: color, moisture, lumps, ulcers, lesions, and edema
  b. Buccal mucosa: color, moisture, lesions, nodules, and bleeding
  c. Gums: lesions, bleeding, edema, and exudate; loose or missing teeth
  d. Tongue: color, symmetry, movement, texture, and lesions

e. Hard and soft palates: intactness, color, patches, lesions, and petechiae

f. Eyes: position, alignment, and general appearance; presence of lesions, nodules, redness, swelling, crusting, flaking, excessive tearing, or discharge; color of conjunctivae; blink reflex; and visual acuity

g. Ears: position, alignment, and general appearance; buildup of wax; dryness, crusting, discharge, or foreign body; and hearing acuity

h. Nose: position and general appearance; patency of nostrils; presence of tenderness, dryness, edema, bleeding, and discharge or secretions

9. a. Hearing aids: Batteries should be checked routinely, and earpieces cleaned daily with mild soap and water. Observe for impacted cerumen, dead batteries.

b. Dentures: Clean dentures daily to reduce plaque and potentially harmful microorganisms by soaking in and brushing with a nonabrasive denture cleanser. Avoid toothpaste as it can be too harsh for denture surfaces. Apply gloves and hold the dentures over a basin of water or a sink lined with a washcloth or soft towel to prevent breakage if they fall. If necessary, grasp the dentures with a 4″ × 4″ piece of gauze to help prevent them from slipping out of your gloved hands. Use cool or lukewarm water for cleansing, hot water may warp the dentures. Rinse dentures thoroughly before reinserting. Offer the patient the opportunity to brush the gums and tongue and rinse the mouth before the dentures are replaced. Assist the patient with care as necessary.

10. Sample answers: Deficient self-care abilities, vascular disease, arthritis, diabetes mellitus, history of biting nails or improper trimming, fungal infections, frequent or prolonged exposure to chemicals or water, trauma, ill-fitting shoes, or obesity

APPLYING YOUR KNOWLEDGE
CRITICAL THINKING QUESTIONS
Sample Answers

1. a. The nurse maintains a professional demeanor, promotes patient comfort and dignity, assesses patient preference in regard to hygiene.

b. The nurse encourages the patient to complete what they are able to, framing this in relation to their goals, such as discharge to home, recovery, and long-term complications.

c. The nurse maintains a matter-of-fact demeanor and explains that urine remaining on the skin can promote breakdown and odor. The nurse attempts to determine the underlying reason for refusing care, such as poor self-esteem or trauma. If able, the nurse could ambulate the patient to a commode or bathroom and assist the patient with perineal care using a washcloth and pitcher of warm water poured over the perineal area.

2. Spinal or back surgery, fractured ribs, pain

3. Answers will vary

REFLECTIVE PRACTICE: CULTIVATING QSEN COMPETENCIES
Sample Answers

1. Patient-centered care/safety: With what assessments and teaching will Sonya and her daughter need help to meet Sonya's hygiene needs?
The nurse should investigate Sonya's feelings about being cared for by her daughter since hygiene is such a personal matter. The nurse should encourage her to take care of as many hygienic practices as possible using her left side. Teaching should include how to adapt a bathroom to the needs of a disabled person, for example: having grab bars installed (if not present), placing a chair in the shower and using handheld showerheads, checking water temperature, ensuring privacy, placing a nonskid mat in the shower/tub, helping the patient get in and out of the shower, keeping the bathroom door unlocked, and helping to wash and dry areas the patient can't reach (such as the back and feet). The nurse informs Sonya's daughter that skin of the older adult becomes dry and daily bathing the entire body may not be necessary. The nurse can teach about caring for her mother's hair, dentures, and hearing aids.

2. Patient-centered care: What would be a successful outcome for this patient?
By next visit, the patient demonstrates washing areas of her body that she can reach. By next visit, the patient's daughter states that she is comfortable with the care plan for hygienic measures instituted for her mother.

3. Patient-centered care/evidence-based practice: What intellectual, technical, and interpersonal competencies are most likely to bring about the desired outcome?
Intellectual: having basic knowledge about hygiene, hygiene measures, and the products and equipment that facilitate safe care. Recognizing skin of older adults will become dry and more fragile with age.
Technical: ability to adapt hygiene care measures and modify the bathroom to meet the needs of an older adult with right-sided paralysis
Interpersonal: ability to encourage patients and their caregivers, as appropriate, in learning new safety and self-care measures related to hygiene

4. Patient-centered care/teamwork and collaboration: What resources might be helpful for Sonya and her daughter?
Home health aide services, information on adaptive devices for people with paralysis, PT consult for strengthening the affected side and safety getting in and out of the shower/tub.

PATIENT CARE STUDY

Answers will vary with student experience.

PRACTICING FOR NCLEX
MULTIPLE-CHOICE QUESTIONS

1. c   2. a   3. a   4. b   5. c
6. d   7. a   8. c   9. c   10. b

ALTERNATE-FORMAT QUESTIONS
Multiple-Response Questions

1. a, b, e
2. b, c
3. d, f
4. a, b, d
5. d, e

Prioritization Question

1. c

CHAPTER 33

ASSESSING YOUR UNDERSTANDING
FILL IN THE BLANKS

1. primary
2. exudate
3. leukocytes, macrophages
4. granulation
5. fistula
6. chloride
7. circular
8. eschar
9. dressing
10. binder

MATCHING EXERCISES
Matching Exercise 1

1. d 2. f 3. e 4. b 5. a
6. c

Matching Exercise 2

1. c 2. e 3. b 4. f 5. d
6. a

Matching Exercise 3

1. b 2. e 3. a 4. d 5. e
6. c

SHORT ANSWER

1. a. Protect the body; immunologic function
   b. Regulate body temperature
   c. Sense stimuli from the environment and transmit these sensations
   d. Absorption and elimination
   e. Help maintain water and electrolyte balance
   f. Produce and absorb vitamin D
2. a. External pressure: compresses blood vessels and causes friction
   b. Friction and shearing forces: tears and injures blood vessels
3. a. Nutrition: Poorly nourished cells are easily damaged (e.g., vitamin C deficiency causes capillaries to become fragile, and poor circulation to the area results when they break).
   b. Hydration: Dehydration can interfere with circulation and subsequent cell nourishment.
   c. Moist skin: Moisture associated with urinary incontinence increases the risk for skin damage more than chemical irritation from the ammonia in urine.

d. Mental status: The more alert a patient is, the more likely it is that they will relieve pressure periodically and manage adequate skin hygiene.
   e. Age: Older people are good candidates for pressure injuries because their skin is susceptible to injury.
   f. Immobility: Causes prolonged pressure on body areas.
4. Sample answer: Provide the caregivers with a simple, easy-to-understand list of instructions and visual aids discussing care of a pressure injury. The nurse helps the patient and family identify the causative factor(s) for the pressure injury before developing the care plan. Additionally, the nurse suggests alternate positions to relieve pressure on the coccyx. The nurse and family consult frequently with the health care provider about applications of products or dressings. The nurse teaches the caregivers proper handwashing technique, the use of clean technique, and reviews signs of infection. They are told to contact the provider or home health nurse about any problems.
5. a. Hemostasis: Hemostasis occurs immediately after the initial injury. Involved blood vessels constrict and blood clotting begins through platelet activation and clustering. After only a brief period of constriction, these same blood vessels dilate and capillary permeability increases, allowing plasma and blood components to leak out into the area that is injured, forming a liquid called exudate.
   b. Inflammatory phase: The inflammatory phase follows hemostasis and lasts about 2 to 3 days. White blood cells, predominantly leukocytes and macrophages, move to the wound. About 24 hours after the injury, macrophages enter the wound area and remain for an extended period. Macrophages are essential to the healing process. They not only ingest debris, but also release growth factors that are necessary for the growth of epithelial cells and new blood vessels. These growth factors also attract fibroblasts that help to fill in the wound, which is necessary for the next stage of healing. Acute inflammation is characterized by pain, heat, redness, and swelling at the site of the injury.
   c. Proliferative phase: The proliferative phase follows the inflammatory phase, beginning on day 2 or 3 of wound development and lasts 2 to 3 weeks. New tissue is built to fill the wound space (action of fibroblasts). Capillaries grow across the wound, fibroblasts form fibrin that stretches through the clot, a thin layer of epithelial cells forms across the wound, and blood flow is reinstituted. Granulation tissue forms the foundation for scar tissue.
   d. Maturation phase: Begins about 3 weeks after injury, possibly continuing for months or years if wound is large. Collagen is remodeled, new collagen is deposited, and avascular collagen tissue becomes a flat, thin white line.
6. Sample answers:
   a. The patient will consume a balanced diet rich in protein and vitamin C and zinc to promote wound healing.

b. The patient will remain free of infection at the site of the pressure injury.

c. The patient will demonstrate/participate in turning and self-care measures necessary to prevent/heal the pressure injury.

7. Sample answers:

a. Overall appearance of skin: Are there any areas on your body where your skin feels paper-thin? How does your skin feel in relation to moisture—dry, clammy, oily?

b. Recent changes in skin condition: Have you noticed any sores anywhere on your body? Do you ever notice any redness over a bony area when you stay in one position for a while?

c. Activity/mobility: Do you need assistance to walk to the bathroom? Can you change your position freely and painlessly?

d. Nutrition: Have you lost weight lately? Do you eat well-balanced meals?

e. Pain: Do you have any painful sores on your body? Do you take any medications for pain?

f. Elimination: Do you have any problems with incontinence? Have you ever used any briefs or pads for incontinence problems?

8. a. Appearance: Assess for the approximation of wound edges, color of the wound and surrounding areas, drains or tubes, sutures, and signs of dehiscence or evisceration.

b. Wound drainage: Assess the amount, color, odor, and consistency of wound drainage. Drainage can be assessed on the wound, the dressings, in drainage bottles or reservoirs, or under the patient.

c. Pain: Assess whether the pain has increased or is constant; pain may indicate delayed healing or infection.

d. Sutures and staples: Assess the presence and type of suture and whether enough tensile strength has developed to hold the wound edges together during healing.

9. Provide physical, psychological, and aesthetic comfort; debride (remove necrotic tissue) if appropriate; prevent, eliminate, or control infection; absorb drainage; maintain a moist wound environment; protect the wound from further injury; and protect the skin surrounding the wound.

10. a. R = red = protect: Red wounds are in the proliferative stage of healing and are the color of normal granulation. They need protection by gentle cleansing, using moist dressings, applying a transparent or hydrocolloid dressing, and changing the dressing only when necessary.

b. Y = yellow = cleanse: Yellow wounds are characterized by oozing from the tissue covering the wound, often accompanied by purulent drainage. They need to be cleansed using irrigation; wet-to-moist dressings; using nonadherent, hydrogel, or other absorptive dressings; and topical antimicrobial medication.

c. B = black = debride: Black wounds are covered with thick eschar, which is usually black but may also be brown, gray, or tan. The eschar must be debrided before the wound can heal by using sharp, mechanical, chemical, or autolytic debridement.

11. a. Hot water bags or bottles: Relatively inexpensive and easy to use; may leak, burn, or make the patient uncomfortable from their weight.

b. Electric heating pad: Can be used to apply dry heat locally; it is easy to apply and relatively safe and provides constant and even heat. Improper use can result in injury.

c. Aquathermia pad: Commonly used in health care agencies for various problems including back pain, muscle spasms, thrombophlebitis, and mild inflammation. Safer than a heating pad but still must be checked carefully.

d. Chemical heat packs: Commercial hot packs provide a specified amount of dry heat for a specific period.

e. Warm moist compresses: Used to promote circulation and reduce edema. Must be changed frequently and covered with a heating agent.

f. Sitz baths: Patient is placed in a tub filled with sufficient water to reach the umbilicus; the legs and feet remain out of the water.

g. Warm soaks: The immersion of a body area into warm water or a medicated solution to increase blood supply to a locally infected area; to aid in cleaning large sloughing wounds, such as burns; to improve circulation; and to apply medication to a locally infected area. Makes manipulation of a painful area much easier because of the buoyancy.

12. Drains may be inserted in or near a wound to promote removal of blood and wound exudate. This promotes wound healing and to reduces the risk of abscess formation.

APPLYING YOUR KNOWLEDGE
CRITICAL THINKING QUESTIONS

1. Sample answer: For all patients (a,b,c), minimize moisture causing skin maceration. Relieve pressure on bony prominences. For adults, pad coccyx, trochanters, areas beneath oxygen tubing. For neonates or comatose patients with feeding tubes, inspect and protect areas around and beneath tubes. Protect reddened areas per facility policy. A premature infant receiving life support may have periods of hypoxemia, decreasing oxygen to the tissues, which promotes skin breakdown. For all patients, consult the dietician to provide adequate protein and calories to prevent tissue damage.

2. Answers will vary.

REFLECTIVE PRACTICE: CULTIVATING QSEN COMPETENCIES
Sample Answers

1. Patient-centered care/evidence-based practice: What nursing intervention would be appropriate to prevent skin irritation and the development of pressure injuries for Sam?

The nurse reviews the electronic health record to determine the cause and extent of the bone infection and risk factors for breakdown, as well as reviewing available photographs. The nurse provides education (e.g., diabetes), protects skin that is at risk, and institutes measures to minimize these risks in the future. The nurse also pays attention to skin folds and areas where moisture can accumulate and cause maceration of the skin, by keeping these areas clean and dry. The nurse encourages the patient to consume a balanced diet to promote healing.

To protect the patient, the nurse implements turning and positioning schedules as well as the use of appropriate support surfaces (tissue load management surfaces) and repositions him at least every 2 hours. The nurse encourages the patient to be out of bed and ambulate as permitted. The nurse monitors and trends the WBC count to assess resolution of the bone infection.

2. Patient-centered care: What would be a successful outcome for this patient?
Decreasing WBCs, cooperation with hygiene, nutrition, positioning and turning as well as getting out of bed if permitted. At follow-up appointment, the patient will have normal WBCs and intact skin free of skin irritations, infections, and wounds.

3. Evidence-based practice: What intellectual, technical, and interpersonal competencies are most likely to bring about the desired outcome?
Intellectual: the nurse is aware that large amounts of subcutaneous and tissue fat (which has fewer blood vessels) may slow wound healing. Fatty tissue is more difficult to suture, is more prone to infection, and takes longer to heal. Knowledge of the phases of wound healing and factors that affect wound healing
Technical: knowledge of administration of antibiotics to heal the bone infection; recognition that bone infections are slow to heal. Ability to correctly use the products, protocols, and equipment necessary to prevent and treat pressure injuries and other skin alterations
Interpersonal: ability to establish trusting professional relationships that enlist patients and their caregivers in a plan to prevent or treat pressure injuries and other skin alterations

4. Teamwork and collaboration: What resources might be helpful for Sam?
Home health care visits, printed and/or AV materials on prevention of pressure injuries

PATIENT CARE STUDY

Answers will vary with student experience.

PRACTICING FOR NCLEX
MULTIPLE-CHOICE QUESTIONS

1. b   2. d   3. a   4. c   5. d
6. c   7. b   8. d   9. d   10. a
11. a   12. a   13. a

ALTERNATE-FORMAT QUESTIONS
Multiple-Response Questions

1. a, b, c, e
2. b, c, e, f
3. a, d, e
4. c, d, e
5. a, b, c
6. b, c, d
7. a, d, e
8. c, d, e
9. a, d, e
10. b, c, f
11. b, d, e

Sequencing Question

1.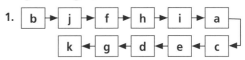

CHAPTER 34

ASSESSING YOUR UNDERSTANDING
FILL IN THE BLANKS

1. skeletal
2. origin, insertion
3. umbilicus; symphysis
4. locomotion
5. Contractures
6. Osteoporosis
7. isokinetic
8. thrombus
9. atrophy
10. flaccidity
11. paresis, paralysis
12. left hand

IDENTIFICATION

1. a. Fowler's position
   b. Supine position
   c. Side-lying or lateral position
   d. Sims' position
   e. Prone position

MATCHING EXERCISES
Matching Exercise 1

1. e   2. c   3. f   4. b   5. a

Matching Exercise 2

1. e   2. f   3. d   4. a   5. b
6. c

Matching Exercise 3

1. a   2. d   3. b   4. e   5. c
6. f

CORRECT THE FALSE STATEMENTS

1. F, irregular bones
2. T
3. T

4. T

5. F, Body mechanics

6. T

7. F, wider

8. F, proprioceptor or kinesthetic

9. F, basal ganglia

10. T

11. T

12. T

13. F, same

14. T

15. F, slide, roll, push, or pull

16. F, circumduction

17. F, hyperextended

18. F, hyperflexion

19. T

20. older adult's

SHORT ANSWER

1.

Body System	Effects of Exercise	Effects of Immobility
Cardiovascular	↑ Efficiency of heart ↓ Resting heart rate and blood pressure ↑ Blood flow and oxygenation of all body parts	↑ Cardiac workload ↑ Risk for orthostatic hypotension ↑ Risk for venous thrombosis
Respiratory	↑ Depth of respiration ↑ Respiratory rate ↑ Gas exchange at alveolar level ↑ Rate of carbon dioxide excretion	↓ Depth of respiration ↓ Rate of respiration Pooling of secretions Impaired gas exchange
Gastrointestinal	↑ Appetite ↑ Intestinal tone	Disturbance in appetite Altered protein metabolism Altered digestion and utilization of nutrients
Urinary	↑ Blood flow to kidneys ↑ Efficiency in maintaining fluid and acid–base balance ↑ Efficiency in excreting body wastes	↑ Urinary stasis ↑ Risk for renal calculi ↓ Bladder muscle tone
Musculoskeletal	↑ Muscle efficiency ↑ Coordination ↑ Efficiency of nerve impulse transmission	↓ Muscle size, tone, and strength ↓ Joint mobility, flexibility Bone demineralization ↓ Endurance, stability ↑ Risk for contracture formation
Metabolic	↑ Efficiency of metabolic system ↑ Efficiency of body temperature regulation	↑ Risk for electrolyte imbalance Altered exchange of nutrients and gases
Integumentary	Improved tone, color, and turgor resulting from improved circulation	↑ Risk for skin breakdown and formation of decubitus ulcers
Psychological Well-Being	Energy, vitality, general well-being Improved sleep Improved appearance Improved self-concept Positive health behaviors	↑ Sense of powerlessness ↓ Self-concept ↓ Social interaction ↓ Sensory stimulation Altered sleep–wake pattern ↑ Risk for depression

2. a. Motion, maintenance of posture
   b. Heat production
   c. Promote venous return
3. a. The afferent nervous system conveys information from receptors in the periphery of the body to the central nervous system (CNS).
   b. Nerve cells called neurons are responsible for conducting impulses from one part of the body to another.
   c. This information is processed by the CNS, and a response is decided on.
   d. The efferent system conveys the desired response from the CNS to skeletal muscles by way of the somatic nervous system.
4. a. Body alignment or posture: The alignment of body parts that permits optimal musculoskeletal balance and operation and promotes healthy physiologic functioning.
   b. Balance: A body in correct alignment is balanced; its center of gravity is close to the base of support, the line of gravity goes through the base of support, and the object has a wide base of support.
   c. Coordinated body movement: Using major muscle groups rather than weaker ones and taking advantage of the body's natural levers and fulcrums.
5. Sample answers:
   a. Develop a habit of maintaining erect posture, begin activities by broadening the base of support while lowering the center of gravity and tightening the abdominal muscles.
   b. Use the weight of the body as a force for pulling or pushing by rocking on the feet or leaning forward or backward.
   c. Slide, roll, push, or pull an object rather than lifting it to reduce the energy needed to move the weight against the pull of gravity.
   d. Use the weight of the body to push an object by falling or rocking forward, and to pull an object by falling or rocking backward.
6. a. Aerobic exercises (running, swimming, tennis): Sustained muscle movements that increase blood flow, heart rate, and metabolic demand for oxygen over time, thereby promoting cardiovascular conditioning.
   b. Stretching exercises (warm-up and cool-down exercises): Movements that allow muscles and joints to be stretched gently through their full range of motion; increase flexibility.
   c. Strength and endurance exercises (weight training): Weight training, calisthenics, and specific isometric exercises can build both strength and endurance, increase the power of the musculoskeletal system, and improve the body as a whole.
   d. Activities of daily living (shopping, cleaning): All activities of daily living have an effect on health and provide increased fitness that does not require a gym.

7. Sample answers:
   a. Increased energy, vitality, and general well-being
   b. Improved sleep
   c. Improved self-concept
   d. Increased positive health behaviors
8. a. Pillows: Pillows are used primarily to provide support or to elevate a part. Pillows of different sizes are useful for different body parts.
   b. Mattresses: A mattress should be firm but should have sufficient "give" to permit good body alignment to be comfortable and supportive. A well-made and well-supported foam-rubber mattress retains a uniform firmness.
   c. Adjustable bed: The head of an adjustable bed can be elevated to the desired degree, and the distance from the floor can be altered to allow the patient to get in and out of bed more easily or to allow health care workers to give care without back strain.
   d. Bed side rails: They help to remind patients that they are not in their usual environment and keep them from falling out of bed.
   e. Trapeze bar: This handgrip suspended from a frame near the head of the bed makes moving and turning considerably easier for many patients and facilitates transfers into and out of bed.
   f. Cradle: A metal frame that keeps the top bedding off the patient's lower extremities while providing privacy and warmth.
   g. Sandbags: Sandbags immobilize an extremity and support body alignment. They are not hard or firmly packed but should be placed so they do not create pressure on bony prominences.
   h. Trochanter rolls: Used to support the hips and legs so that the femurs do not rotate outward.
   i. Hand/wrist splints or rolls: A commercial plastic or aluminum splint is used to hold the thumb in place no matter what position the hand is in.
9. a. Quadriceps setting exercise and drills: Have the patient contract the muscles on the front of the thighs by pulling kneecaps toward hips; hold the position to the count of four; relax muscles for count of four. Frequency: two or three times each hour, four to six times a day.
   b. Pushups: Sitting in bed: Instruct patient to lift hips off the bed by pushing down with hands on the mattress. Lying on abdomen: Instruct patient to place hands near the outstretched body at shoulder level with palms down on the mattress and elbows bent sharply; then have patient straighten elbows while lifting head and shoulders off bed. Wheelchair: Instruct patient to place hands on arms of chair and raise body three or four times a day and increase frequency as upper body strength is increased.
   c. Dangling: Instruct the patient to sit on the edge of the bed with legs and feet dangling over the side. Rest the patient's feet on the floor or footstool.

Have patient assume a marching position. (Remain with patient in case they feel faint.)

10. **a.** Physical assessment: The nurse would assess the following:

General ease of movement: Are body parts moving fluidly and is voluntary movement controlled and coordinated?

Gait: Is head erect? Are the vertebrae straight, knees and feet forward, and arms swinging freely in alternation with leg swings?

Alignment—in standing position: Can a straight line be drawn from the ear through the shoulder and hip?

Joint structure and function: Are there any joint deformities or limitations in full range of motion?

Muscle mass tone and strength: Are they adequate to accomplish movement and work?

Endurance: Is patient able to turn in bed, maintain correct alignment when sitting and standing, ambulate, and perform self-care activities?

b. Diagnosis: Activity intolerance related to decreased muscle mass, tone, and strength.

c. Exercise program: Do range-of-motion exercises twice a day to build up muscles and joint capabilities. Use quadriceps drills two or three times an hour, four to six times a day. Do settings twice a day and pushups three or four times a day.

11. Sample answers:

a. General ease of movement: Normal: Body movements are voluntarily controlled, fluid, and coordinated.
Abnormal: Involuntary movements, tremors, tics, chorea, etc.

b. Gait and posture: Normal: Head erect, vertebrae straight.
Abnormal: Spastic hemiparesis, scissors gait.

c. Alignment: Normal: In the standing and sitting position, a straight line can be drawn from the ear through the shoulder and hip; in bed, the head, shoulders, and hips are aligned.
Abnormal: Abnormal spinal curvatures, inability to maintain correct alignment independently.

d. Joint structure and function: Normal: Absence of joint deformities, full range of motion.
Abnormal: Limitations in the normal range of motion, increased joint mobility.

e. Muscle mass, tone, and strength: Normal: Adequate muscle mass and tone. Abnormal: Atrophy, hypotonicity.

f. Endurance: Normal: Ability to turn in bed, maintain correct alignment.
Abnormal: Weakness, pallor.

APPLYING YOUR KNOWLEDGE
CRITICAL THINKING QUESTIONS

1. Answers will vary.
2. Answers will vary.
3. Answers will vary.

REFLECTIVE PRACTICE: CULTIVATING QSEN COMPETENCIES
Sample Answers

1. Patient-centered care/safety: What patient teaching might the nurse incorporate into the plan of care to help Kelsi's parents minimize the complications of immobility for their daughter?
After reviewing the health record and ensuring there are no injuries to the head, neck, or spine, the nurse demonstrates ROM exercises and encourages the parents to participate in their daughter's care. The nurse explains the purpose of elevating the heels off the bed, applying hand rolls or splints, trochanter rolls, frequent repositioning and turning schedules to prevent reddened areas or pressure injury, as well as stasis of respiratory secretions.

2. Patient-centered care/evidence-based practice: What would be a successful outcome for this patient?
By next visit, Kelsi's parents will demonstrate range-of-motion exercises to help maintain mobility and prevent contractures. Kelsi will be free from pressure injuries, flexion, and stiffness.

3. Patient-centered care/evidence-based practice: What intellectual, technical, interpersonal, and ethical/legal competencies are most likely to bring about the desired outcome?
Intellectual: knowledge of and ability to teach about common problems associated with immobility. Ability to provide emotional support for the parents and information on patients who are unresponsive.
Technical: ability to use correctly the protocols, products, and equipment necessary to promote body alignment and to prevent or treat complications related to immobility
Interpersonal: ability to demonstrate empathy, caring, and support for the parents who are dealing with an unknown outcome. The nurse demonstrates respect for a patient's human dignity and encourages patients to participate in care to maintain functional status.
Ethical/legal: ability to act as a patient advocate to promote the maximum level of patient functioning. The nurse uses veracity, when explaining the plan of care and the patient's response.

4. Teamwork and collaboration: What resources might be helpful for this family?
Psychologist or social worker, PT, printed or AV materials on range-of-motion exercises. If patient is recovering, home health care services, physical rehabilitation services, OT, education to catch up with schoolwork. If Kelsi is not recovering, the nurse could collaborate with the health care team about introducing the idea of discharge, pediatric long-term care, or palliative care.

PATIENT CARE STUDY

Answers will vary with student experience.

PRACTICING FOR NCLEX
MULTIPLE-CHOICE QUESTIONS

1. b	**2.** a	**3.** c	**4.** d	**5.** a
6. c	**7.** b	**8.** c	**9.** d	**10.** c
11. b	**12.** a	**13.** b	**14.** b	**15.** c
16. a				

ALTERNATE-FORMAT QUESTIONS
Multiple-Response Questions

1. c, d
2. a, c, f
3. b, c, d
4. c, f
5. b, c d, f
6. c, e, f
7. b, e

CHAPTER 35

ASSESSING YOUR UNDERSTANDING

FILL IN THE BLANKS

1. Rest
2. sleep
3. reticular, bulbar
4. circadian
5. shift
6. obesity
7. insomnia
8. oxygen
9. delta
10. parasomnia
11. hypersomnia
12. narcolepsy

MATCHING EXERCISES
Matching Exercise 1

1. e	**2.** a	**3.** c	**4.** f	**5.** d
6. b				

Matching Exercise 2

1. b	**2.** a	**3.** d	**4.** a	**5.** c
6. b				

CORRECT THE FALSE STATEMENTS

1. T
2. T
3. F, at stage I, NREM sleep
4. F, 4 or 5
5. F, 12 to 16
6. T
7. F, protein and carbohydrate
8. F, hinders
9. T
10. F, antihistamines
11. False, Sleep apnea

SHORT ANSWER

1. **a.** Restores physical well-being
   b. Relieves stress and anxiety
   c. Restores the ability to cope and to concentrate on activities of daily living

2. **a.** Infants
   Amount of sleep: 12 to 16 hrs/day
   Interventions: place on the back to sleep to prevent SIDS, takes several naps per day
   b. Children
   Amount of sleep: 9 to 11 or 12 hrs/day
   Interventions: relaxed bedtime routine, parental presence
   c. Adults
   Amount of sleep: 7 to 9 hrs/day
   Interventions: avoid electronics; use bed only for sleeping and sex; avoid routine sleep medications
   d. Older adults
   Amount of sleep: may take longer to fall asleep; wake earlier and more frequently during the night
   Interventions: avoid polypharmacy, manage pain

3. **a.** Physical activity: Activity increases fatigue and promotes relaxation that is followed by sleep. It also increases both REM and NREM sleep.
   b. Psychological stress: The person experiencing stress tends to find it difficult to obtain the amount of sleep they need, and REM sleep decreases.
   c. Motivation: A desire to be wakeful and alert helps overcome sleepiness and sleep; when there is minimal motivation to be awake, sleep generally follows.
   d. Culture: Bedtime rituals, sleeping place, and pattern of sleep may vary according to culture.
   e. Diet: Carbohydrates appear to have an effect on brain serotonin levels and promote feelings of calmness and relaxation; protein may actually increase brain energy alertness and concentration.
   f. Alcohol and caffeine: Alcohol in moderation seems to help induce sleep in some people, but large quantities limit REM and delta sleep. Caffeine is a CNS stimulant and may interfere with the ability to fall asleep.
   g. Smoking: Nicotine has a stimulating effect, and smokers usually have a more difficult time falling asleep.
   h. Environmental factors: Most people sleep best in their usual home environments.
   i. Lifestyle: Sleep disorders are the major problem associated with shift work, and developing a sleep pattern is especially difficult if the shift changes periodically. Sleep can be affected by watching some types of television shows, participating in stimulating activity, and level of activity or exercise.
   j. Exercise: Moderate exercise is a healthy way to promote sleep, but exercise that occurs within 2 hours before normal bedtime can hinder sleep.
   k. Illness: Illness is a physiologic and psychological stressor and, therefore, influences sleep.
   l. Medications: Sleep quality is influenced by certain drugs that may decrease REM sleep.

4. The cause of the sleep disturbance, the related signs and symptoms, when it first began and how often it occurs, how it affects everyday living, the severity of the problem and whether it can be treated independently by nursing, how the patient

is coping with the problem, and the success of any treatments attempted

5. **a.** Energy level
   b. Facial characteristics such as bright eyes, or dark circles beneath the eyes
   c. Behavioral characteristics—accurate problem solving, prone to errors
   d. Data suggestive of potential sleep problems
6. Sample answer: Ensure the patient has a comfortable bed with a supportive mattress, with bottom linens tight and clean. The upper linens should allow freedom of movement and not exert pressure. A quiet, darkened room with privacy, proper ventilation, and a comfortable temperature should be provided. Provide a small protein and carbohydrate for insomnia.
7. Sample answers:
   a. Impaired sleep: excessive daytime sleeping related to effects of biologic aging
   b. Impaired sleep: altered sleep–wake patterns related to frequent rotations of shift
8. **a.** Eyes: Dart back and forth quickly
   b. Muscles: Small muscle twitching, large muscle immobility
   c. Respirations: Irregular; sometimes interspersed with apnea
   d. Pulse: Rapid or irregular
   e. Blood pressure: Increases or fluctuates
   f. Gastric secretions: Increase
   g. Metabolism: Increases; body temperature increases
   h. Sleep cycle: REM sleep enters from stage II of NREM sleep and reenters NREM sleep at stage II; arousal from sleep difficult
9. Sample answers:
   a. Usual sleeping and waking times: Do you usually go to bed and wake up around the same time?
   b. Number of hours of undisturbed sleep: Do you have any difficulty falling asleep? Do you wake up during the night?
   c. Quality of sleep: Do you feel rested after the amount of sleep you get?
   d. Number and duration of naps: Do you find yourself falling asleep during the day?
   e. Energy level: Do you feel refreshed after a night's sleep?
   f. Means of relaxing before bedtime: Do you watch television or read before bedtime?
   g. Bedtime rituals: What do you do before going to bed?
   h. Sleep environment: What is your bedroom environment like?
   i. Pharmacologic aids: Do you ever take medications to help you fall asleep?
   j. Nature of a sleep disturbance: What do you think is causing your sleep problem?
   k. Onset of a disturbance: When did you first notice that you had trouble falling asleep?
   l. Causes of a disturbance: Are you doing anything different before bedtime?
   m. Severity of a disturbance: Do you have breathing problems during the night?
   n. Symptoms of a disturbance: Do you grind your teeth at night?
   o. Interventions attempted and results: What measures have you taken to promote a comfortable sleep environment? Have these measures been successful?

10. Explain the different presentations of sleep apnea in children versus adults.
    Adult OSA is characterized by five or more predominantly obstructive respiratory events (the absence of breathing [apnea] or diminished breathing efforts [hypopnea] or respiratory effort-related arousals) during sleep, accompanied by excessive daytime sleepiness, fatigue, insomnia, loud snoring, observed apnea, and/or gasping for air during sleep. Pediatric OSA is defined by the presence of one of these findings: snoring, labored/obstructed breathing, enuresis (urinating during sleep), or hyperactivity or other neurobehavioral problems, sleepiness, fatigue (American Academy of Sleep Medicine, 2014). Children with OSA are more likely to have behavioral problems than daytime sleepiness (MFMER, 2020a). A common underlying cause in children is enlargement of the adenoids and tonsils or have obesity/be overweight (Nierengarten, 2018; MFMER, 2020a).

APPLYING YOUR KNOWLEDGE
CRITICAL THINKING QUESTION

1. Sample answer: Nurses and nursing assistants round at bedtime to assist patients to the bathroom before bed, provide evidence based interventions for noise reduction, and, establish a common time to dim the lights. The nurse collaborates with dietary to stock small carbohydrate and protein snacks and plans to stock sufficient blankets.

REFLECTIVE PRACTICE: CULTIVATING QSEN COMPETENCIES
Sample Answers

1. Patient-centered care/evidence-based practice: What nursing interventions might the nurse employ to help alleviate Charlie's sleep disturbances?
   Nursing strategies for promoting rest and sleep in older adults include encouraging physical activity, maintaining a regular sleep schedule and discouraging napping, providing a cool, dark room arranging an assessment for depression and treatment, reviewing medications, assessing for any side effects of sleep pattern disturbance, and decreasing fluids in the evening. Suggest a warm shower before bed. Restricting the intake of caffeine, nicotine, and alcohol, especially later in the day is advised.
2. Patient-centered care/evidence-based practice: What would be a successful outcome for this patient?
   At next visit, Charlie states he tried some strategies to help alleviate his sleep disturbance.
   In 3 weeks, he reports obtaining 6 undisturbed hours of sleep at night.
3. Patient-centered care/evidence-based practice: What intellectual, interpersonal, and ethical/legal

competencies are most likely to bring about the desired outcome?

Intellectual: knowledge of the factors that affect rest and sleep, including medical conditions and medications and evidence-based interventions to promote and maintain sleep, especially in the older adults

Interpersonal: ability to assist older adults to develop methods to promote adequate sleep and cope with disturbed sleep patterns

Ethical/legal: ability to practice in an ethically and legally defensible manner when providing care to patients experiencing disturbed sleep pattern

4. Teamwork and collaboration: What resources might be helpful for Charlie?

Printed materials on sleep enhancement strategies, relaxation therapy, consultation with a sleep therapist. Consider medical conditions and medications that cause nocturia, that may require collaboration with the health care provider: diuretics, heart failure, enlarged prostate.

PATIENT CARE STUDY

Answers will vary with student experience.

PRACTICING FOR NCLEX

MULTIPLE-CHOICE QUESTIONS

1. b	**2.** a	**3.** a	**4.** b	**5.** a
6. d	**7.** b	**8.** c	**9.** b	**10.** b
11. c	**12.** b			

ALTERNATE-FORMAT QUESTIONS

Multiple-Response Questions

1. a, c, e
2. b, d, e
3. a, d
4. a, b, c
5. b, c, e, f
6. a, b, d, e

CHAPTER 36

ASSESSING YOUR UNDERSTANDING

FILL IN THE BLANKS

1. Pain
2. subjective
3. nociceptive
4. endorphins, enkephalins
5. transmission
6. Acute
7. referred
8. neuropathic
9. chronic
10. quality

MATCHING EXERCISES

Matching Exercise 1

1. b	**2.** f	**3.** d	**4.** e	**5.** a
6. c				

Matching Exercise 2

1. c	**2.** b	**3.** c	**4.** d	**5.** a
6. b				

Matching Exercise 3

1. a	**2.** b	**3.** d	**4.** c	**5.** e
6. f				

SHORT ANSWER

1. Health problem: acute pain, postoperative
   Etiology: surgical incision, cesarean section
   Signs and symptoms: refusal to move, muscle tension and rigidity, and holding lower abdomen and wincing when moving

2. The injured tissue releases chemicals that excite nerve endings. A damaged cell releases histamine, which excites nerve endings. Lactic acid accumulates in tissues injured by lack of blood supply and is believed to excite nerve endings and cause pain or lower the threshold of nerve endings to other stimuli. Bradykinin, prostaglandins, and substance P are also released.

3. Referred pain can be transmitted to a cutaneous site different from where it originated because afferent neurons enter the spinal cord at the same level as the cutaneous site to which the pain has been referred.

4. The theory states that small nerve fibers conduct excitatory pain stimuli toward the brain, exaggerating the effect of the arriving impulses through a positive feedback mechanism. Large nerve fibers appear to inhibit the transmission of pain impulses from the spinal cord to the brain through a negative feedback system (Melzack & Wall, 1965). There is a transmission mechanism that is believed by some to be located in substantia gelatinosa cells in the dorsal horn of the spinal cord. This serves as the gate. Only a limited amount of sensory information can be processed by the nervous system at any given moment. When too much information is sent through, certain cells in the spinal column interrupt the signal as if closing a gate (Pasero & McCaffery, 2011).

5. Sample answers:
   a. Culture/ethnicity: In one culture, it may be acceptable to express pain vocally, whereas in another culture, such vocal expressions of pain are unacceptable.
   b. Family, biologic sex, or age: Spouses may reinforce pain behavior in their partners.
   c. Religious beliefs: In some religions, pain is viewed as suffering and as a means of purification to make up for individual or community sin.
   d. Environment and support people: Caring support people can help a patient cope with the unfamiliar health care environment.
   e. Anxiety and other stressors: Fear of the unknown may compound anxiety and aggravate pain.
   f. Past pain experience: A child may have no fear of pain because he has never experienced pain.

6. Sample answers:
   a. "You are the authority on your pain experience, and you must let your nurse know when you are

in pain or when the medication isn't working anymore."

b. "Physical addiction may occur with chronic opioid use, but this is not the same as the psychological dependence of addiction. Studies suggest that only half of 1% of all people with cancer pain and other severe types of pain will become addicted to opioids."

c. "It is a myth that pain in the older adult is part of the normal aging process. Opioid drugs can be used to manage your pain safely as long as we take the appropriate precautions and conscientiously assess any side effects."

7. Sample answers:

a. Duration of pain: "For how long have you been experiencing this pain?"

b. Quantity and intensity of pain: "How often do you get these attacks? On a scale of 1 to 10, how would you rate the intensity of this pain?"

c. Quality of pain: "How would you describe the pain (sharp, intense, dull, throbbing, etc.)?"

d. Physiologic indicators of pain: "Have you noticed any physical changes since you've been experiencing this pain?"

8. Answers will vary with student experiences and may include the following: Professional organizations including the ANA and American Society of Pain Management Nurses directly oppose the use of placebos outside of clinical trials. Risking the possible consequences of being discovered will decrease the trust and respect of nurses and health care providers involved. Based on nursing ethics, the nurse is obliged to decline/refuse to administer a placebo.

9. **a.** Patient with a cognitive impairment: Many cognitively impaired patients cannot verbally report their pain or express concepts; therefore, nurses must rely on their own careful assessments, their empathetic qualities, and the expectation that this patient will experience pain if a verbal patient usually reports this event as painful.

b. 5-year-old patient: Children cannot always express their pain; the nurse must observe facial expressions, body positions, crying, and physiologic responses. Communication with parents or guardians is vital for accurate pain assessment.

c. Older adult: Nurses should be aware that older adults fear that admitting pain may limit their independence; boredom, loneliness, and depression may affect an older adult's perception of pain and willingness to report it. Also, their choice of terms in describing pain may be deceptive.

APPLYING YOUR KNOWLEDGE
CRITICAL THINKING QUESTIONS
Sample Answers

1. The nurse has assessed the patient's pain as severe. If the patient is due for pain medication, the nurse has parameters to administer 2 mg of morphine. If it is not yet time for a dose of analgesic, the nurse

can attempt repositioning, ice/heat, and other nonpharmacologic methods of relief. If these are ineffective, the nurse contacts the provider for additional prescriptions for a breakthrough dose of medication, a new order with a shortened time frame between doses, or an adjunctive pain medication, such as gabapentin. Recall that patients with chronic pain do not continue to display vital sign changes or outward responses in the same way patients with acute pain might. As a nurse, you recognize that pain is intensely personal and is what the patient says it is when they experience it. Using the nursing process, the nurse first quantifies/scales the pain, determines the quality, location, what has helped in the past, and if this is a change in pattern. The nurse determines what the patient's goal is for pain relief and whether quality of life is more important than duration of life with pain. If assessment reveals the current pain regimen is ineffective, the nurse collaborates with the provider to revise the pain management plan, including adjunctive measures, nonpharmacologic measures (ice). The nurse assures the patient that their report of pain is valid and that you will collaborate with the provider and health care team to discuss alternate strategies for pain relief. If the patient is able, the nurse can reposition the patient, provide support to body parts with pillows, offer a gentle back rub. Note these interventions may need to be deferred until an acceptable level of pain relief has been achieved.

2. Answers will vary.

3. Answers will vary based on tool used and student experience.

REFLECTIVE PRACTICE: CULTIVATING QSEN COMPETENCIES
Sample Answers

1. Patient-centered care/safety: What nursing interventions might the nurse use to help manage this patient's pain associated with diabetic neuropathy? The nurse assesses the precise location, duration, severity/scale, quality of the pain, what has helped in the past and includes its impact on the patient's quality of life. The nurse can elicit more information about the patient's anxiety and fear, by determining what they know about neuropathy and diabetes. The nurse is mindful that stress and fatigue intensify the effects of pain.

For patients with numbness, the nurse discusses safety with ambulation, including wearing well-fitting shoes, having adequate light, removing scatter rugs, and small dogs or other trip hazards. The nurse can assess the patient's overall blood glucose management and provide education related to progression of diabetes if in poor control. Medication safety, blood glucose monitoring, and any pain medications, especially those that are sedating.

2. Patient-centered care/evidence-based practice: What would be a successful outcome for this patient? By next visit, Carla states three interventions she has tried for pain relief, including medications, not holding stress, distraction, among others. She states that she feels a bit less anxious understanding why the numbness and tingling has occurred and is mindful of keeping her blood glucose in good control. She has started on a medication specific to neuropathic pain, and states that it is helpful.

3. Patient-centered care/evidence-based practice: What intellectual competencies are most likely to bring about the desired outcome? Intellectual: knowledge of the pain experience, specifically medications helpful for neuropathic pain, pain process, and factors influencing the pain experience, such as stress and fatigue. Pain scales or questionnaires that evaluate affective and sensory responses to pain can improve pain management. The nurse must have knowledge of diabetes management and treatment of neuropathy. The nurse encourages the patient to follow up with the provider for a filament test.

4. Teamwork and collaboration: What resources might be helpful for Carla? Consultation with an endocrinologist or neurologist if doesn't have one, printed materials on neuropathy and safety. Proper (diabetic) shoes. If she becomes homebound, home care or home health aide could be helpful, especially with bathing/showering with neuropathy.

PATIENT CARE STUDY

Answers will vary with student experience.

PRACTICING FOR NCLEX
MULTIPLE-CHOICE QUESTIONS

1. c	**2.** d	**3.** c	**4.** c	**5.** a
6. c	**7.** b	**8.** d	**9.** a	**10.** c
11. d	**12.** c	**13.** c	**14.** b	**15.** c

ALTERNATE-FORMAT QUESTIONS
Multiple-Response Questions

1. a, c, d
2. c, e, f
3. b, c, d, f
4. c, d, e
5. b, d, e

Prioritization Question

1. c

CHAPTER 37

ASSESSING YOUR UNDERSTANDING
FILL IN THE BLANKS

1. nutrition
2. 27.5 (ratio of weight [in kilograms] to height [in meters])
3. obesity
4. catabolic
5. trans
6. calories
7. A, D, and K
8. proteins, vegetables, starches
9. 45, 65
10. 10, 35
11. 50, 60
12. aspiration
13. Basal
14. Nutrients
15. lack, appetite
16. Trace

MATCHING EXERCISES
Matching Exercise 1

1. b	**2.** a	**3.** b	**4.** c	**5.** b
6. c				

Matching Exercise 2

1. a, dairy
2. d, salt and processed foods
3. b, milk, cola
4. f, salt
5. e, seafood
6. c, liver

Matching Exercise 3

1. c	**2.** e	**3.** f	**4.** a	**5.** d
6. b				

SHORT ANSWER

1. Nitrogen balance is a comparison between nitrogen intake and nitrogen excretion, reflecting catabolism and anabolism. When catabolism and anabolism occur at the same rate the body is in a state of neutral nitrogen. A positive nitrogen balance indicates that nitrogen intake is greater than excretion, such as during tissue growth. A negative nitrogen balance occurs as tissue is breaking down faster than it is being replaced, such as during starvation causing muscle wasting.

2. a. Saturated fatty acids: Saturated fats contain more hydrogen than unsaturated fats. Most animal fats are considered saturated and have a solid consistency at room temperature (e.g., roast beef). Saturated fats raise cholesterol and risk for cardiovascular disease.
   b. Unsaturated fatty acids: most vegetable fats are considered unsaturated, remain liquid at room temperature, and are referred to as oils. Unsaturated fats lower serum cholesterol levels (e.g., vegetable fats). Unsaturated fats help lower serum cholesterol levels.
   c. Trans fats: Trans fats mostly occur in hydrogenated oils, which are solid at room temperature. Trans fats tend to raise LDL ("bad") cholesterol and lower HDL ("good") cholesterol increasing

the risk for heart disease, stroke, and development of type 2 diabetes (American Heart Association, 2017).

3. a. Infancy: The period from birth to 1 year of age is the most rapid period of growth. Nutritional needs per unit of body weight are greater than at any other time in the life cycle.

b. Toddlers and preschoolers. During this stage, the growth rate slows. Mobility, autonomy, and coordination increase, as do muscle mass and bone density. This age group develops an attitude toward food. Appetite decreases and becomes erratic.

c. School-aged children: Nutritional implications focus on health promotion. Increasing energy requirements should be balanced with foods of high nutritional value. The appetite improves but may still be irregular.

d. Adolescents: Nutrient needs increase to support growth. Weight consciousness becomes compulsive in 1 of 100 teenage girls and results in an eating disorder.

e. Adults: Growth ceases, and nutritional needs level off.

f. Pregnant persons: Nutrient needs increase to support growth and maintain maternal homeostasis, particularly during the second and third trimesters. Folate (folic acid) supplementation is needed during pregnancy, which has significantly decreased the risk of children born with neural tube defects. Caloric needs are higher for lactation than for pregnancy.

g. Older adults: Because of the decreases in BMR and physical activity and loss of lean body mass, energy expenditure decreases. The calorie needs of the body decrease.

5. Sample answers:

a. Eat a variety of high-fiber foods daily (whole-grain breads and cereals, fruits, vegetables, dry beans).

b. Drink water: 2,200 to 3,000 mL/day for adults.

c. Substitute high-fiber foods for low-fiber foods (brown rice instead of white).

d. Add bran to diet slowly to decrease likelihood of flatus and distention.

6. a. Anorexia nervosa: Characterized by denial of appetite and bizarre eating patterns; may result in extremely dangerous amount of weight loss; can be fatal. Typical person is adolescent girl, competitive; obsessive; distorted body image.

b. Bulimia: Characterized by gorging followed by purging with self-induced vomiting, diuretics, and laxative use.

7. a. Biologic sex: Men have higher caloric and protein requirements than women because of their larger muscle mass.

b. State of health: The alteration in nutrient requirements that results from illness and trauma varies with the intensity and duration of stress.

c. Alcohol abuse: Alcohol can alter the body's use of nutrients and thereby its nutrient requirements by numerous mechanisms.

d. Medications: Nutrient absorption may be altered by drugs that change the pH of the gastrointestinal tract, increase gastrointestinal motility, damage the intestinal mucosa, or bind with nutrients, rendering them unavailable to the body.

e. Religion: Nurses need to be aware of dietary restrictions associated with religions that

4.

Nutrient	Function	Recommended %
a. Carbohydrates	Supply energy (4 cal/g); also spares protein, helps burn fat efficiently, and prevents ketosis	45–65%
b. Proteins	Maintains body tissues; supports new tissue growth; component of body framework	10–35%
c. Fats	Important component of cell membranes; synthesis of bile acids; precursor of steroid hormones and vitamin D; most concentrated source of energy (9 cal/g); aids in absorption of fat-soluble vitamins; provides insulation, structure, and body temperature control	Saturated <10% Unsaturated <35%
d. Vitamins	Metabolism of carbohydrates, protein, and fat; supports vital functions and prevents deficiency diseases	
e. Minerals	Key components of body structures; regulation of body processes	
f. Water	Essential for all biochemical reactions; participates in many biochemical reactions; helps regulate body temperature, helps lubricate body joints; needed for adequate mucous secretions; supports blood volume and blood pressure	2,200–3,000 mL/day

might affect a patient's nutritional requirements.

   f. Economics: Social determinants of health such as a person's food budget affect dietary choices and patterns.

8. a. Food diaries: The patient records all food and beverages consumed in a specified time period (3 to 7 days).

   b. 24-hour diet recall: This is a 24-hour recall, food frequency record, portion sizes, meal and snack patterns, meal timing, and location where food is eaten. The information may not be reliable, based on patient's memory.

   c. Food frequency record: Food frequency records give a general picture of nutritional consumption. The nurse asks about the average number of times certain foods or food groups are consumed in a given period of time: per day, per week, or per month.

9. Sample answer: The nurse begins by assessing the patient's height and weight, could calculate the BMI, and determines if the patient has a therapeutic diet prescription and their understanding of it. The nurse determines if the patient can prepare a meal and feed themselves. The nurse could assess a 24-hour diet recall, assess appetite, evaluates patient's tolerance for specific types of foods and assess for food–medication interactions. The nurse can monitor albumin levels where available. Interventions are based on this assessment data.

10. Sample answers:

   a. Provide simple verbal instructions to the patient and the person who cooks meals and/or family members when appropriate.

   b. Advise the patient to eliminate any foods that are not tolerated.

   c. Offer support and encouragement, help culturally diverse patients to value and understand the importance of communicating concerns and asking questions about prescribed dietary practices.

11. a. Clear-liquid diet: Only foods that are clear liquids at room temperature, such as gelatins, fat-free bouillon, ice pops, clear juices, etc.; inadequate in calories, proteins, and most nutrients.

   b. Full-liquid diet: All liquids that can be poured at room temperature, such as clear liquids plus milk, plain frozen desserts, pasteurized eggs, cream soups (without solids), cereal gruels; high-calorie, high-protein supplements are recommended if used for more than 3 days.

   c. Low-fiber diet: Limited to <10 g/day. Used before surgeries, in ulcerative colitis, diverticulitis, and Crohn's disease.

12. This tube is passed through the nose into the small intestine or percutaneously inserted, typically in the jejunum. Advantage: Minimal risk for aspiration, bypasses the stomach if there is disease or surgical alterations. Disadvantage: Dumping syndrome may develop.

APPLYING YOUR KNOWLEDGE
CRITICAL THINKING QUESTIONS

1. Sample answer:
Assessing: patient's weight, vital signs, electrolytes, prealbumin and albumin levels, glucose levels, determine when the dressing and tubing need to be changed. Assess the insertion site of the central venous access device and the time the PN was hung, as any remaining solutions must be discarded after 24 hours.
Planning: Obtain an infusion pump, inline filter, when changing tubing, use the same lumen each time.
Intervening: Maintain strict aseptic technique when handling any aspect such as dressings, tubing, filters. Contact the health care provider for fever or symptoms of infection.
(Outcome) Evaluating: weight maintained or increased per plan, free from infection, electrolytes within normal range, albumin level normal/normalizing.

2. Answers will vary.

REFLECTIVE PRACTICE: CULTIVATING QSEN COMPETENCIES
Sample Answers

1. Patient-centered care/safety: What patient teaching might the nurse provide to help William meet his nutritional and exercise needs?
The nurse assesses the patient's height, weight, and eating habits through a diet history. The nurse also assesses what the patient knows about hypertension and hypercholesterolemia and their consequences. The nurse assists the patient to develop a diet plan that is low in sodium, fat, and cholesterol. This, along with exercise will promote weight loss. As he has not exercised regularly, the nurse could recommend walking, which he could adapt to his busy lifestyle or dining out. To promote success, the nurse works with the patient to individualize this plan to the patient's lifestyle, culture, intellectual ability, and level of motivation.

2. Patient-centered care: What would be a successful outcome for this patient?
By the end of the visit, the patient lists recommended allowances of grains, vegetables, fruits, milk, and meat and beans as seen in the MyPlate Food Guide. The patient states sources of sodium to avoid. He states he values his health and plans to begin walking several times weekly.
By next visit, William manifests a weight loss of 2 lb and has lower blood pressure and cholesterol levels.

3. What intellectual, interpersonal, and ethical/legal competencies are most likely to bring about the desired outcome?
Intellectual: knowledge of adult teaching principles, nutrients and nutritional requirements for middle adults; knowledge of hypertension and

high cholesterol, and strategies for managing these conditions, and preventing their consequences.
Interpersonal: special interpersonal competencies to help the executive value changes in lifestyle to maintain/improve his health.
Ethical/legal: ability to act as a trusted and effective patient advocate.

4. What resources might be helpful for this patient? Consultation with a nutritionist, printed materials on hypertension and high cholesterol, exercise programs, American Heart Association.

PATIENT CARE STUDY

Answers will vary with student experience.

PRACTICING FOR NCLEX

MULTIPLE-CHOICE QUESTIONS

1. a   2. b   3. c   4. c   5. b
6. a   7. c   8. b   9. c   10. b
11. d   12. c   13. b

ALTERNATE-FORMAT QUESTIONS
Multiple-Response Questions

1. a, c, e, f
2. a, d, e
3. a, e
4. a, b, c, d
5. c, d, e, f
6. c, d, e
7. a, c, d

Prioritization Question

1. a

CHAPTER 38

ASSESSING YOUR UNDERSTANDING
FILL IN THE BLANKS

1. enuresis
2. micturition
3. 6, 8
4. incontinence
5. diversion
6. nocturia
7. hesitancy
8. midstream
9. stent

MATCHING EXERCISES
Matching Exercise 1

1. c   2. b   3. d   4. a   5. e

Matching Exercise 2

1. a   2. d   3. c   4. b   5. e
6. b

SHORT ANSWER

1. a. Developmental considerations: Newborns have no urinary control. Most children develop urinary control between ages 2 and 5 years. Physiologic changes of normal aging may affect urination in the older adult including nocturia, frequency, and stasis medications.

b. Food and fluid: The kidneys should preserve a careful balance of fluid intake and output. Caffeine has a diuretic effect, increasing urine production. Alcohol promotes renal fluid loss by inhibiting release of antidiuretic hormone. Foods high in water, such as fruits, may increase urine production. High-sodium foods and beverages cause sodium and water reabsorption and retention.

c. Psychological variables: People experiencing stress often find themselves voiding smaller amounts of urine at more frequent intervals. Stress can also interfere with the ability to relax perineal muscles and the external urethral sphincter.

d. Activity and muscle tone: Exercise increases metabolism and optimal urine production and elimination. With prolonged periods of immobility, decreased bladder and sphincter tone can result in poor urinary control and urinary stasis.

e. Pathologic conditions: Various renal or urologic problems can affect both the quantity and quality of urine produced.

f. Medications: Medications, such as nephrotoxic medication can damage the kidney. Abuse of NSAID analgesics can result in nephrotoxicity. Cholinergic medications stimulate bladder contraction promoting urination; anticholinergic medication cause urinary retention. Certain drugs cause urine to change color.

2. a. Ability to communicate needs verbally and follow instructions
b. Shows an interest in the potty
c. The child should be able to hold urine for a period of time without diapers being wet.
d. Physically able to sit and rise from potty chair.

3. a. Infants and young children: It is important to assess whether the child has achieved bladder control and whether a toileting schedule has been established for the child. It is also important to identify the words the child uses to indicate the need to void.

b. Older adults: Decreased bladder tone may be a problem. The nursing history should note how the person handles these problems and the adequacy of the solution.

c. Patients with limited or no bladder control or urinary diversions: The procedures and equipment used should be assessed to make sure they follow accepted guidelines and are not predisposing the person to infection or other risk.

d. Patient receiving dialysis: Patients with severely decreased or total loss of kidney function or kidney failure may receive hemodialysis or peritoneal dialysis as a mechanical means of removing fluid and waste normally excreted through the urine. They may void small amounts or experience anuria.

4. a. Kidneys: Palpation of the kidney requires deep palpation and is generally assessed by an advanced practice nurse or health care provider.

 b. Bladder: The bladder can only be assessed when it is distended above the level of the symphysis pubis. Before palpating, ask when the patient last voided. The nurse palpates the area for tenderness, noting the smoothness and roundness of the bladder. A bedside ultrasound bladder scanner can be used to calculate the volume of urine in the bladder without catheterization.

 c. Urethral orifice: This is inspected for any signs of inflammation or discharge. Foul odors should be noted.

 d. Skin integrity and hydration: The skin of the perineal area is assessed for integrity, color, texture, and turgor. Observe for excoriation related to incontinence.

 e. Urine: Assess for color, odor, clarity, and the presence of sediment. Document abnormalities.

5. Sample answers:

 a. The patient will produce urine output about equal to fluid intake.

 b. After teaching, the patient will wipe from front to back.

 c. The patient will be free from pain or discomfort when voiding.

 d. The patient will be free from skin breakdown.

6. a. Schedule: Some patients report voiding on demand in no apparent pattern; others have inflexible patterns that have developed over the years and become anxious if these are interrupted.

 b. Privacy: Many adults and children cannot void in the presence of another person; privacy should be offered in the health care and home settings.

 c. Position: Helping patients assume normal voiding positions, such as assist a patient with male genitalia to stand to void or women having difficulty voiding on a bedpan may be better able to void using bedside commode.

 d. Hygiene: Patients on bedrest often have difficulty performing their usual perineal/genital hygiene. The nurse should place these patients on a bedpan and pour warm soapy water over the perineal area, followed by clear water. Offer towelettes or soapy washcloth for hand hygiene once this care is complete.

7. Sample answers:

 a. Relieve urinary retention.

 b. Obtain a sterile specimen from a woman.

 c. Empty the bladder before, during, and after surgery.

8. Sample answers:

 a. The patient will state methods to decrease odor of the appliance.

 b. After teaching, the patient will demonstrate cleansing the stomal area and changing the appliance.

APPLYING YOUR KNOWLEDGE
CRITICAL THINKING QUESTIONS

1. Sample answer: Instruct patient, and partner if assisting, to wash their hands. They will use clean nonsterile technique, washing the meatus with soap and water before inserting the catheter. A water-soluble lubricant or anesthetic gel will be needed. Instruct them to grasp the penis with the nondominant hand and place it 90 degrees from the body; they should not let go until the procedure is complete. Remind the patient and partner to use a new, sterile catheter each time.

REFLECTIVE PRACTICE: CULTIVATING QSEN COMPETENCIES

1. Patient-centered care/evidence-based practice/safety: How might the nurse respond to Mrs. Morita's remarks regarding her husband's home care?
 The nurse assesses if the patient takes any medications affecting urination such as diuretics, their feelings regarding the incidents; asks Mr. Morita if he has sensations of needing to void or that he is wet, and assesses the skin. The nurse teaches that having an indwelling catheter decreases bladder tone. Further explaining that catheterization can lead to infection and sepsis and should not be the first line treatment for incontinence. The nurse suggests a toileting schedule, proper use of absorbent products, and perhaps a condom catheter, among other interdependent options. The nurse suggests considering home health care personnel to assist with toileting, frequent skin care. The patient may require a further urinary assessment to uncover underlying causes, either physical or psychological, for the incontinence, if these strategies are unsuccessful.

2. Patient-centered care/evidence-based practice/safety: What would be a successful outcome for this patient?
 By next visit, the couple states two methods to promote urinary continence. The patient remains free from skin breakdown. They were able to procure absorbent products, which they use judiciously. By next visit, Mrs. Morita expresses satisfaction with urinary strategies to promote continence and receives outside help at the home.

3. Evidence-based practice: What intellectual, technical, and/or ethical/legal competencies are most likely to bring about the desired outcome?
 Intellectual: knowledge of regaining bladder function after removal of an indwelling catheter, the current evidence regarding catheter-associated urinary tract infection (CAUTI), and nursing strategies to promote continence.
 Technical: ability to assess the bladder, skin, and available resources.
 Ethical/legal: strong sense of accountability for the health and well-being of patients experiencing urinary problems.

4. Teamwork and collaboration: What resources might be helpful for the Morita family?
Home health care services, printed information on urinary incontinence, and care of urinary catheters

PATIENT CARE STUDY

Answers will vary with student experience.

PRACTICING FOR NCLEX

MULTIPLE-CHOICE QUESTIONS

1. a	2. b	3. c	4. a	5. a
6. d	7. c	8. d	9. a	10. d
11. d	12. c	13. b	14. b	

ALTERNATE-FORMAT QUESTIONS
Multiple-Response Questions

1. b, c, e, f
2. c, f
3. b, e, f
4. a, c, e, f
5. a, b, d, e
6. b, c, d
7. a, c, e

Hot Spot Questions

1. Urethra positions.

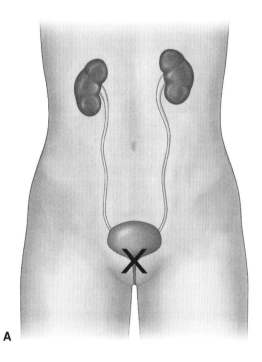

A

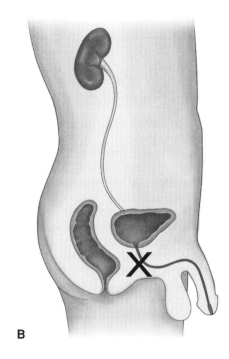

B

2. External sphincter location.

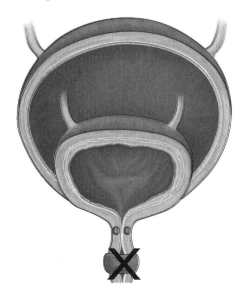

3. Bladder location and size (male).

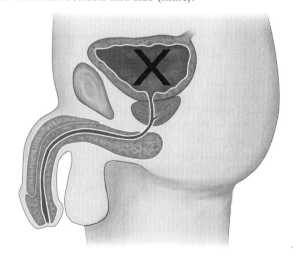

4. Suprapubic catheter position.

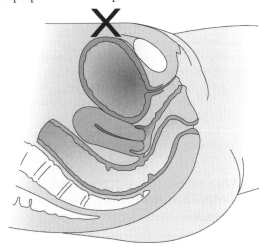

CHAPTER 39

ASSESSING YOUR UNDERSTANDING

FILL IN THE BLANKS

1. anus
2. chyme
3. jejunum, ileum
4. ileocecal
5. peristalsis
6. flatus
7. Valsalva
8. 25, 38
9. ileus

IDENTIFICATION

1. a. Rectum
  b. Internal anal sphincter
  c. External anal sphincter
  d. Anal valve
  e. Anal canal
2. a. Sigmoid colostomy—formed
  b. Descending colostomy—formed
  c. Transverse (single B) colostomy—soft
  d. Ascending colostomy—soft to liquid
  e. Ileostomy—liquid

MATCHING EXERCISES

Matching Exercise 1

1. a   **2.** d   **3.** c   **4.** b   **5.** e
6. f

Matching Exercise 2

1. a   **2.** d   **3.** c   **4.** b

Matching Exercise 3

1. c   **2.** a   **3.** d   **4.** e   **5.** f
6. b

Anatomy Review

1. g	**2.** f	**3.** a	**4.** m	**5.** h
6. b	**7.** n	**8.** c	**9.** i	**10.** q
11. o	**12.** r	**13.** d	**14.** l	**15.** p
16. e	**17.** k	**18.** j		

SHORT ANSWER

1. a. Absorption of water
  b. Production of certain B vitamins and vitamin K
  c. Formation of feces
  d. Expulsion of feces from the body
2. a. The parasympathetic nervous system stimulates movement.
  b. The sympathetic system inhibits movement.
3. a. Inspection: Observes the contour of the abdomen, noting any masses or areas of distension.
  b. Auscultation: The nurse uses a warmed stethoscope to listen for bowel sounds in a systematic, clockwise manner in all abdominal quadrants.
  c. Percussion: Percusses all quadrants of the abdomen in a systematic, clockwise manner to identify any masses, fluid, or air.
  d. Palpation: Performs light palpation in each quadrant while watching the patient's face for nonverbal signs of pain during palpation. The nurse palpates each quadrant in a systematic manner, noting muscular resistance, tenderness, enlargement of the organs, or masses.
4. a. Developmental considerations: The stool characteristics of an infant depend on whether the infant is being fed breast milk or formula.
  b. Daily patterns: Psychological issues such as depression and a change in a person's daily routine may lead to constipation.
  c. Food and fluids: Insufficient fluid and fiber may cause constipation.
  d. Activity and muscle tone: Regular exercise improves gastrointestinal motility.
  e. Lifestyle: A person's daily schedule, occupation, and leisure activities may contribute to a habit of defecating at regular times or to an irregular pattern.
  f. Psychological variables: In some people, anxiety may have a direct effect on gastrointestinal motility, and diarrhea accompanies periods of high anxiety.
  g. Medications: Medications may influence the appearance of the stool—for instance, iron salts result in a black stool from the oxidation of iron.
  h. Diagnostic studies: Patients may need to fast for tests, which may alter elimination patterns.
5. Sample answers: When were you first diagnosed with diverticular disease? How long have you had the pain? Have you ever had this pain before? How often do you move your bowels? What

do your stools look like? Have you noticed any changes in stool lately? What is your regular diet like? Are there any foods you avoid? Are there any foods that help relieve the pain?

6. **a.** Daily fluid intake of 2,000 to 3,000 mL
   b. Increased intake of high-fiber foods
   c. Regular exercise
   d. Acceptance of bowel elimination as a normal process of life

7. Sample answers:
   a. The patient will have a soft, formed bowel movement every 1 to 3 days without discomfort.
   b. The patient will ambulate, increase dietary fiber and fluid intake.
   c. The patient will relate the importance of timing, positioning, and privacy to healthy bowel elimination.

8. **a.** Constipation: Increase intake of high-fiber foods and fluid.
   b. Diarrhea: Prepare and store food properly, avoid highly spiced foods or laxative-type foods, increase intake of low-fiber foods, and replace lost fluids.
   c. Flatulence: Avoid gas-producing foods such as beans, cabbage, onions, cauliflower, and beer.

9. **a.** To relieve constipation or fecal compaction
   b. To prevent involuntary escape of fecal material during surgical procedures
   c. To promote visualization of the intestinal tract by radiographic or instrument examination
   d. To help establish regular bowel function during a bowel training program

10. **a.** Ileostomy: A portion of the ileum is redirected through the abdominal wall and a stoma created. It allows liquid fecal content from the ileum of the small intestine to be eliminated through the stoma.
    b. Colostomy: A portion of the colon is redirected through the abdominal wall and a stoma created. It permits formed feces from the colon to exit through the stoma.

11. **a.** Timing: Patients should be allowed to heed the natural urge to defecate.
    b. Positioning: The squatting position best facilitates defecation.
    c. Privacy: Most patients consider elimination a private act, and nurses should provide privacy for their patients.
    d. Nutrition: Patients with elimination problems may need a dietary analysis to determine which foods and fluids are contributing to their problem.
    e. Exercise: Regular exercise improves gastrointestinal motility and aids in defecation.

APPLYING YOUR KNOWLEDGE
CRITICAL THINKING QUESTIONS

1. Sample answers:
   a. Increase fiber in the diet: salads, raw fruits and vegetables, beans, whole grain foods
   b. Replace lost fluids and electrolytes, low fiber, bland diet for a few days, avoid lactose and high-fiber foods
   c. Offer fruits and vegetables (e.g., prunes, figs, dates), foods containing bran or whole grains.

2. Answers will vary.

REFLECTIVE PRACTICE: CULTIVATING QSEN COMPETENCIES
Sample Answers

1. Patient-centered care/evidence-based practice: What nursing interventions might the nurse implement for this patient?
   The nurse should address methods to prevent and resolve the constipating effects of the opioid medication including teaching about foods that stimulate peristalsis. The nurse encourages increased fluid intake and patient movement (e.g., walking as tolerated). Laxatives may be indicated, or an oil retention enema if a fecal impaction is found.

2. Patient-centered care/evidence-based practice: What would be a successful outcome for this patient?
   By next visit, the patient lists three foods to include in his diet to prevent constipation and that he walks as much as possible. He states he drinks 2.5 quarts of liquid daily.
   By next visit, Leroy verbalizes having regular, pain-free bowel movements.

3. Evidence-based practice: What intellectual, technical, interpersonal, and ethical/legal competencies are most likely to bring about the desired outcome?
   Intellectual: knowledge of the anatomy and physiology of bowel elimination, pharmacology related to bowel function and opioid analgesics, evidence-based interventions to relieve pain and constipation
   Technical: competency with abdominal and dietary assessment
   Interpersonal: ability to interact in a nonjudgmental and professional manner when interacting in situations involving bowel elimination, a typically private matter
   Ethical/legal: adherence to safety and quality when performing nursing interventions to promote bowel elimination

4. Teamwork and collaboration: What resources might be helpful for this patient?
   Consultation with a dietitian, pain management consultation if needed, printed or AV materials discussing the effect of medications and diet, and appropriate interventions

PATIENT CARE STUDY
Answers will vary with student experience.

PRACTICING FOR NCLEX
MULTIPLE-CHOICE QUESTIONS
1. d   **2.** d   **3.** b   **4.** a   **5.** d
6. c   **7.** b

ALTERNATE-FORMAT QUESTIONS
Multiple-Response Questions

1. c, d, f
2. b, c, f
3. c, d, f
4. b, e, f
5. a, c, d, e
6. c, d, e
7. a, c, e
8. b, d, e

Sequencing Question

1.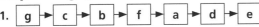

Prioritization Question

1. b

CHAPTER 40

ASSESSING YOUR UNDERSTANDING
FILL IN THE BLANKS
  1. breathing
  2. exchange
  3. atelectasis
  4. resistance
  5. Compliance
  6. thoracentesis
  7. surfactant
  8. sinoatrial
  9. dysrhythmia (arrhythmia)
10. output

IDENTIFICATION
1. a. Frontal sinus
  b. Nasal cavity
  c. Epiglottis
  d. Right lung
  e. Right bronchus
  f. Terminal bronchiole
  g. Diaphragm
  h. Left lung
  i. Mediastinum
  j. Trachea
  k. Esophagus
  l. Larynx and vocal cords
  m. Laryngeal pharynx
  n. Oropharynx
  o. Nasopharynx
  p. Sphenoidal sinus

2. a. Cuff
  b. Outer cannula
  c. Inner cannula
  d. Obturator

MATCHING EXERCISES
Matching Exercise 1
1. b   **2.** e   **3.** d   **4.** a   **5.** c
6. f

Matching Exercise 2
1. e   **2.** b   **3.** f   **4.** c   **5.** a
6. d

Matching Exercise 3
1. f   **2.** b   **3.** f   **4.** c   **5.** a
6. d

SHORT ANSWER
1. a. Integrity of the airway system to transport air to and from the lungs
  b. Properly functioning alveolar system in the lungs to oxygenate venous blood and remove carbon dioxide from the blood
  c. Properly functioning cardiovascular system to carry nutrients and wastes to and from body cells
2. a. Upper airway: the nose, pharynx, larynx, and epiglottis. Its main function is to warm, filter, and humidify inspired air.
  b. Lower airway: trachea, right and left mainstem bronchus, segmental bronchi, and terminal bronchioles. The major functions are conduction of air, mucociliary clearance, and production of pulmonary surfactant.
3. Sample answers:
  a. ABG: This test measures the adequacy of oxygenation, ventilation, and perfusion through the base excess or deficit of arterial blood.
  b. Creatine kinase (CK): Cardiac biomarkers reflect injury to tissues such as the heart muscle.
  c. Troponin: Protein found in skeletal and cardiac muscle fibers and released after injury to the heart. These biomarkers are used to monitor cardiac injury and myocardial infarction.
  d. Cytologic study: This involves a microscopic examination of sputum and the cells it contains. It is done primarily to detect cells that may be malignant, determine organisms causing infection, and identify blood or pus in the sputum.
4. a. Any change in the surface area available for diffusion will have a negative effect on diffusion of oxygen or carbon dioxide.
  b. Incomplete lung expansion or lung collapse (atelectasis) prevents pressure changes and exchange of gases by diffusion in the lungs.
  c. Any disease or condition that results in thickening of the alveolar–capillary membrane makes diffusion of oxygen or carbon dioxide more difficult.

d. The partial pressure, or pressure resulting from any gas in a mixture depending on its concentration, can also affect diffusion.

5. a. Dissolved in plasma (2%)
   b. Carried by red blood cells in the form of oxyhemoglobin (98%)

6. a. Infant: Respiratory activity is abdominal. The chest wall is so thin that the ribs, sternum, and xiphoid process are easily identified.
   b. Preschool- and school-aged child: Some subcutaneous fat is deposited on the chest wall, so landmarks are less prominent than in an infant; preschool child's eustachian tubes, bronchi, and bronchioles are elongated and less angular than in an infant, so the number of routine colds and infections decrease until the child enters school.
   c. Older adult: Bony landmarks are more prominent; kyphosis contributes to appearance of leaning forward and can limit respiratory ventilation. Barrel chest deformity may develop, senile emphysema may be present; power of respiratory and abdominal muscles are reduced.

7. Before: Collect baseline respiratory and related assessment and ensure informed consent is signed. Teach the patient that a local anesthesia will be administered, instruct patient they may be asked to sit on edge of the bed or lie on the back, to remain still, and follow provider's instructions for breathing; administer analgesics as ordered.
During: Observe patient for reactions or complication such as pneumothorax or hypotension. Report any deviation from normal color, pulse, and respiratory rates to health care provider; ensure that specimens, if obtained, are taken to the laboratory immediately.
After: Observe patient for changes in vital signs, particularly respirations; obtain chest radiograph.

8. The inhalation of cigarette smoke increases airway resistance, reduces ciliary action, increases mucus production, causes thickening of the alveolar–capillary membrane, and causes bronchial walls to thicken and lose their elasticity. It is the major risk factor for COPD and cardiopulmonary diseases including cancer, coronary heart disease, emphysema, chronic bronchitis. E-cigarette or vaping-associated lung injury (EVALI), is an emerging health issue of concern, or cancers.

9. a. Deep breathing: The nurse instructs the patient to make each breath deep enough to move the bottom ribs. The patient should start slowly, inspiring deeply through the nose and expiring slowly through the mouth.
   b. Incentive spirometry: The patient takes a deep breath and observes the results of their efforts as they register on the spirometer as the patient sustains maximal inspiration.

c. Pursed-lip breathing: While sitting upright, the patient inhales through the nose while counting to three and then exhales slowly and evenly against pursed lips while tightening the abdominal muscles. During exhalation, the patient counts to seven. To purse the lips, the patient should pucker the lips as though they are whistling or using a straw.
   d. Diaphragmatic breathing: The patient places one hand on the stomach and the other on the middle of the chest. The patient breathes in slowly through the nose, letting the abdomen protrude against their hand as far as it will go. Then the patient breathes out through pursed lips while contracting the abdominal muscles, with one hand pressing inward and upward on the abdomen. Perform the steps for 5 to 10 minutes, three to four times daily, followed by relaxation.
   e. Voluntary coughing: The nurse encourages the patient to cough voluntarily combined with deep breathing. Coughing upon arising, before meals, and at bedtime is suggested. For a patient with neuromuscular disorders, assisted cough is used.

10. a. Avoid open flames in the patient's room.
   b. Place "No Smoking" signs in conspicuous places in the patient's room.
   c. Check to see that electric equipment is in good working order.
   d. Avoid wearing and using synthetic fabrics, which build up static electricity.
   e. Avoid using oils in the area.

11. a. Oropharyngeal/nasopharyngeal airway: Semicircular tube of plastic or rubber inserted into the back of the pharynx through the mouth or nose in a spontaneously breathing patient; used to keep the tongue clear of the airway and to permit suctioning of secretions; often used for postoperative patients until they regain consciousness.
   b. Endotracheal tube: Polyvinylchloride tube that is inserted through the nose or mouth into the trachea using a laryngoscope as guide; used to administer oxygen by mechanical ventilator, to suction secretions easily, or to bypass upper airway obstructions.
   c. Tracheostomy tube: The curved tracheostomy tube is inserted into a surgical opening in the trachea. This may be used to replace an endotracheal tube, provide a method to mechanically ventilate the patient, bypass an upper airway obstruction, or remove tracheobronchial secretions.

12. Nursing responsibilities include assisting with insertion and removal of a chest tube. Once the tube is in place, monitor the patient's respiratory status and vital signs, maintain an occlusive dressing, and maintain the patency and integrity of the drainage system. Assess drainage quality and quantity.

13. Sample answers:
   a. Help the patient assume a position that allows free movement of the diaphragm and expansion of the chest wall to promote ease of respiration.
   b. Encourage the patient to drink 1.5 to 2 L of fluids daily to thin secretions.
   c. Provide humidified air.
   d. Promote breathing exercises, incentive spirometer, and controlled coughing.
   e. Use chest PT, percussion, vibration, and postural drainage.
   f. Suction as appropriate.

14. Put on PPE, including goggles or face shield. Suction the airway prior to replacing a disposable inner cannula or cleaning a nondisposable one. Regularly change dressings and ties. Site care is performed per policy with saline to remove secretions and crusting at site and on faceplate. Keep a spare tube and obturator (the same size as the patient's) at the bedside. Document care and alterations.

15. a. Angina: a type of myocardial ischemia; stable angina is a temporary imbalance between the amount of oxygen needed by the heart and the amount delivered to the heart muscles, causing chest pain or discomfort.
   b. Myocardial infarction: one type of acute coronary syndrome characterized by the death of heart tissue due to lack of oxygen, is also known as a heart attack.
   c. Dysrhythmia also referred to as arrhythmia: a disturbance of the rate and/or rhythm of the heart caused by an abnormal rate of electrical impulse generation from the SA node, or from impulses originating from a site or sites other than the SA node. They can occur with heart disease, hypertension, damage to the heart, in the presence of various drugs, with decreased oxygenation of the heart tissues, and with trauma. Symptoms may include decreased blood pressure, dizziness, palpitations, weakness, or fainting.
   d. Heart failure: occurs when the heart is unable to pump a sufficient blood supply, resulting in inadequate perfusion and oxygenation of tissues. Chronic hypertension, coronary artery disease, and disease of the heart valves are risk factors. Symptoms include shortness of breath, edema (swelling), and fatigue.

APPLYING YOUR KNOWLEDGE

CRITICAL-THINKING QUESTIONS

1. Sample answers:
   a. Assess oxygenation and breathing sounds to determine if suction is needed.
   b. Perform chest PT or administer bronchodilators.

   c. Administer an antibiotic and a corticosteroid.
   d. Administer oxygen; help the patient correlate smoking with lung damage and inflammation.

2. Sample answers: Triggers or activity at the time, what usually relieves it, do they wear/need oxygen, assess the pulse oximetry, ABG if indicated by signs and symptoms, underlying disease process.

REFLECTIVE PRACTICE: CULTIVATING QSEN COMPETENCIES

Sample Answers

1. Patient-centered care/evidence-based practice/ teamwork and collaboration: How might the nurse respond to Ms. McIntyre's request not to provide resuscitation if she stops breathing?
   The nurse first ensures the patient is competent to make decisions. The nurse would ask the patient or check the chart for advance directives, living will, or DNR and if one is not executed, the nurse could encourage the provider to speak with the patient and create the DNR. The nurse encourages the patient to discuss the decision with family members as appropriate. A palliative care or hospice consultant, health care provider could be called in to facilitate the process. The nurse should take into consideration age-related changes that may be increasing Ms. McIntyre's symptoms and that may respond to appropriate treatment and therapy.

2. Patient-centered care: What would be a successful outcome for this patient?
   The patient vocalizes understanding of, and signs, an advance directive and DNR to direct her care and protect her rights as a patient.

3. Patient-centered care/evidence-based practice/ teamwork and collaboration: What intellectual, technical, and ethical/legal competencies are most likely to bring about the desired outcome?
   Intellectual: knowledge of developmental and pathophysiologic variables affecting respiratory function; knowledge that CPR and mechanical ventilation does not cure the underlying disease.
   Technical: ability to manage the patient's airway and mechanical ventilation. The equipment and protocols necessary to diagnose and treat respiratory problems.
   Ethical/legal: knowledge of patients' and families' rights related to refusal of care

4. Teamwork and collaboration: What resources might be helpful for Ms. McIntyre?
   A progress meeting with the patient (family if available) and health care team to discuss preparation of an advanced directive stating 'allow natural death' or 'do not resuscitate'. Determination of competency by psychiatrist or psychologist where indicated, advance directives, and living wills, legal counsel could also be helpful.

PATIENT CARE STUDY

Answers will vary with student experience.

PRACTICING FOR NCLEX
MULTIPLE-CHOICE QUESTIONS

1. c	**2.** a	**3.** b	**4.** a	**5.** d
6. c	**7.** c	**8.** a	**9.** d	**10.** b
11. d	**12.** a	**13.** d	**14.** a	**15.** b

ALTERNATE-FORMAT QUESTIONS
Multiple-Response Questions

1. a, b, e
2. b, c, e
3. b, c, d, e
4. a, b, e
5. a, b, e, f
6. b, d, e
7. b, e

Sequencing Questions

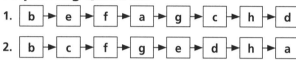

1. b → e → f → a → g → c → h → d
2. b → c → f → g → e → d → h → a

Prioritization Question

1. a

CHAPTER 41

ASSESSING YOUR UNDERSTANDING
FILL IN THE BLANKS

1. homeostasis
2. Intracellular
3. Extracellular
4. Insensible
5. Sensible
6. Electrolytes
7. ion
8. cations
9. anions
10. Solvents
11. osmosis
12. isotonic
13. hypertonic
14. hypotonic

MATCHING EXERCISES
Matching Exercise 1

1. a	**2.** c	**3.** a	**4.** a	**5.** c
6. b	**7.** d			

Matching Exercise 2

1. a	**2.** c	**3.** a	**4.** b	**5.** b
6. a	**7.** c			

Matching Exercise 3

Name of Acid–Base Disturbance	Characteristics
1. Respiratory acidosis	Low pH, high $PaCO_2$, normal HCO_3^-
2. Metabolic acidosis	Low pH, normal $PaCO_2$, low HCO_3^-
3. Respiratory alkalosis	High pH, normal $PaCO_2$, high HCO_3^-
4. Metabolic alkalosis	High pH, low $PaCO_2$, normal HCO_3^-

Matching Exercise 4

1. g	**2.** f	**3.** d	**4.** a	**5.** b
6. e	**7.** c	**8.** h		

CORRECT THE FALSE STATEMENTS

1. T
2. F, electrolytes
3. F, hypotonic solution
4. T
5. F, hydrogen
6. F, alkali
7. F, alkaline
8. F, lungs
9. T
10. F, hypernatremia
11. F, disproportionate
12. T

SHORT ANSWER

1. **a.** 7.35 to 7.45
   b. 35 to 45 mm Hg
   c. 22 to 26 mEq/L
   d. >80 mm Hg
   e. >95%
2. **a.** Osmosis: water, a solvent, passes from an area of lesser solute concentration to an area of greater solute concentration until an equilibrium is established.
   b. Diffusion: Tendency of solutes to move freely throughout a solvent, from an area of higher concentration to an area of lower concentration, until an equilibrium is established.
   c. Active transport: A process that requires energy for the movement of substances through a cell membrane from an area of lesser concentration to an area of higher concentration.
3. **a.** Ingested liquids: Fluid intake is regulated by the thirst mechanism and is stimulated by intracellular dehydration and decreased blood volume.
   b. Food: The amount of water depends on the food (e.g., melons have a higher water content than bread).

c. Metabolic oxidation: Water is an end product of oxidation that occurs during the metabolism of carbohydrates, fats, and protein (food).

4. a. Kidneys as urine
   b. Skin as perspiration
   c. Insensible water loss

5. a. Kidneys: Approximately 180 L of plasma is filtered daily in the adult, and 2 L of urine is excreted. They selectively retain electrolytes and water and excrete wastes.
   b. Cardiovascular system: The heart and blood vessels are responsible for pumping and carrying nutrients and water throughout the body and perfusing the kidney.
   c. Lungs: The lungs regulate oxygen and carbon dioxide levels of the blood.
   d. Thyroid: Thyroxine, released by the thyroid gland, increases blood flow in the body. This in turn increases renal circulation, which results in increased glomerular filtration and urinary output.
   e. Gastrointestinal tract: The GI tract absorbs water and nutrients that enter the body through this route.
   f. Nervous system: The nervous system acts as a switchboard and inhibits and stimulates mechanisms that influence fluid balance; pituitary gland inhibits or releases ADH.

6. a. Acidosis: Characterized by a high concentration of hydrogen ions in ECF, which causes the pH to fall below 7.35
   b. Alkalosis: Characterized by a low concentration of hydrogen ions in ECF, which causes the pH to exceed 7.45

7. a. Respiratory acidosis: decreased alveolar ventilation and resulting in the retention of carbon dioxide and an excess of carbonic acid in ECF. As the carbonic acid concentration increases, the kidneys retain more bicarbonate and increase their excretion of hydrogen. Note the lungs, which are causing the acidosis cannot compensate (for the rise in carbonic acid levels).
   b. Respiratory alkalosis: A deficit of carbonic acid in ECF caused by increased alveolar ventilation and resulting in a decrease in carbon dioxide. Respiratory rate and depth increase because carbon dioxide is being excreted faster than normal; depression or cessation of respirations can occur. The kidneys attempt to alleviate this imbalance by increasing bicarbonate excretion and hydrogen retention. Note that the lungs are unable to compensate for the alkalosis, as they are the cause of the disturbance.
   c. Metabolic acidosis: A deficit of bicarbonate in ECF resulting from an increase in acidic components or an excessive loss of bicarbonate. The lungs (the unaffected system) attempt to increase the rate of carbon dioxide excretion by increasing the rate and depth of respirations; the kidneys attempt to compensate by retaining

bicarbonate and excreting more hydrogen. May result in loss of consciousness and death.
   d. Metabolic alkalosis: An excess of bicarbonate in ECF resulting from loss of acid or ingestion or retention of base. The body attempts to compensate by retaining carbon dioxide through the unaffected system. Respirations become slow and shallow, and periods of apnea may occur. The kidneys excrete potassium and sodium along with excess bicarbonate and retain hydrogen within carbonic acid.

8. a. Increased hematocrit: severe dehydration and shock (when hemoconcentration rises considerably)
   b. Decreased hematocrit: acute, massive blood loss; hemolytic reaction following transfusion of incompatible blood
   c. Increased hemoglobin: hemoconcentration of the blood
   d. Decreased hemoglobin: anemia, severe hemorrhage, and following a hemolytic reaction

9. a. Urine pH and specific gravity: Specific gravity is a measure of the kidney's ability to concentrate urine. Normal range: 1.005 to 1.030. Both may be obtained by dipstick measurement on a fresh voided specimen or through lab analysis.
   b. Serum electrolytes: Indicate plasma levels of select electrolytes
   c. Arterial blood gases: Indicate the adequacy of oxygenation and ventilation and acid–base status

10. Handling all equipment, performing dressing changes, assessing patient for evidence of infection or other complications, and maintaining the supplies necessary to continue home infusion.

APPLYING YOUR KNOWLEDGE
CRITICAL THINKING QUESTIONS

1. Sample answers:
   a. Exercise causes excess perspiration and respiratory fluid losses due to rapid breathing. Replacement with water and/or isotonic sport beverages should be encouraged.
   b. Ingesting excessive sodium bicarbonate, a base, will cause metabolic alkalosis. The high-sodium load could lead to high(er) blood pressure.
   c. The infant requires isotonic fluid replacement with electrolytes such as potassium and sodium.
2. Sample answer: Foods low in sodium include fresh fruits and vegetables and proteins and other foods cooked without added salt. Foods to avoid include canned or processed meats, cheeses (except lower sodium), fast foods.

REFLECTIVE PRACTICE: CULTIVATING QSEN COMPETENCIES
Sample Answers

1. Patient-centered care, tatient-centered care, teamwork and collaboration: Based on the data in this scenario, what body systems are involved in Mr. Park's fluid volume excess? What interventions would be appropriate?

Fluid volume excess has developed causing the bounding pulse, distended neck veins, and abnormal lung sounds. The nurse raises the head of the bed to permit respiratory expansion and ease dyspnea. The nurse collaborates with the provider, recommending IV fluids be held for a period of time. The patient may need to avoid sodium-containing foods or fluids. The nurse records the assessment data and interventions in the electronic health record.

2. Patient-centered care/evidence-based practice: What would be a successful outcome for Mr. Park? By end of shift, the patient states the reasons for fluid restrictions and that he is breathing more easily following cessation of IV fluids and positioning.

3. Evidence-based practice/safety: What intellectual, technical, and ethical/legal competencies are most likely to bring about the desired outcome? Intellectual: knowledge of assessing, interpreting, and intervening when the patient displayed signs of fluid volume excess or possible speed shock. The nurse follows up on the error of the IV rate with the nurse manager, health care provider, and patient (per policy). An event (incident or variance report) will be completed. The nurse evaluates the interventions, observing for the expected outcome of stopping the IV infusion.
Technical: ability to use the equipment, such as IV pump and protocols necessary to administer IV antibiotics.
Ethical/legal: strong sense of accountability for the health and well-being of patients and willingness to hold themselves or colleagues accountable for safe quality practice.

4. Teamwork and collaboration: What resources might be helpful for this patient?
Patient teaching and printed materials on fluid volume excess.

PATIENT CARE STUDY

Answers will vary with student experience.

PRACTICING FOR NCLEX
MULTIPLE-CHOICE QUESTIONS

1. c	**2.** c	**3.** b	**4.** d	**5.** b
6. c	**7.** b	**8.** b	**9.** b	**10.** a
11. b	**12.** a	**13.** c	**14.** d	**15.** c

ALTERNATE-FORMAT QUESTIONS
Multiple-Response Questions

1. a, b, d, f
2. b, d, f
3. d, e, f
4. a, b, c
5. b, d, f
6. a, b, e
7. c, d, e
8. b, c, d

Chart/Exhibit Questions

1. c	**2.** a	**3.** d	**4.** a	**5.** b
6.				

pH	PaCO$_2$	HCO$_3^-$	Acidosis or Alkalosis	Respiratory or	Metabolic	Comp Y/N	Complete (C) or Partial (P)
7.28	63	25	Acidosis	×		N	
7.20	40	14	Acidosis		×	N	
7.52	40	35	Alkalosis		×	N	
7.16	82	30	Acidosis	×		Y	P
7.36	68	35	Normal pH-↑ pCO$_2$	× acidosis		Y	C (pH is normal)
7.56	23	26	Alkalosis	×		N	
7.40	40	26	Normal	Normal	Normal	N/A	
7.56	23	26	Alkalosis	×		N	
7.26	70	25	Acidosis	×		N	
7.52	44	38	Alkalosis		×	N	
7.32	30	18	Acidosis		×	Y	P
7.49	34	26	Alkalosis	×		N	

Hint: Compensation occurs in the unaffected system. Complete compensation returns the pH to normal; partial compensation occurs when the pH remains outside the normal range.

Hot Spot Questions

1.

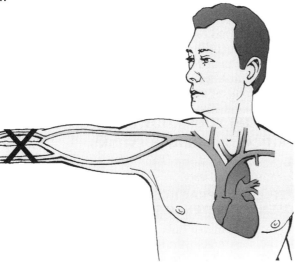

2.

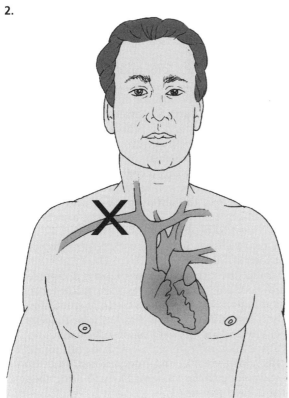

CHAPTER 42

ASSESSING YOUR UNDERSTANDING
FILL IN THE BLANKS
1. actualization
2. concept
3. global
4. ideal
5. false

6. identity
7. disability
8. loved
9. 6, 7
10. substance

MATCHING EXERCISES
Matching Exercise 1
1. a   **2.** d   **3.** e   **4.** f   **5.** c
6. b

Matching Exercise 2
1. d   **2.** b   **3.** c   **4.** d   **5.** b
6. a   **7.** a

SHORT ANSWER
1. Sample answer: Nurses interacting with older adults must first identify their attitudes and feelings about aging and older adults. Then measures such as addressing older adults respectfully, communicating that you take their concerns seriously, adjusting your communication style to accommodate sensory or cognitive deficits, noticing and affirming their personal strengths, and advocating for needed services are used.
2. Answers will vary with student experiences.
3. Sample answers:
   a. Significance: Do you feel loved and appreciated by the key people in your life?
   b. Competence: Does anything interfere with your ability to do the things that are important to you?
   c. Virtue: How would you describe your ability to follow your moral code?
   d. Power: Do you feel you are in control of your life?
4. Sample answers:
   a. Developmental considerations: A teenager needs guidance and trust to make good choices that affect their life.
   b. Culture: As a child internalizes the values of parents and peers, culture begins to influence their sense of self.
   c. Internal and external resources: Social determinants such as income may influence one's self-concept.
   d. History of success or failure: A child who repeatedly fails in school may have difficulty succeeding in life.
   e. Stressors: Self-concept determines the way a person perceives stressors in their life and reacts to them.
   f. Aging, illness, or trauma: Paralysis after a traumatic injury will most likely affect self-concept.
5. Sample answers:
   a. Dispel the myth that it is necessary to know all there is to know about nursing to be a good nurse: Nurses must constantly learn new theories and procedures to keep up with medicine.
   b. Realistically evaluate strengths and weaknesses: A periodic review of one's skills, strengths, weaknesses, and goals should be undertaken.

c. Accentuate the positive: Nurses recall what they do correctly and learn from their mistakes.

d. Develop a conscious plan for changing weaknesses into strengths: Focus on developing needed technical skills, research best practices, consider joining a nursing organization related to your practice.

e. Work to develop team self-esteem: Recognize or congratulate colleagues and celebrate when the nursing team is successful. Seek certifications as a group or for yourself.

f. Actively demonstrate your commitment to the nursing profession and concern about the nursing profession's public image: Be aware of nurses' impact on society; the image they project should be consistent with professional standards.

6. Answers will vary with student experiences.

7. Sample answers:

a. Personal identity: How would you describe yourself to others?

b. Patient strengths: What special talents and abilities do you have?

c. Body image: What are your positive physical attributes?

d. Self-esteem: What do you like most about yourself?

e. Role performance: What major roles describe you?

8. a. Encourage patients to identify their strengths.

b. Notice and reinforce patient strengths.

c. Encourage patients to reach for the strengths they admire in others and to try them on.

9. a. Use looks, touch, and speech to communicate worth.

b. Speak respectfully to the patient and addressing the patient by preferred name.

c. Move the patient's body respectfully when providing care.

10. Sample answers:

a. Help them find meaning in the experience, regain mastery to the extent that this is possible, and realistically evaluate the adequacy of their coping strategies. Encourage them to develop a "game plan" for confronting anxiety-producing situations. Identify and secure interventions for treatable depression. Address treatable causes of self-identity disturbances, such as pain or substance abuse.

b. Notice and affirm positive physiologic characteristics of the patient. Teach preventive self-care measures that reduce uncomfortable signs of aging. Explore new activities (which may include old hobbies) that are within the changing physical abilities of the patient.

c. Help patient identify and use personal strengths. Let them know that you value them for who they are. Use their preferred name. Ask questions about their life, interests, and values. With PT and OT, engage them in activities in which they can be successful. Empower them to meet their needs by providing necessary knowledge, teaching new behaviors, and instilling the belief that they can change.

d. Explore with patient the many roles the older adult has fulfilled throughout their lifetime. Encourage her to reminisce. Facilitate grieving over valued roles that she can no longer perform. Assess for depression, pain, and other problems that may create impatience.

APPLYING YOUR KNOWLEDGE

CRITICAL THINKING QUESTIONS

1. Answers will vary.
2. Answers will vary.

REFLECTIVE PRACTICE: CULTIVATING QSEN COMPETENCIES

1. Patient-centered care: What interventions might the nurse employ to try to resolve Anthony's self-image disturbance?

   The nurse assesses each component of Anthony's self-concept to determine how they fit with his role expectation and function as a "whole" man. The nurse assesses the major stressors that place anyone at relative risk for maladaptive responses, such as withdrawal, isolation, depression, extreme anxiety, substance abuse, or exacerbation of physical illness. The nurse also assesses his previous coping, strengths, and self-concept prior to surgery. Using this data, the nurse can assist with glucose control, pain management, and adaptation to the loss of their leg. Setting a goal of ambulating with a prosthesis may be helpful in promoting adaptation to the loss and restoring self-image.

2. Patient-centered care: What would be a successful outcome for this patient?

   By next visit, the patient lists three positive aspects of their self-image.

   Prior to discharge, the patient reports he appreciates poor glucose control was a risk factor for the amputation. The patient successfully ambulates short distances with new prosthesis. He suggests an activity he looks forward to after discharge.

3. Patient-centered care/teamwork and collaboration/safety: What intellectual, interpersonal, and ethical/legal competencies are most likely to bring about the desired outcome?

   Intellectual: knowledge of postoperative care of patient with amputation, measures to manage diabetes, pain management, and self-concept for a middle-aged man

   Interpersonal: strong interpersonal skills to establish a trusting relationship with a middle-aged man after an amputation; work as a team on pain management, glucose control, and home safety with a prosthesis

   Ethical/legal: commitment to patient advocacy, including getting the patient needed assistance with glucose control and pain management to achieve his health goals.

4. **Teamwork and collaboration: What resources might be helpful for this patient?**
Exercise or yoga classes, web-based meditations, identifying triggers for GI upset, printed or AV materials on stress reduction techniques

PATIENT CARE STUDY
Answers will vary with student experience.

PRACTICING FOR NCLEX
MULTIPLE-CHOICE QUESTIONS
1. a	**2.** c	**3.** a	**4.** b	**5.** a
6. d	**7.** c	**8.** a	**9.** a	**10.** d
11. c	**12.** b	**13.** c		

ALTERNATE-FORMAT QUESTIONS
Multiple-Response Questions

1. b, d, f
2. d, e
3. c, e, f
4. c, d, f
5. a, e, f

Sequencing Question

1.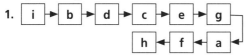

CHAPTER 44

ASSESSING YOUR UNDERSTANDING
FILL IN THE BLANKS
1. perceived
2. Bereavement, mourning
3. outcome
4. dysfunctional
5. brain
6. palliative
7. Hope
8. Hospice
9. dignity
10. natural

MATCHING EXERCISES
Matching Exercise 1
1. e	**2.** a	**3.** d	**4.** c	**5.** f
6. b				

Matching Exercise 2
1. d	**2.** a	**3.** e	**4.** b	**5.** c
6. f				

CORRECT THE FALSE STATEMENTS
1. F, unresolved grief
2. F, anger
3. T
4. F, durable power of attorney for health care
5. T

6. F, no-code or do-not-resuscitate
7. T
8. F, mortician
9. F, nurse

SHORT ANSWER
1. **a.** Care of the body: Place body in normal anatomic position; remove soiled dressings and tubes (unless an autopsy is being performed); place ID tags on shroud, ankle, and prostheses.
   b. Care of the family: Be an attentive listener; attend funeral (if family permits); make follow-up call to assess family's well-being.
   c. Discharging legal responsibilities: The mortician assumes responsibility for handling and filing the death certificate with proper authorities. A clinician's signature is required on the certificate (check your state law to see if nurses can sign death certificates), as well as that of the pathologist, the coroner, and others in special cases. The nurse is responsible to ensure that the death certificate is signed.
2. **a.** Denial and isolation: The patient denies that they will die, may repress what is discussed, and may isolate themselves from reality.
   b. Anger: The patient expresses rage and hostility and adopts a "why me?" attitude.
   c. Bargaining: The patient tries to barter for more time.
   d. Depression: The patient goes through a period of grief before death.
   e. Acceptance: The patient feels tranquil; they have accepted death and are prepared to die.
3. As soon as possible, the patient should be told her diagnosis and prognosis, how the disease is likely to progress, and what this will mean for her. *Cultural influences may dictate how much information is desired and which family members are to be informed.*
4. Answers will vary with student experiences.
5. Nurse's role is to participate in the decision-making process by offering helpful information about the benefits and burdens of continued ventilation and description of what to expect if it is initiated. Supporting the patient's family and managing sedation and analgesia are critical nursing responsibilities.
6. Sample answers:
   a. Communicate openly with patients about their losses and invite discussion of the adequacy of their coping mechanisms.
   b. Respond genuinely to the concerns and feelings of dying patients and their families; do not be afraid to cry with the patient and to allow feelings to show.
   c. Value time spent with patients and family members in which supportive presence is the primary intervention.
7. Sample answers:
   a. The patient will make health care decisions reflecting their values and goals.

b. The patient will experience a comfortable and dignified death.

c. The patient and family will accept the need for help as appropriate and use available resources.

8. Sample answers:

a. In favor of: It is a beneficent and compassionate act. It takes the matter outside the reach of "medical power" and scrupulosity. It respects autonomy by preserving the patient's control of the manner, method, and timing of death.

b. Against: It undermines the value of, and respect for, all human life. A focus on euthanasia will divert attention from other valuable palliative techniques. If legalized, it is predicted that patients will feel a subtle pressure to conform in order to relieve the economic and emotional burdens they impose on family and friends.

9. **a.** No-code: The nurse validates the health care provider has written DNR on the chart of a patient, the patient or surrogate has expressed a wish that there be no attempts made to resuscitate the patient in the event of a cardiopulmonary emergency. The nurse continues to provide comfort measures and any medications or treatments specified.

b. Comfort measures only: Nurses should be familiar with the forms used to indicate patient preferences about end-of-life care. The goal of a comfort measures only order is to indicate that the goal of treatment is a comfortable, dignified death and that further life-sustaining measures are no longer indicated.

c. Do-not-hospitalize orders: These orders are used by patients in long-term care facilities and other residential settings who have elected not to be hospitalized for further aggressive treatment. The nursing responsibilities would be the same as for comfort measures only.

d. Terminal weaning: The nurse's role is to participate in the decision-making process by offering helpful information about the benefits and burdens of continued ventilation and a description of what to expect during terminal weaning.

10. **a.** Durable power of attorney: Nurses must facilitate dialog about this advance directive, which appoints an agent the person trusts to make decisions in the event of the appointing person's subsequent incapacity.

b. Living will: Nurses must also facilitate dialog about this advance directive, which provides specific instructions about the kinds of health care that should be provided or avoided in particular situations.

c. POLST form: A Physician Order for Life-Sustaining Treatment form, or POLST form, is a medical order indicating a patient's wishes regarding treatments commonly used in a medical crisis. It must be completed and signed by a health care professional in close consultation with the patient. As a medical order, it cannot be filled out by a patient. These forms are not available in all states.

APPLYING YOUR KNOWLEDGE
CRITICAL THINKING QUESTIONS

1. Sample answers:

a. Allow patient to grieve for future dreams. Assess patient's strengths and goals. Help manage pain and promote mobility.

b. Allow patient to grieve for future dreams, perhaps of children or more children. Assess patient's strengths and goals. Refer patient to support groups.

c. Anticipate the patient's anger, followed by depression. Assess what is important to the patient and support her in achieving it. Provide pain management if needed.

2. Answers will vary according to student experiences.

REFLECTIVE PRACTICE: CULTIVATING QSEN COMPETENCIES
Sample Answers

1. Patient-centered care/evidence-based practice: How might the nurse react to Yvonne in a manner that respects her right to privacy while at the same time helping her through the grief process?
The nurse should realize that this patient is experiencing anticipatory loss and use this knowledge to help her cope with the potential loss of her baby. To develop meaningful communication the nurse needs to use open-ended questions to elicit information and listen to the patient, recognizing both her verbal and nonverbal cues. The nurse should also be encouraging without giving false reassurances. If she agrees to participate, Yvonne would benefit from grief counseling.

2. Patient-centered care/evidence-based practice: What would be a successful outcome for this patient?
By next visit, the patent vocalizes her fears for her baby and herself and lists the benefits of grief counseling.

3. Patient-centered care/teamwork and collaboration: What intellectual, interpersonal, and/or ethical/legal competencies are most likely to bring about the desired outcome?
Intellectual: ability to identify the impact that loss, grief, and death and dying have on the patient and their family members
Interpersonal: ability to establish trusting relationships, even in times of great crisis related to anticipatory loss
Ethical/legal: commitment to safety and quality, strong sense of responsibility and accountability, and strong advocacy skills

4. Teamwork and collaboration: What resources might be helpful for Yvonne?
Grief counseling, information on premature babies

PATIENT CARE STUDY

Answers will vary with student experience.

PRACTICING FOR NCLEX

MULTIPLE-CHOICE QUESTIONS

1. c	**2.** b	**3.** a	**4.** b	**5.** d
6. b	**7.** b	**8.** b	**9.** a	**10.** a
11. a	**12.** c			

ALTERNATE-FORMAT QUESTIONS

Multiple-Response Questions

1. a, c, f
2. b, c, d, e
3. d, e, f
4. a, c, d
5. a, d, e, f
6. b, d, e, f

Prioritization Question

1. d

CHAPTER 45

ASSESSING YOUR UNDERSTANDING

FILL IN THE BLANKS

1. perception
2. reception
3. Kinesthesia, proprioception
4. Stereognosis
5. adaptation
6. deprivation
7. overload
8. processing
9. presbycusis

MATCHING EXERCISES

Matching Exercise 1

1. d	**2.** a	**3.** c	**4.** b	**5.** e
6. f				

Matching Exercise 2

1. a	**2.** c	**3.** b	**4.** d	**5.** b
6. a				

SHORT ANSWER

1. **a.** A stimulus, an agent, act, or other influence capable of initiating a response by the nervous system.
   b. A receptor or sense organ must receive the stimulus and convert it into a nerve impulse.
   c. The nerve impulse must be conducted along a nervous pathway from the receptor or sense organ to the brain.
   d. A particular area in the brain must receive and translate the impulse into a sensation.
2. Sample answers:
   a. Environment: A patient with AIDS in isolation is at high risk for sensory deprivation.
   b. Impaired ability to receive environmental stimuli: A patient who is visually impaired is at high risk for sensory deprivation.
   c. Inability to process environmental stimuli: A patient who is confused cannot process environmental stimuli.

3. **a.** Perceptual responses: inaccurate perception of sights, sounds, tastes, smells, and body position; poor coordination and equilibrium; mild to gross distortions in perception, ranging from daydreams to hallucinations
   b. Cognitive responses: inability to control the direction of thought content; decreased attention span and ability to concentrate; difficulty with memory, problem solving, and task performance
   c. Emotional responses: inappropriate emotional responses: apathy, anxiety, fear, anger, belligerence, panic, depression; rapid mood changes
4. Sample answers:
   a. A patient is disoriented by the strange sights, odors, and sounds in a CCU.
   b. A burn victim is in constant pain and cannot concentrate on their environment.
   c. A confused patient panics at the sight of doctors and nurses probing their body.
5. Sample answers:
   a. Infant: soothing sounds, rocking, holding, and changing position, changing patterns of light and shade
   b. Adult: use of music, poetry, drama to alleviate boredom
   c. Older adult: use of art classes or organizing a book club in a long-term care facility
6. Sample answers:
   a. Patient will report feeling safe and in control of their environment.
   b. Patient will acknowledge or verbalize acceptance of the sensory deficit.
7. Sample answer:
   This patient is likely suffering from sensory deprivation. Measures should be taken to stimulate as many senses as possible. The curtains could be opened to allow light into the room; soft music could be played to stimulate auditory functioning; flavorful meals could be prepared to stimulate taste; flowers, cards, and pictures could be displayed to stimulate visual functioning.
8. **a.** Avoid damage from UV rays.
   b. Use caution with aerosol sprays.
   c. Have regular eye examinations and tests for glaucoma.
   d. Know the danger signals that indicate serious eye problems.
9. Sample answers:
   a. Visual: Read different types of books to the child; limit television watching; plan various outings.
   b. Auditory: Teach the child songs; play records; join a storytelling group.
   c. Olfactory: Have the child identify different odors; prepare enticing meals and savor the aromas.
   d. Gustatory: Encourage the child to experiment with different foods with varying colors, tastes, shapes, and textures; introduce finger foods into diet.
   e. Tactile: Use games and sports to increase body contact with child; demonstrate affection by hugging, holding child in lap, etc.

10. Sample answers:
   a. Visually impaired patients: Acknowledge your presence in the patient's room, identify yourself by name, and speak in a normal tone of voice.
   b. Hearing-impaired patients: Avoid excessive noise, avoid excessive cleaning of ears, and know the symptoms of hearing loss.
   c. Unconscious patients: Be careful of what is said in the patient's presence; assume the person can hear you and speak to the person before touching them.

APPLYING YOUR KNOWLEDGE
CRITICAL THINKING QUESTIONS

1. a. Answers will vary.
   b. Stereognosis; answers will vary.
   c. Answers will vary.
2. Answers will vary.

REFLECTIVE PRACTICE: CULTIVATING QSEN COMPETENCIES
Sample Answers

1. Patient-centered care/safety: What nursing interventions might be appropriate for Dolores' spouse? Sensory deprivation can lead to perceptual, cognitive, and emotional disturbances. Therefore, the nursing care plan should include sensory stimulation for the couple. The nurse should also investigate if hearing aids would help the patient with their hearing loss. The nurse should assess the family to see how they are coping with the changes in their social environment. Safety in the home and community is also an issue that needs to be addressed. The nurse should incorporate knowledge of the guidelines for communicating both with persons with reduced vision and hearing when developing a teaching plan to assist Dolores in dealing with her husband's condition.
2. Patient-centered care/safety: What would be a successful outcome for this patient? By next visit, the patient states that they are adapting to their condition and receiving new sensory stimulation from their environment. The patient remains free from falls or injury.
3. Patient-centered care: What intellectual and interpersonal competencies are most likely to bring about the desired outcome? Intellectual: Knowledge of the arousal mechanism and how the body responds, including sensoristasis and adaptation; ability to integrate knowledge of sensory alterations, including factors contributing to disturbed sensory perceptions. Interpersonal: Demonstration of the ability to empathize and communicate with patients with sensory deficits and interact effectively with patients and their caregivers. Normalize the experience for older adults.
4. Teamwork and collaboration: What resources might be helpful for the patient and partner?

Social services, printed materials on sensory deficits, community services

PATIENT CARE STUDY
Answers will vary with student experience.

PRACTICING FOR NCLEX
MULTIPLE-CHOICE QUESTIONS
1. c **2.** d **3.** b **4.** a **5.** a
6. d **7.** b **8.** b **9.** a

ALTERNATE-FORMAT QUESTIONS
Multiple-Response Questions
1. b, c, e, f
2. a, b, d, f
3. a, c, e
4. d, e, f
5. b, d, f
6. c, e, f

CHAPTER 46

ASSESSING YOUR UNDERSTANDING
FILL IN THE BLANKS
1. Sexuality
2. Gender
3. orientation
4. premenstrual
5. erogenous zones
6. transdermal
7. Rape
8. trafficking
9. knowledge, behavior

MATCHING EXERCISES
Matching Exercise 1
1. f **2.** d **3.** b **4.** a **5.** c
6. e

Matching Exercise 2
1. f **2.** b **3.** a **4.** e **5.** c
6. d

SHORT ANSWER
1. Sample answers:
   a. Chronic pain: Teach altered or modified positions for coitus.
   b. Diabetes: Some men may be candidates for a penile prosthesis; pharmacologic management of erectile dysfunction may be indicated.
   c. Cardiovascular disease: Teach gradual resumption of sexual activity, comfortable position for affected partner.
   d. Loss of body part: Allow patient to discuss the change in body image.
   e. Spinal cord injury: Encourage stimulation of other erogenous zones.
   f. Mental illness: Provide counseling for depression.
   g. Sexually transmitted infections (STIs): Educate the public about the prevention and treatment of STIs.

2. Sample answer:
The nurse recommends safer sexual practices for all patients and at least annual testing. Higher risk in those who engage in needle-sharing and sexually active gay, bisexual, and other MSM. Additionally, the nurse recommends testing for all pregnant persons in the United States at the first prenatal visit and/or when another STI is diagnosed. The nurse discusses considering PrEP and PEP with any STI diagnosis; begin ART and behavioral/psychosocial services as soon as possible with HIV infection. The nurse teaches signs and symptoms of HIV infection or AIDS including an asymptomatic period, fatigue, diarrhea, weight loss, enlarged lymph nodes, fever, anorexia, and night sweats.

3. a. Any inpatient or outpatient who is receiving care for pregnancy, an STI, infertility, or conception
b. Any patient who is currently experiencing a sexual dysfunction or problem
c. Any patient whose illness will affect sexual functioning and behavior in any way

4. Sample answers:
a. "Could you describe what happens?"
b. "What do you think caused the problem, or what was happening when you first noticed it?"
c. "Have you tried anything in the past to correct the problem?"

5. Complete the following table, listing the advantages and disadvantages associated with contraceptive methods.

APPLYING YOUR KNOWLEDGE
CRITICAL THINKING QUESTIONS

1. Sample answers:
a. An 18-year-old female victim of date rape who is brought to the emergency room for testing and treatment: "Can you tell me what happened? Is there someone, a partner you'd like to call? Are you using contraception? Is there any chance you could be pregnant?"
b. A 5-year-old girl who presents with soreness and redness in the genital area: "Can you show me where you hurt? Did anyone touch you in your private areas?"

2. Sample answers:
a. Male undergoing radiation treatment for colon cancer reports of impotence: "Has something like this ever happened before? Many men experience episodes of impotence with changes in health or fatigue. Have you discussed this with your oncologist?"
b. Menopausal female reports vaginal dryness and pain during intercourse: "What have you tried for this issue? How are you and your partner dealing with this?"
c. Sexually active teenager reports a burning sensation during urination: "Are you using protection with sexual activity? Is it possible your partner has an infection or STI?"

Method	Advantages	Disadvantages
a. Behavioral	Methods can be effective in avoiding pregnancy if mutual understanding, support, and motivation exist between sexual partners. There are no side effects (as in hormonal methods) and no messy devices to insert. Periodic abstinence and fertility awareness methods are two methods of contraception that involve charting a female's fertility pattern. The best approach to monitoring fertility is a combination of temperature methods, cervical mucus method, and calendar method, called the symptothermal method.	Requires abstinence during ovulation and a complete understanding of the signs and symptoms of ovulation. Continuous abstinence involves not having any sex with a partner at all. It is 100% effective in preventing pregnancy and STIs. However, people may find it difficult to abstain for long periods of time.
b. Barrier methods	Condoms help to prevent STIs; appropriate for women with sensitivity to the pill; effective when used correctly; relatively inexpensive methods.	Devices must be applied before intercourse; not all people can wear them; threat of toxic shock syndrome with vaginal sponge.
c. Intrauterine devices	High rate of effectiveness; little care or motivation on part of patient is necessary; excellent method for females who have completed their families but are not ready for sterilization.	Serious side effects and complications.
d. Hormonal methods	Many beneficial noncontraceptive effects, for example, protecting females against development of breast, ovarian, and endometrial cancer; almost 100% effective when taken as directed.	Cost may be prohibitive to some; compliance is necessary; some females should not take the pill due to physiologic disorders or diseases.
e. Sterilization	After initial surgery and recheck, no further compliance is necessary; almost 100% effective.	Should be considered permanent and irreversible.

REFLECTIVE PRACTICE: CULTIVATING QSEN COMPETENCIES
Sample Answers

1. Patient-centered care/interprofessional collaboration: What issues might the nurse address in the care plan for Jefferson? What patient teaching should be incorporated into the care plan?
The nurse should review the effects of Jefferson's conditions on sexual function and assess his current status as well as the effect of the medications he is taking to see if they are a contributing factor. The nurse could consult with the primary health care provider to see if an adjustment in the medications might alleviate the problem. The nurse should also explore the emotional and psychological effects of the dysfunction on Jefferson and his wife and consult with other members of the health care team to develop an effective care plan. Patient teaching could include information about medications to treat impotence and the possibility of having a penile implant.

2. Patient-centered care: What would be a successful outcome for this patient?
Following an adjustment to his medications, Jefferson vocalizes an improvement in his sexual functioning.

3. Patient-centered care/safety: What intellectual and interpersonal competencies are most likely to bring about the desired outcome?
Intellectual: ability to integrate knowledge about sexual health into nursing care, including the ability to identify areas of sexual dysfunction for the patient with a history of diabetes and hypertension experiencing impotence. Ability to monitor side effects of antihypertensive and diabetes medications (e.g., hypotension, hypoglycemia).
Interpersonal: strong interpersonal skills to establish trusting relationships and build rapport with a patient experiencing impotence

4. Teamwork and collaboration: What resources might be helpful for Jefferson?
Counseling, printed materials on impotence and preventative/corrective measures, information on the effect of medications on sexual functioning

PATIENT CARE STUDY

Answers will vary with student experience.

PRACTICING FOR NCLEX
MULTIPLE-CHOICE QUESTIONS

1. a	**2.** c	**3.** c	**4.** b	**5.** d
6. c	**7.** b	**8.** c		

ALTERNATE-FORMAT QUESTIONS
Multiple-Response Questions

1. b, c, f
2. b, c
3. d, e, f
4. b, d, e
5. c, d, e, f
6. a, b, e

Sequencing Question

1. 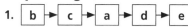 b → c → a → d → e

Prioritization Question

1. d

CHAPTER 47

ASSESSING YOUR UNDERSTANDING
FILL IN THE BLANKS

1. alienation
2. distress
3. forgiveness
4. guilt
5. Witnesses
6. atheist, agnostic
7. Parish (faith community)
8. parents
9. Suffering

MATCHING EXERCISES
Matching Exercise 1

1. a	**2.** d	**3.** c	**4.** b	**5.** d
6. c				

Matching Exercise 2

1. a	**2.** d	**3.** c	**4.** b	**5.** a
6. d				

SHORT ANSWER

1. **a.** Need for meaning and purpose
   b. Need for love and relatedness
   c. Need for forgiveness
2. Sample answers:
   a. Offering a compassionate presence
   b. Assisting in the struggle to find meaning and purpose in the face of suffering, illness, and death
   c. Fostering relationships with God/humans that nurture the spirit
   d. Facilitating the patient's expression of religious or spiritual beliefs and practices
3. **a.** Life-affirming influences: enhance life, give meaning and purpose to existence, strengthen feeling of self-worth, encourage self-actualization, and are health giving and life-sustaining
   b. Life-denying influences: restrict or enclose life patterns, limit experiences and associations, place burdens of guilt on people, encourage feelings of unworthiness, and are generally health denying and life inhibiting
4. Sample answers:
   a. Many religions prescribe dietary requirements and restrictions.
   b. Some religious faiths restrict birth control practices.
5. Sample answers:
   a. As a guide to daily living: Religions may specify dietary requirements or birth control measures.

b. As a source of support: It is common for people to seek support from religious faith in times of stress; this support is often vital to the acceptance of an illness. Prayer, devotional reading, and other religious practices often do for the person spiritually what protective exercises do for the body physically.

c. As a source of strength and healing: People have been known to endure extreme physical distress because of strong faith; patients' families have taken on almost unbelievable rehabilitative tasks because they had faith in the eventual positive results of their effort.

d. As a source of conflict: There are times when religious beliefs conflict with prevalent health care practices; for example, the doctrine of Jehovah's Witnesses prohibits blood transfusions. For some, illness is viewed as punishment for sin and is inevitable.

6. a. Developmental considerations: As a child matures, life experiences usually influence and mature their spiritual beliefs. With advancing years, the tendency to think about life after death prompts some people to reexamine and reaffirm their spiritual beliefs.

b. Family: A child's parents play a key role in the development of the child's spirituality.

c. Ethnic background: Religious traditions differ among ethnic groups. There are clear distinctions between Eastern and Western spiritual traditions, as well as among those of individual ethnic groups, such as Native Americans.

d. Life events: Both positive and negative life experiences can influence spirituality and in turn are influenced by the meaning a person's spiritual beliefs attribute to them.

7. Answers will vary with student experience.

8. a. Basis of authority or source of power

b. Scripture or sacred word

c. An ethical code that defines right and wrong

d. A psychology and identity that allow its adherents to fit into a group and the world to be defined by the religion

e. Aspirations or expectations

f. Some ideas about what follows death

9. Sample answers:

a. Spiritual pain: "This seems to be a source of deep pain for you...."

b. Spiritual alienation: "Does it seem like God is far away from your life?"

c. Spiritual anxiety: "You seem afraid that God might not be there for you when you need Him?"

d. Spiritual anger: "I sense you are very angry with God for taking away your child. Can you share more about this?"

e. Spiritual loss: "Tell me more about how your inability to get to the synagogue is affecting you."

f. Spiritual despair: "So you are saying that no matter how hard you try, you'll never be able to be close to God?"

10. Health Problem: Hopelessness, Etiology: related to the belief that God doesn't care
Sample interventions: The nurse should offer a supportive presence, facilitate the patient's practice of religion, counsel the patient spiritually, or contact a spiritual counselor.

11. Sample answers: The room should be orderly and free of clutter. Place a seat for the counselor at the bedside or near the patient. The bedside table should be free of items and covered with a clean, white cover if a sacrament is to be administered. Close the bed curtains for privacy, or move the patient to a private setting.

APPLYING YOUR KNOWLEDGE
CRITICAL THINKING QUESTIONS

1. Answers will vary based on student belief and experience. While it is acceptable to pray with a patient, if you are uncomfortable, you may offer to sit quietly while the patient prays.

2. Answers will vary.

REFLECTIVE PRACTICE: CULTIVATING QSEN COMPETENCIES
Sample Answers

1. Patient-centered care/safety: How might the nurse use blended nursing skills to provide holistic, competent nursing care for Margot and her husband? Margot is in need of assistance and education to help her care for her husband at home. The nurse could check with social services or look into community services that would allow her to attend her church services and other community support groups. The nurse will emphasize safety as appropriate for using the stove, wandering, falls and toileting or preventing skin breakdown, if incontinent.

2. Patient-centered care: What would be a successful outcome for this patient/family?
By next visit, Margot receives some assistance with her husband and vocalizes a connectedness with her church and community.

3. Patient-centered care/safety/evidence-based practice: What intellectual and interpersonal competencies are most likely to bring about the desired outcome?
Intellectual: ability to identify spirituality as a source of patient support, strength, or conflict, incorporating this information into the patient's care plan. Knowledge of Alzheimer's disease, caregiver role strain, and home safety.
Interpersonal: ability to establish trusting relationships, even in times of distress, crisis, and conflict. Ability to demonstrate respect, empathy, and caring for the patient.

4. Teamwork and collaboration/safety: What resources might be helpful to Margot and her husband? Respite care, adult day care, meals-on-wheels, parish nursing, community support groups

PATIENT CARE STUDY

Answers will vary with student experience.

PRACTICING FOR NCLEX
MULTIPLE-CHOICE QUESTIONS

1. c   **2.** d   **3.** c   **4.** a   **5.** b
6. d   **7.** b

ALTERNATE-FORMAT QUESTIONS
Multiple-Response Questions

1. a, b, d, e
2. d, e
3. b, d, e
4. b, c

Prioritization Question

1. c

Appendix A Nursing Process Worksheet-Instructions

Medical Problem or Diagnosis *State the reason for admission or the encounter with a provider. You may state a medical diagnosis such as "exacerbation of COPD" or as a "rule out" diagnosis (e.g., R/O MI).* *For purposes of learning, this diagnosis may or may not directly reflect the problem(s) identified by the nurse.*	**Expected Outcomes** *Outcomes should be clear, measurable, and time focused.* *Begin the statement, "the patient will," followed by the outcomes the patient will achieve to indicate resolution or prevention of the actual or potential problem or need.* *Stating two or three outcomes for each actual or potential problem or need is common.*
Actual or Potential Health Problem or Need *Identify actual or potential problems that are addressed by the nurse **or** the interprofessional team.* *Base these on the critical thinking care study or your initial and ongoing patient assessments.*	**Nursing Interventions** *Clearly state what the nurse will do. Use action verbs such as assess, provide, administer, assist, teach, and consult.* *Begin the intervention with, "the nurse will." Include nursing actions in addition to assessments to effect change.*
Possible Etiologic Factors *State the underlying cause(s) of the actual or potential problem or need.* *Avoid using a medical diagnosis as the cause, rather state a problem the nurse can treat, such as weakness and inability to expectorate mucus.*	
Potential Signs and Symptoms *State the signs and symptoms, also called clinical manifestations or cues, that the nurse uses to identify the actual or potential problem or need.* These are the signs and symptoms the patient displays (not the etiology). Include subjective and objective data. Example: if identifying a problem related to airway clearance, describe the mucus and cough; for a problem related to gas exchange, include a pulse oximetry reading and arterial blood gas results.	**Evaluative Statement** *This statement clearly addresses the patient's progress toward the identified outcomes. The statement(s) may include revisions to the original interventions to better facilitate achievement of the goals, problem resolution, or prevention of the actual or potential problem or need.* Note: every outcome may not be achieved in a single shift or even week depending on the patient and the complexity of the problem.

Follow your professor's instructions regarding a nursing care plan versus an interprofessional plan of care.

Nursing Process Worksheet

Medical Problem or Diagnosis	Expected Outcomes
↓	
Actual or Potential Health Problem or Need	↓
↓	Nursing Interventions
Possible Etiologic Factors	
↓	↓
Potential Signs and Symptoms	Evaluative Statement

Although many care plans are interprofessional, this format focuses on use of the nursing process.
Follow your professor's guidelines for completing this worksheet.

Additional Nursing Process Worksheets available on thePoint

QUADM0324